Illness narratives in practice

Illness narratives in practice
Potentials and challenges of using narratives in health-related contexts

Edited by

Gabriele Lucius-Hoene
Department of Rehabilitation Psychology
and Psychotherapy, University of Freiburg, Germany

Christine Holmberg
Institute of Social Medicine and Epidemiology,
Medical School Theodor Fontane, Brandenburg/Havel, Germany

Thorsten Meyer
Rehabilitation Sciences, Faculty of Public Health, University of Bielefeld,
Germany

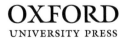

OXFORD
UNIVERSITY PRESS

OXFORD

UNIVERSITY PRESS

Great Clarendon Street, Oxford, OX2 6DP,
United Kingdom

Oxford University Press is a department of the University of Oxford.
It furthers the University's objective of excellence in research, scholarship,
and education by publishing worldwide. Oxford is a registered trade mark of
Oxford University Press in the UK and in certain other countries

Published in the United States of America by Oxford University Press
198 Madison Avenue, New York, NY 10016, United States of America

British Library Cataloguing in Publication Data

Data available

Library of Congress Control Number: 2018941860

ISBN 978–0–19–880666–0

9 8 7 6 5 4 3 2 1

Printed and bound by
CPI Group (UK) Ltd, Croydon, CR0 4YY

Acknowledgements

We sincerely thank all the people who helped us create this book: Margret Xyländer and Daniel Nowik for their exceptional and unremitting organizational support, their patience in networking with the editors and authors, and their helpful overview of the many tasks; Johanna Meyer for her extensive and skillful language adaptions of the manuscripts; Anke Desch for her careful editorial help in getting the manuscripts to print; Jürgen Bengel from the Department of Rehabilitation Psychology, Freiburg University, and Cornelia Helfferich, Protestant University of Applied Sciences, Freiburg, who provided the means for the language revisions. At Oxford University Press, we found appreciative and patient help and guidance for our many questions. Last but not least, we would like to thank all the contributors to this book. It was a pleasure to work with all of you!

Contents

Section 9 **Illness narratives in the media**

Abbreviations

ACMG	American College of Medical Genetics		JAMA	Journal of the American Medical Association
ADHD	Attention-deficit hyperactivity disorder		MCAD	Medium-chain acyl-coa dehydrogenase
AEBCD	Accelerated experience-based co-design		MPH	Methylphenidate hydrochloride
			MS/MS	Tandem mass spectrometry
CAQDAS	Computer-assisted qualitative data analysis software		NBS	Newborn screening
CFS	Chronic fatigue syndrome		NIHR	National Institute of Health Research
CIHI	Canadian Institute for Health Information		PCORI	Patient-Centered Outcomes Research Initiative
CIHR	Canadian Institutes for Health Research		PKU	Phenylketonuria
CPES	Canadian Patient Experience Survey		PREMs	Patient-reported experiences
			PROMs	Patient-reported outcomes
CPX	Clinical performance examination		PSA	Prostate-specific antigen
EBCD	Experience-based co-design		QoL	Quality of life
FFT	Friends and Family Test		RfPB	Research for patient benefit
GP	General practitioner		SDA	Structural dream analysis
HCAHPS	Hospital Consumer Assessment of Healthcare Providers and Systems		SPD	Social Democratic Party of Germany
HERG	Health Experiences Research Group		SPOR	Strategy for Patient-Oriented Research
HPV	Human papilloma virus		USPSTF	US Preventative Services Task Force
HS&DR	Health Service & Delivery Research		VAERS	Vaccine Adverse Event Recording System
ICU	Intensive care unit		VET	Vocational education and training
IRB	Institutional review board		WHO	World Health Organization

Contributors

Manna Alma, Senior Researcher, Department of Health Sciences, University Medical Center Groningen, University of Groningen, Netherlands

Yong Ik Bak, Medical Humanities, University of Konyang, Korea

Matthias Bandtel, Director of the Educational Programme kompass, Mannheim University of Applied Sciences, Germany

Martina Breuning, Scientific Associate, Department of Rehabilitation Psychology and Psychotherapy, University of Freiburg, Germany

Jens Brockmeier, Professor of Psychology, The American University of Paris, France

Sabine Corsten, Professor of Therapy and Rehabilitation Sciences (Speech and Language Therapy), Catholic University of Applied Sciences, Mainz, Germany

Amos Fleischmann, Class A Senior Lecturer, Graduate School of Education, Achva Academic College, Israel

Peter Frommelt, Specialist in Neurology and Psychiatry, Neurorehabilitation Private Practice, Berlin, Germany

Rachel Grob, Director of National Initiatives; Clinical Professor at the Center for Patient Partnerships and Senior Scientist at the Department of Family Medicine and Community Health, University of Wisconsin-Madison, USA

Elisabeth Gülich, Professor, Faculty of Linguistics and Literature, Bielefeld University, Bielefeld, Germany

Hille Haker, Richard McCormick, S. J., Endowed Chair of Moral Theology, Loyola University Chicago, USA; President of Societas Ethica, European Society for Research in Ethics

Friedericke Hardering, Senior Researcher, Institute for Sociology, Goethe-University, Frankfurt, Germany

Chris Heape, Design Research Consultant, SDU Design, University of Southern Denmark, Denmark

Cornelia Helfferich, Emeritus Professor, Sociology, Evangelische Hochschule Freiburg, Freiburg, Germany

Wolfgang Himmel, Professor of Health Sciences, Department of General Practice, University Medical Center Göttingen, Göttingen, Germany

Lisa Hinton, Medical Sociologist, Health Experiences Research Group (HERG), University of Oxford, Oxford, UK

Christine Holmberg, Institute of Social Medicine and Epidemiology, Medical School Theodor Fontane, Brandenburg/Havel, Germany

Lars-Christer Hydén, Professor of Social Psychology, and Director of Center for Dementia Research (CEDER), Linköping University, Linköping, Sweden

Yeonok Jeoung, Professor of Nursing Science, Kyundong University, Republic of Korea

Ernst von Kardorff, Professor Emeritus of Rehabilitation Sciences, Humboldt University of Berlin, Germany

Alexander Kiss, Professor of Psychosomatic Medicine, University Hospital Basel, Basel, Switzerland

Janka Koschack, Psychologist, University Medical Center Göttingen, Germany

Joyce Lamerichs, Assistant Professor and Senior Researcher, Department of Language, Literature & Communication, VU University Amsterdam, Netherlands

Henry Larsen, Professor of Participatory Innovation, SDU Design, University of Southern Denmark, Denmark

Maya Lavie-Ajayi, Senior Lecturer, Spitzer Department of Social Work, Ben-Gurion University of the Negev, Beersheba, Israel; Chair of the Israeli Center for Qualitative Research of People and Societies

John Lavis, Canada Research Chair in Evidence-Informed Health Systems and Professor, Department of Health Evidence and Impact (HEI), McMaster University, Ontario, Canada

Susan Law, Director of Research and Scientist, Trillium Health Partners; Institute for Better Health Associate Professor, Institute for Health Policy, Management and Evaluation, University of Toronto Director, Health Experiences Research Canada

Louise Locock, Professor of Health Services Research, University of Aberdeen, Scotland, UK

David Loutfi, MSc, PhD Student, Department of Family Medicine, McGill University

Gabriele Lucius-Hoene, retired Professor of Rehabilitation Psychology, Department of Rehabilitation Psychology and Psychotherapy, University of Freiburg, Germany

Eleonora Massa, Independent Researcher, Rome, Italy

Paula McDonald, GP, Seven Dials Health Centre, Brighton, UK

Maria I. Medved, Professor of Psychology, The American University of Paris, France; Adjunct Professor of Psychology, University of Manitoba, Canada

Thorsten Meyer, Integrative Rehabilitation Research Unit and Institute of Epidemiology, Hannover Medical School, Germany

Erez C. Miller, Senior Lecturer of Psychology and Special Education, Achva Academic College, Israel

Ora Nakash, Associate Professor, Baruch Ivcher School of Psychology, Interdisciplinary Center in Herzliya, Israel and School for Social Work, Smith College, Northampton, MA

Ilja Ormel, MSc-PH, PhD Student, Department of Family Medicine, McGill University Research Program Coordinator, Health Experiences Research Canada

Alexander Palant, Sociologist and Health Science Researcher, Department of General Practice, University Medical Center Göttingen, Göttingen, Germany

Christian Roesler, Professor of Clinical Psychology, Catholic University of Applied Sciences, Freiburg, Germany; Lecturer of Analytical Psychology, University of Basel, Switzerland

Merja Ryöppy, PhD Research Fellow, SDU Design, University of Southern Denmark, Denmark

Mark Schlesinger, Professor of Health Policy, Chair of the Department of Health Policy and Management, School of Public Health, Yale University, USA

Victoria A. Shaffer, Associate Professor, Departments of Health Sciences and of Psychological Sciences, University of Missouri, USA; Director of the Medical Decision Research Lab, Department of Health Sciences, University of Missouri, USA

Valentina Simeoni, Independent Researcher, Castelfranco Veneto, Italy

Claudia Steiner, Dipl. Phil. II, Psychosomatic Medicine, University Hospital Basel, Basel, Switzerland

Margret Xyländer, Scientific Associate, Faculty of Health Sciences, Bielefeld University, Bielefeld, Germany

Sue Ziebland, Professor of Medical Sociology and Director of the Health Experiences Research Group (HERG), Nuffield Department of Primary Care Health Sciences, University of Oxford

Brian J. Zikmund-Fisher, Associate Professor of Health Behavior and Health Education, and Research Associate Professor of Internal Medicine, University of Michigan, Michigan, USA

Section 1

Introduction

Chapter 1

Introduction

Chances and problems of illness narratives

Gabriele Lucius-Hoene, Christine Holmberg, and Thorsten Meyer

Since the 1960s, oral storytelling as a social and discursive practice has re-emerged as a way of dealing with subjective, social, and cultural developments and experiences (Polkinghorne, 1988). In the wake of this revival, illness narratives have become increasingly popular. Accounts of personal experiences of illness and encounters with the medical world, their impact on biography and daily life, and patients' efforts to cope with illness have moved out of the private or literary realm, and into the common discourse. When Arthur Kleinman coined the term 'illness narratives' in 1983, it was welcomed as a window into the experiences of patients, thus offering a new perspective in medicine via the social sciences that bridged the gap between physicians' and patients' outlooks on the nature of suffering from illness (Cassell, 2004; Toombs, 1992). Narratives may provide privileged insights into the patients' 'lifeworld' or the 'world of illness' (in contrast to the 'world of medicine'; see Mishler, 1984), their subjective illness or curative theories, their adherence strategies, choices, and actions, or their coping endeavours. This makes narratives valuable not only in medicine, but also in social and cultural sciences and psychology, showing how illness experiences are intertwined with psychological, cultural, socio-economic, and political conditions. Patients' experiences, often collected in interviews, have come to play a significant role in health care (Ziebland et al., 2013).

The narrative approach promises to reshape doctor–patient communication, where each take a more equal role based on understanding of how doctors honour their patients' subjectivity, and re-introduce talking and listening into medicine and medical education (Greenhalgh and Hurwitz, 1998; Charon et al., 2017). With the growing acceptance of interpretative methods, illness narratives are acknowledged as a valid form of research data across a wide range of disciplines (Hurwitz et al., 2004), linking subjective suffering with medical practice, identities, social meanings, and cultural significance. Making illness stories eminent is also about rediscovering that the narrative scheme has always been at the core of clinical practice, diagnostics, and treatment, whether the professional players have been aware of it or not (Mattingly, 1998). Not only is individual experience grasped in stories, but they also pervade professional and institutional developments and social practices of dealing with health and illness, and their influences on each other.

The use of illness narratives of all kinds have also become teaching material for students and practicing health care providers, sources of information and support, helpful tools for other patients, therapists, and planners of medical support and health services, or resources to educate the public. The media exploit the appeal of stories of suffering, healing, resistance, despair, or newly found integrity in the face of severe illness. They also create their own stories, combining on a meta-level many different sources, discourses, and enactments of dealing with both physical and mental illness.

Illness stories do not always have to be told or written. They may exist as subplots to clinical and institutional practice, or exert a major influence on public opinions about health, illness, and professional care as unspoken, but all-pervasive, interpretative blueprints.

Looking closer, 'illness narrative' is an umbrella term for very different kinds of stories. They may be told, written, enacted, or implicitly underlie public discourses without being fixed in language. Narratologists agree that narrative is 'a fundamental way of organizing human experience and a tool for constructing models of reality', and that trying to define a narrative by distinctive features quickly leads to highly conflicting views about where to draw the line (Ryan, 2005, p. 345). A more constructive approach than defining is to describe what people do when they tell a story. According to Kohler Riessman,

> ... in everyday oral storytelling, a speaker connects events into a sequence that is consequential for later action and for the meaning that the speaker wants listeners to take away from the story. Events perceived by the speaker as important are selected, organized, connected, and evaluated as meaningful for a particular audience (2008, p. 3).

Thus, from a subjective point of view, stories help define for the storyteller what has happened and what the experience has meant, creating a version of the experience for the listener. When narratives are used as data, researchers must be explicit about what kind of 'reality' the narratives represent and how to relate these 'realities' to the purposes of research (Riessman, 2008, p. 183; see also Chapter 2 of this book). Polkinghorne suggests that 'To ask of a narrative, "What really happened?" is to assume that plots are simply representations of extralinguistic realities and that they can be investigated empirically by recapturing those extralinguistic realities ... ' (1988, p. 159). Alternatively, they may be taken as the teller's subjective interpretations of what happened as her personal view of reality. However, it is important to consider that the teller of events organizes her story from the present, but interprets it with hindsight, to explain how things happened from the standpoint of a 'retrospective teleology' (Brockmeier, 2001). The construction of stories is always a co-production between teller and a real or imagined audience as a combination of voices drawing on many cultural resources, and thus '... the power of narrative (is) to impart a vision of reality ... that is at once socially positioned and culturally grounded' (Garro and Mattingly, 260).

The narrative product is not only created to make listeners take up certain information and a specific meaning, but telling a story also enables the teller to give meaning to the—sometimes overwhelming—events encountered. Telling a story means connecting events in causal or final chains of sentences and thus building an understanding and a sense of what has happened for both the listener and the storyteller (Herman 2002, 2009).

Illness narratives in research and in the public arena vary greatly in many dimensions, e.g., whose voice is heard as the teller, who is meant to be the audience, which kind and range of illness experience is addressed, whose illness is being narrated, for what purpose, and with what consequences. Their conditions of origin—whether they are told spontaneously, elicited by health professionals or researchers, aimed at the media, or carefully elaborated as literary achievements—provide both opportunities and restrictions for their use and impact.

According to these outlines, a substantial part of data which are in use in social science and its adjacent fields are partly or wholly narratives. Interview-based research, as soon as it asks for personal experiences, mostly offers open questions, refrains from forcing answers, and obtains its data as verbalized memories and their surrounding attitudes and evaluations. So, quite independent of the research topic and aim, the temporal structure of interviewees' utterances transforms them into narratives and encompasses the aforementioned epistemological features. Whereas many research projects tend to ignore these narratological qualities, others play them out and derive special insights by analysing them.

Narratives possess unique communicational properties of creating realities and engaging the audience, which explains why they add a special persuasive power to the content they convey and why they serve many purposes across different areas of health and illness. Advocates of a holistic approach in medicine are enthusiastic about illness narratives as easily obtainable, highly intriguing, and widely successful across disciplines. However, narratives by no means provide straightforward and uncomplicated data. The intrinsic value of narratives may disguise the additional dangers present if the epistemological characteristics of stories, their context and condition of origin, their properties as linguistic constructions of experiences, and the effects of storytelling on listeners are not taken into account. The often-used naïve approach to treat patient narratives as simple renderings of a given event ignores that they are not a representation of reality.

This book provides a critical reflection on narratives in practice. It comprises some basic considerations and examples of how illness narratives have found their place in the media, counselling and psychotherapy, teaching and training for students and professionals, and in diagnostics and decision-making. It asks how scholars should make use of narratives and how to respond to this use. It argues that the use of narratives in applied contexts raises many questions about what kind of tools these narratives are, and what epistemological foundations, communicational properties, and pragmatic effects they comprise when shifted from research material to clinical, educational, and/or instructive instruments in various settings. It also addresses how this shift raises ethical concerns and reflections. Generally, the book aims to sensitize professionals who use illness narratives in the field of medicine for their problems, challenges, and opportunities.

The first part, methodological and epistemological challenges, begins with general and basic considerations concerning status and methodological questions of illness narratives. In Chapter 2, Gabriele Lucius-Hoene, Martina Breuning, and Cornelia Helfferich focus on the necessary decisions concerning the relationship between narrative data, researchers' or users' aims, and the kind of reality to which they contribute. In Chapter 3, Janka Koschack and Wolfgang Himmel show how scientists inevitably change narrative data when preparing them for use, e.g., on an Internet platform meant to inform and support other patients. Lars-Christer Hydén points out in Chapter 4 how narrative norms work in the background of researchers' expectations; as a consequence, stories of tellers who are not able to match these norms run the risk of not being understood and consequently neglected. In Chapter 5, Thorsten Meyer and Margret Xyländer examine how cases and parts of illness narratives are selected for a specific use in practice. They take the perspective of qualitative researchers and apply ideas of sampling and generalizability in research on narrative, criticizing the widespread tendency of qualitative researchers to use only those narratives in the presentation of their data which fit into their argumentation or have a special appeal.

Part two addresses ethical and communicational aspects of using narratives in medicine. In Chapter 6, Hille Haker explores ways to integrate a narrative ethics approach as part of the ethical counselling, ensuring that both individual experiences and the normative dimensions of actions are included in the conversations. By means of a single case intake interview, Maya Lavie-Ajayi and Ora Nakash show in Chapter 7 how the stories of doctor and patient clash, and argue that the battle of narratives is a political battle about power in defining diagnoses and treatment recommendations.

Narratives can be regarded as a very important material in counselling and psychotherapy. Patients talk about their experiences, problems, and symptoms, which are all interwoven closely with crucial events, their biographical situations, and their theories about personal and illness developments. As a form of psychotherapy, narrative therapy addresses the underlying narrative character of patients' utterances and also regards the therapeutic process as an unfolding narrative, using its structure and dynamics as a guideline. The third part, narratives in psychotherapy, rehabilitation and vocational training, shows examples of narratives in therapeutic, neurological, and workplace rehabilitation. Especially for patients with severe disabilities, telling and understanding stories may support identity work and the work towards increased quality of life. In a project with aphasia patients, Sabine Corsten and Friedericke Hardering implement an adopted biographic-narrative intervention aiming at identity renegotiation and social participation, discussed in Chapter 8. Chapter 9 by Peter Frommelt, Maria Medved, and Jens Brockmeier discusses how a narrative approach combining patients' stories and narrative practice can help with meaning making and support patients in existentially devastating situations after brain injury. In Chapter 10, Ernst von Kardorff shows how patient narratives help to understand their endeavours to cope with their illnesses at the workplace and in vocational training.

Narratives have become popular and useful tools to help teach and train medical students and professionals. Mainly they are used to provoke a shift of perspective from the professional view that is 'outside' the illness to the 'inside' of lived experiences. Illness stories can give insight into the worlds of being ill and suffering, but also into patients' motives for using medical institutions, choosing between diagnostic or therapeutic options, ways of cooperation and adhering, and managing their lives. They are also meant to induce empathy and reflections about the role of practitioners toward patients. Part four presents many different approaches and projects of using narratives in training of students and medical staff. Alexander Kiss and Claudia Steiner report in Chapter 11 on how they use narratives, especially in terms of novels and movies, in medical training for students in Switzerland across the whole study curriculum. Yeonok Jeoung, Gabriele Lucius-Hoene, and Yong Ik Bak expand this idea in Chapter 12 toward the use of narratives in doctors' training in Korea. Here, they shed special light on eastern philosophical traditions and a contrasting habitus of physicians in Korea today. In Chapter 13, Alexander Palant and Wolfgang Himmel give examples of how to use illness narratives in medical education with material from the German DIPEx website of patients' experiences, www.krankheitserfahrungen.de. While they work with authentic stories from patients collected in interview projects, Paula McDonald uses a different approach to make medical students visit websites and other sources of patients' experiences with illness. She offers courses where students have to create narratives of a fictional patient. In Chapter 14 she demonstrates this approach, and shows how her students feel that this task enhances their empathy and understanding.

An unconventional approach towards using illness narratives is presented by Chris Heape, Henry Larsen and Merja Ryöppy from Denmark in Chapter 15. They try out participatory theatre methods to change healthcare practice both for professionals as well as for persons affected by illnesses. In Chapter 16, Joyce Lamerichs and Manna Alma report on a project from the Netherlands, in which they developed an educational module for intermediate vocational education for students to learn about patients with dementia. They provide an insight into the lessons, how the students have picked up different aspects of the narratives they were confronted with, and how they related it to their own experiences with patients.

Part five of the book, narratives in diagnostics, shows how patients' use of language strategies bringing their experiences into stories may play a decisive role for diagnostic purposes. By using conversational analysis methods on transcripts of patients' stories about their seizures and experiences of intensive fear, Elisabeth Gülich demonstrates in Chapter 17 how a close analysis of their narrative practices can deliver criteria for differential diagnosis. In Chapter 18, Christian Roesler introduces Structural Dream Analysis (SDA) as a method to investigate the meaning conveyed in dream series from analytical psychotherapies and to connect dreams with the psychopathology of the patient and processes in psychotherapy.

Part six, narratives in decision-making, deals with the roles that experience and storytelling play as patients must make increasingly complex and seldom clear-cut health care decisions. Christine Holmberg in Chapter 19 demonstrates the concerted effort to reduce the influence of personal experiences and provide patients and providers with epidemiological data to help them base decisions on valid scientific knowledge. She argues that such efforts are crucial, but need to be carefully balanced with patients' experiences, and to do so, she investigates the principal nature of experience. She further solicits a recognition of narratives in clinical encounters as fundamentally true, not as scientific knowledge but rather as phenomenological and radically subjective knowledge of active agents in the health care encounter. In Chapter 20, Victoria Shaffer and Brian Zikmund-Fisher show a route of including narratives in patient decision-aids without hampering decision-aids' scientific validity. They present a range of criteria on how to decide which narratives to use in decision-aids in order to stay true to the richness of experience and the scientific evidence presented.

Part seven of the book, narratives in health care, returns to the use of narratives as information sources and scientific data in order to promote change. Lisa Hinton and colleagues present in Chapter 21 different formats of how the elicitation of individuals' health experiences may be used to improve health care delivery. In the same vein, in Chapter 22 Susan Law and colleagues reflect on strategies of how analyses derived from narrative data may be incorporated into evidence-based health policy approaches. Chapter 23, Rachel Grob and Mark Schlesinger's investigation into the problematic singling out of particular and singular stories in media reports, completes this part of the book. Grob and Schlesinger strengthen the importance of presenting the complexities and variety of experiences to understand health care delivery and health care experiences, particularly when the aim is to change practice.

The public space of the media, especially the Internet with its means of communication and participation, adds a new dimension to the impact of personal stories and to the definition and significance of health problems and their management. In addition to the presentation of biographical narratives which cover a broader time frame, Internet platforms write their own meta-stories by contrasting contributions and bringing together different voices and perspectives. In Chapter 24, Eleonora Massa and Valentina Simeoni show how Facebook structures and contextualizes socially acceptable stories of being pregnant and becoming a mother. While these experiences tend to support each other and share common grounds, in Chapter 25 Erez Miller and Amos Fleischman work out the controversies and opposing world views which are negotiated on the Internet. They discuss how, when revealed on platforms documenting patients' experiences with anti-ADHD drugs, professionals' and patients' voices clash. By picking up, commenting, discussing, and debating illness experiences, the media may exact disclosure of public persons' health status. In Chapter 26, Matthias Bandtel shows how the media impose normative expectations and moral questions of power and control on the body presentations of politicians when they suffer from severe illness, thus usurping and dominating their pathographies in the name of political responsibility.

Throughout, the reader encounters a wide array of topics, arguments, and reflections on how illness narratives are used in practice—and how they might be used in a better or more sensitive way. In critically following the lines of arguments of the different authors, it is hoped that this book will reach its aim: to increase the sympathy of those professionals who use illness narratives in the field of medicine for their problems, challenges, and opportunities.

References

Brockmeier, J., 2001. From the end to the beginning: Retrospective teleology in autobiography. In: J. Brockmeier and D. Carbaugh, eds. *Narrative and identity. Studies in autobiography, self and culture.* Amsterdam: John Benjamins Publishing. pp. 247–280.

Cassell, E. J., 2004. *The nature of suffering and the goals of medicine.* Oxford: Oxford University Press.

Charon, R., DasGupta, S., Hermann, N., Marcus, E. R., and Spiegel, M., eds., 2017. *The principles and practice of narrative medicine.* Oxford: Oxford University Press.

Garro, L. and Mattingly, C., 2000. Narrative turns. In: C. Mattingly and L. Garro, eds. *Narrative and the cultural construction of illness and healing.* Berkeley: University of California Press. pp. 259–269.

Greenhalgh, T. and Hurwitz, B., eds., 1998. *Narrative based medicine. Dialogue and discourse in clinical practice.* London: BMJ Books.

Herman, D., 2002. *Story logic. Problems and possibilities of narrative.* Lincoln, NE: Nebraska University Press.

Herman, D., 2009. *Basic elements of narrative.* Chichester: Wiley-Blackwell.

Hurwitz, B., Greenhalgh, T., and Skultans, V., eds., 2004. *Narrative research in health and illness.* London: Wiley Blackwell.

Mattingly, C., 1998. *Healing dramas and clinical plots. The narrative structure of experience.* Cambridge: Cambridge University Press.

Mishler, E., 1984. The discourse of medicine: The dialectics of medical interviews. Norwood, NJ: Ablex.

Polkinghorne, D. E., 1988. *Narrative knowing and the human sciences.* Albany, NY: State University of New York Press.

Riessman, C. K., 2008. *Narrative methods for the human sciences.* Los Angeles: Sage.

Ryan, M-L., 2005. Narrative. In: D. Herman, M. Jahn, and M-L Ryan, eds. *Routledge encyclopedia of narrative theory.* New York: Routledge. pp. 344–348.

Toombs, S., 1992. *The meaning of illness. A phenomenological account of the different perspectives of physician and patient.* Dordrecht: Springer.

Ziebland, S., Coulter, A., Calabrese, J. D., and Locock, L., eds., 2013. *Understanding and using health experiences. Improving patient care.* Oxford: Oxford University Press.

Section 2

Methodological and epistemological challenges

Chapter 2

Illness narratives in practice

Which questions do we have to face when collecting and using them?

Gabriele Lucius-Hoene, Martina Breuning, and Cornelia Helfferich

Introduction: the hidden agenda behind the use of illness narratives

Lately, illness narratives, i.e., first-person stories about experiences with illness and its personal consequences, gained a significant place within research data and as practical instruments. These narratives were discovered and exploited in many health-related contexts, e.g., in medical education, media information, health politics, and health markets, and their basis for use in these contexts is strong: they are informative, interesting, highly suggestive, and emotionally entrancing. When people come in touch with illness, these experiences are shared, and in this sharing, gain worth.

Illness narratives are much more than what they initially seem to be. They deal with events and experiences as constructions of inner and outer worlds (Herman, 2009, 108–136), seemingly telling 'what has happened'. They are not independent from their creation—the act of telling itself. Telling a story is an ordinary and ubiquitous activity, but it is highly complex and has many effects on both the tellers and listeners. The product, the story, and the activities of telling and listening are inseparable from their cultural context, as well as from the psychological and social aspects of the persons involved (Brockmeier, 2015; Polkinghorne, 1988). In contexts of research and use, the many facets of personal narratives, the complex relationships between the act and the text, the conditions of creation, and the effects they carry on are deeply confounded, but rarely considered (Langellier, 1989).

Illness narratives come along as omnipresent, self-explanatory, fairly easy to find and understand, and seemingly useful for many purposes (Meisel and Karlawish, 2011). But those who listen to stories may experience moments of doubt concerning the credibility of both the story and the storyteller. When looking at the conditions that surround the stories' formation, as well as into the users' goals, serious questions arise. The answers enable or limit the ways the stories themselves can be used. Primarily, they refer to the epistemological status of a narrative, i.e., to the question of what a narrative actually *is*, and how it is constituted. For example, a narrative might be considered as a reflection or representation of something that happened and was experienced before or as a more or less arbitrary fiction. These questions are not adding unnecessary complexity to the strategies of using illness narratives, but they are unavoidable because they make us consider practical problems as well as ethical implications. Additionally, academic probity requires disclosure of the methodological assumptions that are underlying the use of illness narratives. Transparency is obligatory when evaluating the methodical choices, discussing limitations of the data, and judging the generalizability and scope of results and conclusions.

But there are different answers to these questions. For some purposes, illness narratives may be considered reliable and 'true enough' accounts of 'what has happened' as to their specific use, e.g., for educational purposes. In other cases, the transformation of experience into narrative via its complicated construction processes involving memory, intention, and language may be crucial; this approach is based on the presumption that it is impossible to capture the truth of former experiences. In either case, there should be an awareness of the underlying questions and transparency-related decisions that are part of the process.

This chapter hopes to shed light on the underlying questions faced when working with illness narratives in practical or research contexts. These considerations are meant to help others specify their own point of view and their assumptions concerning the methodological status, the purpose of use of narratives, and the relationship between goals and data. However, the authors neither favour nor advocate specific answers or methodological points, special research approaches, or conceptions about data. Neither do they take methodological sides nor contribute to epistemological controversies about illness narratives. Instead, the chapter adopts a rather pluralistic and pragmatic view. Many of the issues raised may be salient for some readers and their purposes, but irrelevant for others.

The questions posed throughout may be applied to illness narratives which are already available and have been told, collected, and used for other purposes, e.g., illness stories from the literature or on the media. They also may be applied to illness narratives which have to be raised as data by researchers and users themselves.

Which questions do we have to consider?

The intentions, research questions, and aims related to narrative use

♦ Why do we (as researchers or professionals working with narrative data) want to use illness narratives (and not any other kind of data)—what do we expect from them?

♦ Which are the questions we expect narratives to shed light on, or which effects are they meant to have when we use them? Do we need information about real life processes or are we mainly interested in subjective illness experiences of patients or other persons? Or do we want to know how these experiences are put into language and what linguistic strategies reveal about processes like coping or identity work and reality constructions of tellers? Do we expect certain intrapsychic or social effects from the acts of telling or listening to stories?

The answers to these questions are the starting point for all following choices. The methodological status that will and can reasonably be ascribed to illness narratives has to fit to the purpose of the use that is made of them, which is discussed in the section Reflections on research intentions, questions, and aims as a context of use.

What is the meaning of 'truth' and 'reality'?

- ◆ Do we hold the stories we work with for 'true', and what do we mean by 'true', respectively?
- ◆ Can we take what patients or others tell us about illness experiences as veridical, i.e., as direct representations of a 'reality' beyond the text we want to explore, or are we not concerned about 'truth' because we want to reconstruct subjective experiences or world views as given in the story?
- ◆ Do we have to consider the question of veridicality at all, or can we just take what is told and use it like any other kind of information?

These questions touch the relationship between the illness experience, its formation into a narrative, and its relation to the events which it depicts. It looks at its epistemological stance and the epistemological stance the user wants or needs to apply (re: the question of truth and narrative, see Riessman, 2008, pp. 183–200). This topic is discussed in the section Epistemological aspects and the problem of veridicality.

Social aspects of storytelling

- ◆ Did the storytellers have control over the conditions of their narration or are the illness narratives in some ways pre-fabricated, e.g., by restricting strategies of data acquisition using tight questionnaires?
- ◆ Do we listen rather more to the voice of the researcher or user instead of to the voice of the storytellers?

These questions turn to the conditions of the production of the narratives and deal with social or research related constraints that influence the emergence of an illness narrative. To tell a story is a social activity that is embedded in a social context. In most cases the storyteller cannot just tell anything that comes into his or her mind, as limitations are unavoidable. These problems are treated in Narrative space and narrative constraints.

Motivation behind the storytelling

- ◆ Can we rely on a general readiness to speak about one's own illness?
- ◆ What do we know or suspect about stakes and interests of storytellers?
- ◆ What kind of effect do specific intentions, motives, and purposes have on the narrative, and how may they be related to our research question or purpose of use?

These questions are directed towards the aims and agendas of the storyteller and the hidden agenda behind his or her cooperativeness to share the personal experience of illness with others. They tackle problems of selectivity, generalizability, and interpretation of illness narratives as data and as published opinions, and these are discussed more in the section Motives and agendas.

The storyteller and listener relationship

- ◆ Can we trace the broader context of the emergence of an illness narrative and what can we find about the mutual calibrations?
- ◆ How do teller and listener match their expectations concerning their roles, their tasks and their encounter?

These questions deal with the interaction of the storyteller and the listener. The emergence of an (illness) narrative is a co-production and involves negotiation of roles, expectations and aims which influence what is told. These aspects are treated in the section Interaction and negotiation.

It is important to remember that these questions are interconnected. According to the intended use they may be more or less salient and complex for a specific enterprise.

This chapter analyses aspects of these points and suggests under what conditions they may be relevant. Throughout are questions concerning what to be aware of when illness narratives are put to use in a certain context. Readers can apply them to their own research or practical intentions and to the narratives they rely on.

Reflections on research intentions, questions, and aims as a context of use

To get an overview and a rough taxonomy of the different research and scientific approaches using narratives, the focus can be on several dimensions of stories or acts of storytelling which can be all or partially relevant for a project.

The first differentiation between research programmes is whether the researchers and users are aware that their data are narratives. They must decide whether they want to exploit and make use of the specific narratological properties of their texts purposefully, or whether the narrative character of their data has no significance for them. In the first case, using and interpreting narratives is often connected with a narratological or text theory which supplies assumptions about the character of narratives as constructions. In the second case, the constructive character of the data is often ignored, and narrations are treated as veridical testimonies of events (see futher on in this chapter regarding the 'naturalistic' or 'experiential' versus the 'performative' approach).

On a second level, it is important to consider the purpose behind collecting narratives. When deciding to use stories as research data or as material for practical use, the expectation is that their narrative character adds a surplus value to the aims of the researcher. According to the many domains using narratives, which are discussed in Chapter 1, narratives may be used:

- because they offer privileged insights into events, experiences, inner worlds, or cultural constructions, thus revealing new and distinctive features for research or for information;
- because their creation in the interaction between teller and listener gives rise to positive effects concerning support, coping, or trust for the tellers;
- because they are expected to elicit empathy and induce convincing, emotionally entrancing, or relieving effects on recipients which are used to educate, support, entertain, or manipulate.

It is important

also to consider how, for what aims, and for which audiences narratives are taken into the public sphere: whether they are meant for a scientific community, for professional use, for other patients, for the media public, etc. Each of these different uses puts certain limits and constraints on dealing with them, as well as different challenges and claims concerning presentability, methodic rigour, ethical considerations, or manageability.

At a further level, it is important to consider the origin of the narratives: in what kind of context are they found, elicited, or told, and it what context may they be listened to or read? Besides the common, but rather artificial, situation of an interview in which a researcher uses leading questions, narratives in professional use can also stem from everyday conversation, from literature, or from the many varieties of public media. The influence of their origin is discussed later in this chapter.

Considerations

- Which properties, effects and aspects of narratives (as representations of events, as constructions of inner or outer worlds, as linguistic devices, as interactional and social tools, as performances …) are important for our project? What is the surplus value we hope to get?
- Are our narratives suitable for the kind of effect and presentation we pursue?
- What kind of handling do the purpose of use, the audience and the origin of the narratives require or allow?
- Is the origin or source of our narratives sufficiently clear and known?

Epistemological aspects and the problem of veridicality: truth, experience, and construction

Narratology offers a broad range of approaches to what narratives are about and displays a varied and complex epistemological background. Social constructionism, backed by empirical evidence from psychology of memory and cognitive science, points out that whenever stories are told about 'what happened to us', reality is constructed, rather than represented (in the sense of 'what has really happened'), and the teller creates her own conceptions of events from rather vague memories, earlier experiences, standpoints, and agendas, and all are aligned with the reactions of the listeners and adapted to the situation.

It is due to these reasons that dealing with narratives quickly leads to the highly debated question about narrative reference and validity: how does narrative correspond to a reality outside the text? Do or can narrators tell the 'truth' about what has happened in an external world, or what kind of 'truth' do they reveal, respectively? Alternatively, do they just supply subjective views with highly personal distortions, 'fictions of factual representations' (White, 1978, p. 121), which accounts for their negative image in positivistic methodology as unreliable and invalid data? The epistemological status of narratives has been discussed in extenso in the comparison of 'narrative truth' and 'historical truth' or truth as correspondence (Riessman, 2008, pp. 186–188) working out the different visions and aspects of reality they refer to.

Thus, in many cases the crucial question is not whether the narrative data are or can be adequate representations of reality per se, but instead whether they fit those aspects of reality the project aims for. The user must decide if 'factual truth' is important or whether the correspondence of the story to a historical truth may remain indeterminate (Riessman, 2008, pp. 183–200).

There are three main ways of dealing with the relationship between stories and reality: First, events in the world 'out there' or second, subjective experiences as an 'inner world' in particular situations are supposed to be a taken-for-granted reality and stories represent a source of information. Third, the narrative language, the narrative data are the starting point, deriving the kind of questions for which they may be suitable: what can these narratives tell us about which kind of world? These differences in the relationship between stories and reality establishes what kind of narratives we need, how we can acquire them, and which epistemological status we can assign to them. In both cases, the main consideration is the matching between what kind of knowledge is sought, and on what ground the narratives will meet the necessary requirements. Thus it is important to look closely at the conditions that have formed the data. How much does the context of storytelling, the audience, or the interviewer and his/her techniques influence the story, and is there any need to be concerned about it?

With these questions in mind, there are roughly three different approaches which parallel three different kinds of research aims.

The 'naturalistic' approach

When people want to know about how things happened in the world, a story can be used as a document of evidence. Similarly, the storyteller is often considered a witness of the events being described. This is called a 'naturalistic' approach, as the listener accepts the content of the story at face value and uses it as a supply of information.

Narratives used in this way have become popular in applied contexts when first-person perspectives are needed, e.g., in the evaluation of services or the course of diseases. Information can be extracted from these stories, for example, the experienced symptoms, the course of the illness, the quality of treatment and procedures, and the patient's interaction with professionals.

Relying on the 'naturalistic' approach, however, does not mean that the question whether we can take the story's content as adequate or good-enough image of what 'really happened' can be ignored. Can the listener presume that the teller's view of what happened is fairly objective and not biased by misjudgments or prejudices? Must the story's reliability or adequacy be confined to its use?

Thus it must be decided if the informants are acceptably trustworthy and capable of offering an adequate report of the incidents in focus. Of course, this depends strongly on the kind of events that have piqued interest and on the kind of scientific information needed: precise facts about procedures or behaviours (e.g., court testimonials) or inner worlds and experiences. It is also important to consider the possibility of a personal bias and blurring of the stories in contrast to a presumed 'outer reality', as well as the kinds of questions asked, if the informants can talk freely, and whether they are or have been in a position to observe correctly what has happened. For instance, the quality of the information obtained can fall when storytellers are too young or too ill, if they fear negative consequences for themselves or others in case of complaints, or when their language skills are hampered.

The 'experiential' approach

A second approach that sees narratives as correct 'testimonials' focuses on stories as an expression of patients' or tellers' subjective experiences, private worlds, and identities, and looks at them 'from the inside' (for more on this see Ziebland et al., 2013). In this case, the question of 'truth' is not a question of the teller's capacities to render correct and unbiased observations of an outer world, but of the person's readiness to expose what he or she has come to see as genuine personal experiences. These stories can be highly informative for the listener who wants to understand about being 'inside' living with an illness, of the impact of personal relationships with professionals, of belief systems, or of coping endeavours.

In this approach, researchers do not judge whether the story is 'right' or 'wrong', but whether it is trustworthy and adequately consistent.

The 'performative' approach

The performative approach focuses on the use and consequences of linguistic and interactional activities. This involves discerning how tellers use language, what aims they want to achieve by narrating the way they do, and the kinds of discourses they use and construct (Gwyn, 2002). There is no need to judge veridicality, trustworthiness, or authenticity; instead the listener can concentrate on what the storytellers achieve by telling things by using the currency of identity construction, negotiation of social relations, and of world views. As an example, Lucius-Hoene, Thiele, and colleagues (2013b) explore linguistic strategies of 'voicing the doctors' in a sample of chronic pain and diabetes stories where the narrators use their own voices to reconstruct the doctors' characteristics, and thus reconstructing the doctors themselves.

Considerations

- Are we interested in outer or in subjective worlds?
- What kind of status do our narratives have in relation to what kind of reality?
- How much are we concerned with the question of truthfulness of our narratives, and if we are, do we have methods at our disposal to test it?
- How much accuracy or trustworthiness of our tellers do we need?
- How can we assess whether our data meet the required standard?

Narrative space and constraints: whose voice do we hear?

Usually, storytellers are encouraged and invited to speak freely, and the floor is open even for the disclosure of shameful aspects and unusual and extraordinary experiences. The story should not only be true, but 'authentic', too, which means it should represent the 'voice' of the storyteller himself and should not be shaped and distorted by external constraints. Again, this idea of authenticity is as fictional as the 'truth' of a story. Telling a story is a fundamentally social activity embedded in a social context and a real or imagined interaction. The same story told to the doctor on the last day of a hospital stay would perhaps be told differently in an online forum for patients. Therefore, the listener should be sensitized to whether or to what degree a storyteller has control over the process of telling the story, and can just let it emerge, or whether he or she is restricted and forced in any way when relating the story. Again, there are different ways to handle the question of whose voice we hear.

As in the 'experiential' approach, one stance may be to take the illness narrative as the genuine voice of the teller without acknowledging any constraints. Because of the deeply ingrained and commonly shared rules and norms of conversation and cooperation in every society (see, for instance, Grice, 1975), there may be no need to scrutinize or doubt the storyteller's 'voice' and 'ownership' (Shuman, 2015) of the story. If there is no opposing information, it is implied that the speaker was able to talk freely, had an open space to express herself, was involved in a correct interviewing practice, and had nothing to fear by talking. Furthermore, researchers' respect towards their data or participants may forbid them to doubt the seriousness and honesty of the storyteller's presentation of self. It is necessary to decide whether the fiction of an authentic or 'authentic enough' story is justifiable and acceptable, and if the conditions of its genesis can, at least partly, be ignored.

Alternatively, as in the 'performative' approach, the social constraints forming the discourse or narrative on illness may be of high importance, as they may touch the core of research interests. Researchers may be interested in the rules about what to reveal to whom about such an intimate bodily experience as illness. For example, comparative studies show rules of decency and, most prominently, the importance of mutual expectations in the social communication on illness. For instance, the storyteller might omit stressing and traumatic experiences in order to save the listener from harm. Sometimes illness narratives may be 'pre-fabricated' in the sense that culturally accepted blueprints of these experiences exist which may dominate throughout the data.

Whichever approach is chosen, it has to be justified by the aim of its use. The impact and effects which the context exerts on the telling of a story should be known, reflected, and weighted. The use of narratives, especially in scientific (qualitative) research, demands methodological considerations about the quality of the data. It must be determined to what extent the researcher 'created' his or her data by influencing or forcing the contents and shape of stories during data collection, data analysis, or data edition (see also Chapter 5). Generally, in most kinds of illness narrative uses, these types of context-related influences and restrictions on illness narratives are necessary for practical reasons. For instance, they must be useful only for a narrow and specific purpose, or a responsible editor may decide to omit parts of an illness narrative for ethical reasons before it is published in the media.

Usually, the storyteller is asked to contribute to the aims of the researcher or user by focusing on those aspects that are relevant for the use of the narrative. He or she might, for instance, be asked to describe the experience of pain, but it makes a difference whether pain is mentioned when *answering* such a question or whether a patient talks unprompted about pain as an important part of the illness' experience. Asking for a narrowly focused narration by using a catalogue of leading questions is generating another illness narrative. This is entirely different from an unspecific and broad invitation to a patient to divulge information about their experience that the patients themselves consider important, and giving the storyteller space for their own relevancies.

Considerations

- How much do we know about the circumstances and the methodical impact of the data acquisition?
- If we did not acquire the stories ourselves, how did the stories come about? Can we trust the source by methodical or ethical standards?
- Do we focus on the story as a personal testimony independent of its context of origin, or do we need some more information beyond the person of the teller?

Motives and agendas: why do people cooperate to tell their stories?

In comparison to the rich methodical considerations and data about researchers' and interviewers' aims and experiences when doing narrative research, much less is known about the motives, hidden or open stakes, and interests of participants taking part in the research. Participation in a project that uses illness narratives is usually voluntary. The storyteller's motivation is nourished by a personal agenda that makes telling a story useful or rewarding to the teller. For example, storyteller motivation may include supporting science, being remunerated, helping fellow sufferers, political motives, or crusades for or against treatment methods or institutions. Participants may be glad to find an audience for their complaints or thanks, get support and confirmation from others, or gain recognition as an illness expert who supplies valuable information to others. Talking about the illness may help people cope with it, which is the basis for narrative approaches to therapy. The motivation or strategic aims of participants influence what is collected as data, story, or text. The selective participation of a group of persons with a specific motivation and agenda can easily result in a bias, when only a specific way of experiencing illness is transmitted, analysed, published, and generalized. To avoid this bias, researchers should understand more about patients' motives to share their experiences (e.g., Lucius-Hoene, Groth, et al., 2013a; Mazanderani et al., 2013), and about the effects of patient agendas and interests on the narration.

Considerations

- How much do we have to know about the storyteller's motives for cooperation?
- Can the storyteller's personal agenda or strategic use of the interview situation exert positive/negative effects on the story?
- How can we trace these effects in the story, i.e., how much do we need to know about the person's background?

Interaction and negotiation: illness narratives as a co-production

The fifth question addresses illness narratives as the result of a co-production between the listener, especially the interviewer, and the storyteller. Telling a story is a situated activity, depending on, as well as shaping, the narrative occasions (Herman, 2009, p. 37). Narrative as talk-in-interaction (Goodwin, 2015) has extensively been picked up, explored, and put into methodical recommendations by interview research (Slembrouck, 2015). The co-production is shaped by the interviewer's instructions, the assigned roles, the mutual expectancies, the sharing of goals, the readiness to cooperate, the individual agendas, and displays of dominance or pliability. Both partners negotiate these aspects in the course of the communication or the interview on illness via various verbal or extra-linguistic means presented in the acts of telling and listening. The role ascribed to the storyteller by the researcher or user may differ from the role the storyteller prefers as his or her favourite self-presentation, and both may misinterpret the expectations and aims of the other. The effects of these negotiations, cooperative endeavours, or misunderstandings may leave their traces in the text and shape of the resulting story, restricting and/or enriching it (Wengraf, 2001; Lucius-Hoene et al., 2015).

Even if the listener maintains a passive role in the exchange, his or her virtual or real presence and attributes (e.g., gender, age, race) and the minute and often subconsciously conveyed signals as an auditor influence the emerging illness narrative. The teller calibrates his story to the anticipated or experienced reactions of the listener as a presentation of a self who has experienced illness. When the project intends to use and publish the story for a broader audience, e.g., via the Internet, the teller's 'listener orientation' may be influenced by the idea of the narrative recipient as a huge community, rather than the immediate individual listener. This influence may result in a presentation quite different to one that documents illness experiences in a diary addressed to an imaginary listener. Traces of the listener orientation and the kind of audience the teller has envisaged may be reflected in the text and identified by linguistic analysis.

Considerations

◆ To what extent do we take into account the interpersonal influence in the interview situation?

◆ How robust or easily manipulated is the storyteller? Does he stick to his own agenda and follow his own themes, or does he comply with the interviewer, or willingly digress?

◆ Which hints do we have about the influence of fictive listeners on the storyteller? Does this influence affect the scope and significance of our data?

The aspects discussed in the previous three sections melt together in the overarching question about what kind of influence the context exerts on what is told and understood. How much of the formation conditions are accessible? How many of them must be present in order to decide on the validity and meaning of the data? How much of this knowledge is necessary for a careful fit of research intentions and the quality of the data? When is it important and necessary to consider the conditions that shaped the illness narrative? Finally, does the use of the narrative justify relying on what was said, allowing the influence of the context to be ignored?

Conclusion: what to be aware of

This chapter has worked through several questions that must be asked by anybody dealing with oral or written stories. They ask how to determine the relationship between narrative data, the researchers' or users' aims, and the kind of reality to which these narratives contribute. The questions are interconnected and ought to be considered and decided successively, as each question leads to the next aspect concerning context, origin, and characteristics of the data available.

Users of illness narratives should be aware that illness narratives are not (only) a plain representation of the storyteller's experience of illness. Without any idea of the properties of illness narrations and of the process by which they become narratives, and without reflecting on the purpose for which illness narratives are used, there is no appropriate way to handle the questions concerning validity.

Therefore, it is the decision of the researcher to determine what kind of reality the narrative represents. They can depict what happened as subjective experiences, as coping efforts, or as arbitrary imaginative constructions. How they are interpreted is not an integral quality or property inherent in the narratives, but it is the researchers or users who decide. Reasonable arguments must exist for this decision and the guiding question must ask for what purpose are illness narratives put to use?

The first question asks whether or not to take into account and exploit the special narrative character and impact of the data beyond the content on a purely informative level. Thus, it is necessary to argue through the consecutive questions and choose a suitable methodology for analysis (e.g., Riessman, 2008; De Fina and Georgakopoulou, 2015); however, they can be ignored and any other methodology which deals with information can be chosen for data management.

In the second case of ignoring the narratological properties, this chapter discussed some adequate purposes of use and audiences that fit this decision. For instance, if narratives are used for the purpose of drawing conclusions and learning from them in order to improve treatment, to spread knowledge about the development of symptoms, or to organize better support, it makes sense to trust in the storyteller and to rely on the facts he or she presents. The naturalistic approach implies that the narratives are regarded as true enough for this use. If there is no trust in the storytellers' ability to present 'true enough' information, it makes no sense to start such a project at all.

In contrast to the information-oriented 'naturalistic' approach, the aim to demonstrate the diversity of personal experiences of illness allows an experiential approach. Here, the question of an objective 'truth' is not crucial as narratives are taken as 'subjective truths'. Presupposing that they represent the 'real voice of the storyteller', it is important to rather reflect on whether the narratives are 'authentic enough' for this purpose. Listeners, e.g., other patients or learners in health care services, want to hear this voice, even if this entails highly idiosyncratic testimonies. In both cases of purpose it is necessary to take into account the selectivity and instability of memories, the influence of social rules (e.g., decency) of how to speak about illness, and even some hidden agenda on the side of the storyteller before considering the narratives as true and/or authentic enough for purpose.

When following the 'performative approach', it is not necessaryto focus on the question of truth or authenticity. However, according to the linguistic methodology chosen, it is imperative to decide on how much context to consider. The narrative is taken as a record of communicational activities presenting a wide array of questions like narrative identity constructions, social strategies, or the co-production of teller and listener; accordingly, the linguistic devices displayed in the emergence of the narration are analysed.

The third aspect—generally, independent of the use of narratives—is how narratives depend on their origin, and this chapter has mentioned some of these aspects to consider that frame and shape the narrative: the influence of the social context, the agenda and motivation of the storyteller, and the interaction between teller and listener. This has a twofold implication: firstly, the situation and environment within which the storytelling takes place must establish the best conditions for the story to come out as true and authentic as possible and necessary for purpose. Secondly, ethical considerations, especially rules of scientific probity, oblige researchers to provide transparency, to reflect the process of emerging narratives, and to clarify whether there may be a bias or misuse of narratives by directing and/or leading the storyteller. While this is a general requirement for the use of narratives, it depends on the purpose of use whether it is decided that the origin is 'good enough' to accept the narration as it is (related to an naturalistic or experiential approach), or whether there is a special interest in the context-dependency of the emergence of illness narrations (performative approach).

To realize that illness narratives are not true or authentic in an absolute sense of these words and to be aware of the social character of narratives neither devaluates nor impairs or blemishes their usefulness. It does not imply mistrust of storytellers, but rather provides a realistic sense of what can be expected of them. It enables researchers to handle the use of illness narratives in a responsible way; that is, to face up to a deliberate decision on their status justified by the purpose of use, to create the best conditions for the telling of the story, and to provide necessary transparency. It provides guidelines to judge that status and why a narrative is true enough, authentic enough, and the context is conducive enough for using it, and to decide on difficult questions of using, editing, and presenting illness narratives.

References

Brockmeier, J., 2015. *Beyond the archive. Memory, narrative, and the autobiographical process.* Oxford: Oxford University Press.

De Fina, A. and Georgakopoulou, A., eds., 2015. *The Handbook of narrative analysis.* Chichester: Wiley Blackwell.

Goodwin, C., 2015. Narrative as talk-in-interaction. In: **A. De Fina** and **A. Georgakopoulou**, eds. *The handbook of narrative analysis.* Chichester, Wiley Blackwell. pp. 195–218.

Grice, H. P., 1975. Logic and Conversation. In **P. Cole** and **J. L. Morgan**, eds. *Syntax and Semantics, Vol. 3: Speech acts.* New York, NY: Academic Press. pp. 41–58.

Gwyn, R., 2002. *Communicating health and illness.* London: Sage.

Herman, D., 2009. *Basic elements of narrative.* Chichester: Wiley-Blackwell.

Langellier, K. M., 1989. Personal narratives: perspectives on theory and research. *Text and Performance Quarterly*, **9**, 243–276.

Lucius-Hoene, G., Groth, S., Becker, A. K., Dvorak, F., Breuning, M., and Himmel, W., 2013a. Wie erleben Patienten die Veröffentlichung ihrer Krankheitserfahrungen im Internet? *Die Rehabilitation*, **52**(3), 196–201.

Lucius-Hoene, G., Thiele, U., Breuning, M., and Haug, S., 2013b. Doctors' voices in patients' narratives. Coping with emotions in storytelling. *Chronic Illness*, **8**, 163–175.

Lucius-Hoene, G., Adami, S., and Koschack, J., 2015. Narratives that matter. Illness stories in the 'third space' of qualitative interviewing. In: F. Gygax and M. A. Locher, eds. *Narrative matters in medical contexts across disciplines.* Amsterdam: John Benjamins. pp. 99–116.

Mazanderani, F., Locock, L., and Powell, J., 2013. Biographical value: towards conceptualisation of the commodifications of illness narratives in contemporary health care. *Sociology of Health & Illness* **35** (6), pp. 891–905.

Meisel, Z. F. and Karlawish, J., 2011. Narrative vs evidence-based medicine. *JAMA*, **306**(18), 2022–2023.

Polkinghorne, D. E., 1988. *Narrative knowing and the human sciences*. Albany, NY: State University of New York Press.

Riessman, C. K., 2008. *Narrative methods for the human sciences*. Los Angeles, Sage.

Slembrouck, S., 2015. The role of the researcher in interview narratives. In: A. De Fina and A. Georgakopoulou, eds. *The handbook of narrative analysis*. Chichester: Wiley Blackwell. pp. 239–254.

Shuman, A., 2015. Story ownership and entitlement. In: A. De Fina and A. Georgakopoulou, eds. *The handbook of narrative analysis*. Chichester: Wiley Blackwell. pp. 38–56.

Wengraf, T., 2001. *Qualitative research interviewing: biographic narrative and semi-structured methods*. Los Angeles: Sage.

White, H., 1978. *The tropics of discourse, Essays in cultural criticism*. Baltimore, MD: Johns Hopkins University Press.

Ziebland, S., Coulter, A., Calabrese, J. D., and Locock, L., 2013. (eds). *Understanding and Using Health Experiences. Improving Patient Care*. Oxford: Oxford University Press.

Chapter 3

The researchers' role in re-constructing patient narratives to present them as patient experiences

Janka Koschack and Wolfgang Himmel

Introduction

According to Arthur W. Frank (2013), illness is a call for stories. Indeed, there are many studies that underpin the power of storytelling as a way of 'meaning making' (not only) for ill people (Rosenthal, 1993). In medicine, there are several reasons where storytelling—or a narrative perspective—has become increasingly important.

Firstly, it can be useful for doctor–patient encounters. Narratives of illness provide a framework for approaching a patient's problems holistically (Mansel, 2014). Narratives may uncover diagnostic and therapeutic options and offer a method for addressing existential qualities such as inner hurt, despair, hope, grief, and moral pain, which frequently accompany, and may even constitute, people's illnesses (Greenhalgh, 1998; 1999). Patient narratives are no less important in medicine than evidence based on scientific research—for several reasons. To begin with, the evidence from randomized trials and cohort studies cannot be mechanistically applied to individual patients whose behaviour is contextual and idiosyncratic and who experience their illness in a unique way. Vice versa, 'evidence-based' clinicians recognize the value of case expertise, i.e., the stories of illness scripts and clinical anecdotes before they select a medical maxim for a clinical decision (Greenhalgh, 1999). A narrative perspective helps doctors in the consultation to focus on the patient, to strengthen professional curiosity, to relieve them from the pressure to issue too many prescriptions and referrals, all of which can improve clinical outcomes (Easton, 2017; Overcash, 2003). Narrative inquiries may enhance the assessment of care needs and narrative stories may be translated into plans for practice and service developments (Hsu and McCormack, 2012).

Secondly, meaning making can support healing when sufferers can tell a story to reflect and express their experiences and when these experiences are heard and acknowledged by others (Collie and Long, 2005). In this case, storytelling has the function of emotional processing, social integration of experiences, and re-establishing them to an organized whole (Boothe, 2010; Romanoff and Thompson, 2006). Especially in psychotherapy, patient narratives can be helpful to recognize patterns of recurring conflicts and the patient's position in these conflicts (Boothe, 2010).

Lastly, there is some evidence that listening to illness stories of others has a positive effect also on fellow patients (Ville and Khlat, 2007; Rosenthal, 2002).

No doubt, the narrative approach is promising, and it seems self-evident as stories and narratives are integrated into our lives from early childhood. Telling stories is an anthropological constant (Straub, 2010). When illness narratives are used in the scientific world e.g. to help patients or other sufferers, there is something that happens which may change the nature of the narratives. This chapter discusses several aspects of storytelling and narratives in use, especially to reflect the authors' own actions and attitudes when engaged in narrative medicine projects. There are four aspects around which this chapter focuses:

◆ What the features of illness narratives are.

◆ How scientific collections of individual patient experiences use illness narratives and how they are presented.

◆ What the features are of such collections of narrative-based patient experiences.

◆ What patients are looking for when visiting a website presenting narrative-based patient experiences.

Storytelling as construction and its functions

Humans are able, and forced, to arrange, order, and interpret stimuli from the outer and the inner environments to create a coherent, meaningful, and manageable world. Although fascinating, this ability often has negative consequences, including misconception, cognitive bias, or social stereotyping (Kahneman, 2003). When looking at Figure 3.1, some readers will see black circles with some white bars, while others will see the white outline of a cube. There are many similar psychological experiments that aim to demonstrate the hypothesis of perception as a mental process of construction. One of the core principles

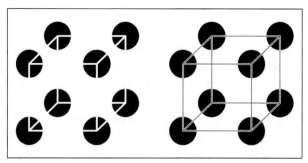

Figure 3.1 What you (do not) see.
Reproduced courtesy of Bernard Ladenthin.

of Gestalt psychology, or Gestalt theory, was developed by Max Wertheimer, Kurt Koffka, Wolfgang Köhler, and Kurt Lewin in the beginning of the twentieth century. From its very beginning, Gestalt theory described the core principle of how humans perceive auditory and visual stimuli. Later, it influenced wide areas of experimental psychology as well as social and cognitive psychology (Read et al., 1997).

Not unlike the organization of auditory and visual stimuli, storytelling, too, is a mental process of construction. In particular, this construction comprises the construction of time and its change, i.e., the chronological order of events. Paul Ricœur (1979) made us aware that—while we normally take it for granted that 'narratives occur *in* time', i.e. within a given temporal framework—narrativity is the mode of discourse through which the mode of being which we call temporality, or temporal being, is brought to language. This process of storytelling has several functions, especially a narrative constitution of time and change, thus being a practice of 'meaning making' by addressing, transforming, and thus reducing contingency (Lucius-Hoene, 2010; Straub, 2010). Illness narratives are the outcomes of this mental process concerning the experiences of illness.

So far, this is a short summary of storytelling as a process of construction—seen from the perspective of the teller. For the listener, however, the sense and significance of the narrative is not merely a matter of, and completed in, the text of a story, but is also the result of an interaction between the world of the text (i.e., the storyteller) and the world of the reader or listener (Irvine and Charon, 2017). In the end, a listener needs a more or less full story to understand its personal meaning (Irvine and Charon, 2017). This may be a challenge for researchers who want to prepare patient narratives for other sufferers in a manageable and condensed form. However, in preserving the meaning of a story, neither can they reduce its content to analysable data in fragmented pieces, nor can they extract its meanings from a story as if they existed separate from its form. As Figure 3.2 shows, the narrative or story can be described as a 'gestalt', the arrangement of its parts comprise a meaning (a); this meaning may get lost when parts are removed

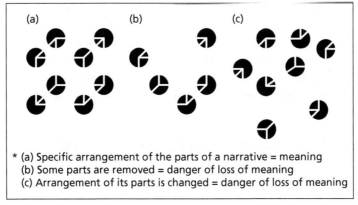

* (a) Specific arrangement of the parts of a narrative = meaning
(b) Some parts are removed = danger of loss of meaning
(c) Arrangement of its parts is changed = danger of loss of meaning

Figure 3.2 The narrative as a 'gestalt'.
Reproduced courtesy of Bernard Ladenthin.

(b), or the parts are arranged in a different way (c). Thus, any work on the text is always an intervention and is inevitably accompanied by changes and shifts of meaning which have to be reflected.

Characteristics of illness narratives

To better understand the characteristics of illness narratives and what is happening when researchers collect illness narratives and process them into patient experiences for publication, we refer to what is known as a DIPEx, or a Database of Individual Patients' Experience of illness; e.g., the German DIPEx website krankheitserfahrungen.de (in English: *illness experiences*). DIPEx websites may be understood as a prototype for patient-orientated websites, and in contrast to many other patient-orientated websites, there are no commercial interests at play behind the website's construction or use. The first and still most well-known version of a DIPEx-Website is the British website www.healthtalk.org, formerly www.dipex.org.

Box 3.1 shows a short illness narrative from a person interviewed for the health issue inflammatory bowel disease bowel disease (in German, Chronisch-entzündliche Darmerkrankungen). When reading this narrative, the reader should remember that storytelling is a mental process of construction. This patient's narrative is about having children or not, presented by a woman suffering from inflammatory bowel disease. Especially two characteristics are noteworthy:

- The narrative is constructed by the teller in the course of her telling. She scans for the right words, she hesitates, she remembers, and she emphasizes (what we can *hear* on krankheitserfahrungen.de, but not *see* in this book).

- Each narrative shows some kind of 'sense', even in instances without any sense, as in the case of an illness. The teller typically looks for an 'ending' that helps the listener to understand the narrative as it is meant. Schütze (2014) calls this need for an ending 'Gestaltschließungszwang'. In this example, the patient completes her story with 'after all, it is good how it went'.

These two characteristics of a narrative—the construction and the 'Gestaltschließungszwang'—underline the Gestalt psychology's credo: that the 'whole' is different from the 'sum of its parts' (Tuck, 2010). If parts of a narration are removed or re-arranged, i.e., experiences that are important for the teller, the meaning the teller intended for the story may be changed. This is illustrated by the 'cube' in Figure 3.1. The meaning of the whole, here the three-dimensional cube, would no longer be visible if parts were missing or interchanged.

Collecting illness narratives and presenting them as patient experiences

Having in mind the characteristics of narratives, this section discusses in more detail how DIPEx researchers collect illness narratives and present them as patient experiences on the website (Ziebland and Herxheimer, 2008). It is important to emphasize here that, of

Box 3.1 Svea Hauck's narrative* about having children

I was pregnant while I was ill, when I had a severe acute episode. The doctors had told me that I would not become pregnant anyway because I was underweight and almost never had my monthly period. Well, exactly that just happened. And then I just had to decide to have an abortion because, first of all, I simply could not imagine being severely ill and raising a child on my own, because, the father, he didn't know either that I was ill. That was just some—when you finally have a chance to experience something, at least, because, I had been in hospital for years, you know. So, there was no chance of affairs with men, and great emotional adventures in a relationship or something like that, of course. All that happened exactly when finally anything at all happened in my life with a partner.

And that's why I decided against the child, also because at that time I was treated with powerful medication. And I was much too afraid. It was a medical indication, it was no problem. Well, I did not bear children since then. I am in a stable relationship, I have even been married for 15 years now, in a, well, multicultural, uh, binational marriage. My partner is from Africa.

The subject of having kids is certainly important in a relationship, and it was a subject of debate for us as well, but first, I was no longer young when we met, and added to this, there were the scientific results I was afraid, well, that it is hereditary, that hereditary transmission can be important. And for me, the most terrible thing to imagine is that my child would have to live through what I lived through, that is, being a sick child.

Also, I know that it doesn't necessarily need to be Crohn, it can be any other illness, you see, I even participated in studies myself. Other illnesses like Type 1 diabetes, that's what my niece has got, or psoriasis, that's what my brother and my mother have. And depression, too. I participated in a study on depression a month ago, conducted by the Max Planck Society. Because of that, well, that was the reason why I said to myself, 'This thought would make me ill'.

Meanwhile, I am of the opinion, I mean, I just never had such a terrible yearning for children. And, also I think you can care for kids without them being your own. And that's what I do, especially in Africa, that's where I do something for kids. I prefer this. So after all, it is good how it went.

* Only parts from this interview can be seen (heard) on krankheitserfahrungen.de

course, researchers are not required for patient stories and experiences to be created and published. For example, women with breast cancer often report their own stories and publish them in books, blogs, or similar media (one of many examples is the Patient Stories section of the website of the Breastlink Breast Cancer Centers: http://www.breastlink.com/breast-cancer-stories). It is noteworthy that there are many fewer published experiences if those who are ill are at risk of being stigmatized or blamed for their condition, for example, in the case of lung cancer.

DIPEx websites present systematic collections and analyses of interviews with people about their experience of illness. It is essential to use open-ended and semi-structured interview methods to ensure not only that the themes the researchers anticipate are addressed; additionally, it is important that unanticipated themes, concerns, and priorities of the respondents are addressed, rather than the agenda of the health researcher. Each collection of interviews is called a 'health issue', and health issues are available across various health conditions like diabetes, pain, epilepsy, different forms of cancer, etc., as well as for patient experiences with the health care system, e.g., access to, and use of, medical rehabilitation measures. Currently, www.healthtalk.org contains more than 100 health issues. As a core principle for each health issue of the website, the researchers analyse 40 to 50 interviews with patients suffering from one health problem, e.g., diabetes or pain. The interview partners are selected carefully according to the principles of maximum variation of illness experiences and social characteristics. Based on the interviews, the project teams identify salient themes and write detailed summaries about each main theme; each theme is then provided online and includes examples from the interviews as video or audio clips to illustrate the different experiences described (Health Experience Research Group, 2014, 2017; Ziebland and McPherson, 2006). Each person presented on the website is introduced with a brief outline of his or her personal profile and experiences, also called 'My story'. The whole process is guided by a detailed 'Researcher Handbook' (Health Experience Research Group, 2014; Health Experience Research Group, 2017) and accompanied by an Advisory Board. This board consists of experts within the respective health issue, including those suffering from the health condition. The advisory board provides input on the literature review, ideas on key areas for sampling categories, topics for the interview guideline, and helps find interview partners.

As a next step, the DIPEx researchers code the interviews and look for themes with the aim of turning illness narratives from interviews into thematically arranged small pieces of stories or patient experiences, comprising several steps.

- First, the interview is cut into pieces, that is, units of meaning. See, for example, the phrase in the middle of Box 3.1: ' … there were the scientific results, I was afraid, well, that it is hereditary, that hereditary transmission can be important'.

- Using a computer-assisted qualitative data analysis software (CAQDAS), such as Atlas ti, segments from the interviews are coded, e.g., in this instance, as 'Afraid of passing on to own children'.

- Based on the coded pieces of many narratives, themes are identified, in this case, as 'Children and family'.

- These themes are arranged under main themes, in this example, as 'Consequences for everyday life and social life'.

- In a last step, pieces of different interviews within a theme are selected for presentation on the website to cover the whole range of experiences within a theme.

Simply put, the website shows (i) the themes that the researchers identified and selected from the different patient narratives, and (ii) how different people talk about the same theme.

The whole process comprises essential elements of qualitative data analysis (Ziebland and McPherson, 2006) to ensure that all common themes and the full range of experiences are shown. However, it is important to highlight two particular aspects of this process.

Firstly, many qualitative approaches explore unknown phenomena and try to reconstruct the studied phenomenon and, by doing so, to receive a deeper understanding and develop theories and models (see, e.g., Smith, 2015; Schreier, 2012). Scientific methods are used to show the range of patient experiences as completely as possible. In other words, it is the perspective and experiences of individuals—rather than the discursive construction of social reality—that matters.

Secondly, the work of DIPEx teams largely follow a bottom-up strategy similar to most qualitative methods. Inevitably, however, there are some points in the production of DIPEx websites where the researchers have to make top-down decisions. For example, more or less all interview partners should be presented on the site—as a gesture of politeness—even if their contributions are nothing more than repetitions of others' experiences. When illustrating themes by audio or video clips, the teams typically try to find a 'positive' clip to start and finish on. Some obviously 'wrong' statements will not be presented on the website or are gently put into perspective, not the least to protect the interview partners. Additionally, some interview partners or experiences are over-represented because they are especially encouraging, interesting, or entertaining, while other interview partners may be very difficult to understand or their experiences are too shocking and are therefore omitted. Some of these rules are explicitly mentioned and frankly discussed in the *DIPEx Handbook* (Health Experiences Research Group, 2014).

Even if all these steps to produce a health issue are performed as carefully as possible, the selection and preparation of the material is subject to a new arrangement and the project teams are, on principle, at risk of losing the gestalt and gist of the patients' stories. Indeed, researchers sometimes feel pressure or are interested in giving a person's story a narrative, dynamic, and positive form, even if such elements did not fully develop within the story, as von Müller und Wermeling (2016) recently showed in their analysis of presentation strategies of illness experiences on krankheitserfahrungen.de.

In other words, the presentation of interview excerpts is a 'sample' arranged from the original patient narratives. Recalling the cube in Figure 3.1, the excerpts are re-narrations of patient stories by the researchers, demonstrating their powerful role and remind the viewer that patient experiences on the DIPEx websites are a (re)construction: by de-constructing the original patient narratives.

In the end, both similarities and differences are visible in the way patients or, more generally, people with a health problem, and researchers act in the case of illness narratives. Both patients and researchers are 'creators': patients trying to construct their experiences into a coherent narrative—a 'gestalt'—and researchers trying to de-construct the patient narratives into a collection of patient experiences (see Figure 3.2). While the ultimate aim of the narrative is to make sense, researchers want to objectify the experiences, i.e., to deploy a large variety of similar experiences, thus showing their range.

What do patients expect from websites that present patient narratives?

After two decades of evidence-based medicine, the expert patient has become the ideal of modern medicine (Donaldson, 2003). The ideal expert patient looks for information to make an informed choice. In the meantime, it is clear that experiential information is as important as scientific information to promote the deliberation of the subjective pros and cons, resulting in a choice that is consistent with the decision-maker's personal values (Ubel and Loewenstein, 1997; Koschack et al., 2015). In the ideal world, this experiential information would be given in a way that is as objective as possible. A scientific database of patient experiences collected by a maximum variation approach (Sandelowski, 1995) seems to be the solution for both requirements, i.e., to make informed choices and to use, for that purpose, experiential information. To receive information in the forefront of a decision, expert patients may visit websites and other sources to collect an exhaustive list of alternatives with pros and cons. To return to the example in Box 3.1, visiting a DIPEx website enables patients to make informed choices about having or not having children when suffering from Morbus Crohn and taking medication.

This *may* happen but there are several problems. Social psychology shows that humans' selection of information is also driven by unconscious processes—to seek information that supports their knowledge and their value system while simultaneously neglecting information that contradicts their knowledge and their value system. This process of which they are not aware is called dissonance reduction (Festinger, 1957).

Additionally, studies on decision-making show that it is important for patients to minimize the decisional conflict that may occur after making decisions. Decisional conflicts may result in situations when a decision is not consistent with a patient's value system. It is possible that visiting a DIPEx website may even increase the risk of a decisional conflict. It may be disturbing for the observer to listen to someone who seems to share her sociodemographic features or to evoke positive feelings, but unfortunately tells about things that are inconsistent with her own values.

Furthermore, Mazanderani and colleagues (2012) describe how people with motor neurone disease or Parkinson's disease, both lifelong conditions with seriously debilitating symptoms, demonstrate a somehow related conflict, and were torn between resistance to sharing their experiences with fellow sufferers and recognizing that they have the same diagnosis, resulting in an attitude and experience of being 'differently the same'.

Figure 3.3 illustrates a fictitious visitor to the website who may be interested in inflammatory bowel diseases (Chronisch-entzündliche Darmerkrankungen) and wants to find out more about the respective patient experiences. Clicking on the chosen topic, the visitor gets a pop-up menu of main topics, for example 'Consequences for everyday

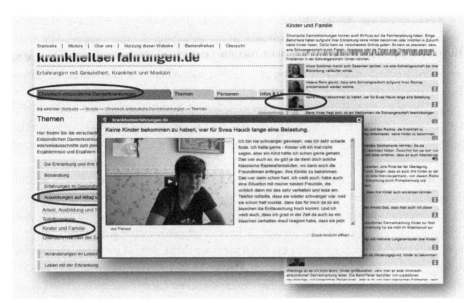

Figure 3.3 How to find an illness narrative on a DIPEx website.
Reproduced courtesy of Wolfgang Himmel.

life and social life' (Auswirkungen auf Alltag und soziales Umfeld). The user can now click on a subtopic, for example 'Children and Family' (Kinder und Familie), and another list opens presenting individuals talking about this issue. For each individual, a strap line gives a résumé about the content. When the user chooses one individual (for example, Svea Hauck), a window opens and a video starts where the observer can hear[*] the person telling his or her experiences with the respective issue. With this process in mind, researchers must ask what patients are looking for when visiting a website that presents such collections of patient experiences, and how well researchers' work and patients' expectations match. What follows are some data and ideas that may shed light on this question.

To date, there is little information about how patients actually use DIPEx websites and how they may turn other patients' experiences into a source of knowledge and support (Mazanderani et al., 2012). Based on our own collection of DIPEx data and using so-called *log* files, preliminary results from a small evaluation study analyzed follow-up on how a sample of 119 visitors explored, i.e., 'surfed' on, krankheitserfahrungen.de (Schierholz, 2016). Patients were asked to explore the website for at least 15 minutes in a way they preferred. Nearly 60% of them used the option to see/hear excerpts (three on average) from the original interviews. The study found that users with a chronic condition did not look at nor explore all experiences in a thematic area. Rather, it showed they selected a sample

---

[*] Many of the interviewees for this website project gave informed consent to show video sequences from the interview, some gave only consent for an audio, and others only for the text of the interview.

of patients or patient stories, although there was no detected specific pattern of choice. Conversations with patients after their visit of the website about their impressions indicated that users with a chronic condition recalled own illness experiences and started to narrate their own story while listening to experiences of others. It seems that patients look for confirmation to avoid cognitive dissonance. This interpretation is also supported by a focus group discussion with users of krankheitserfahrungen.de, initiated by the Berlin DIPEx group (Engler et al., 2016). Users searched for people on the website in similar situations and with similar characteristics to themselves, but not so much for contrasting or entirely different experiences.

The fear of decisional conflict, feelings of cognitive dissonance, or the identity tension of being 'differently the same' seem to result in a behaviour that avoids, instead of looks for, information. In spite of trying to make informed choices, patients may seek confirmation to avoid cognitive dissonance. Of course, people may use a database of patient experiences the way that promises maximal yield for them. But, in this case, they would no longer use the database with the aim to learn more about other patients' ideas and experiences and/or to come to an informed decision in their own case.

Discussion

> True stories are … nutritious and sustaining. They feed the mind with information and the heart with hope and strength. Nature and medical science together can do a great deal to help our bodies and minds heal themselves, but the real experiences of others who have been through the same troubles give us the nourishment that sustains us in the meantime (Philip Pullman, quoted in Elliott, 2006).

To date, patient experiences and the sharing of these experiences are recognized as a source of knowledge and support. But we can only speculate what happens to the listener of patient experiences derived from illness stories, prepared by researchers, and presented as a sample of illness experiences.

This chapter showed that patient-orientated websites that are based on patient narratives follow a process of construction, and deconstruction, thus showing presenting a double 'gestalt' deconstruction or a double 'gestalt'. Narratives are the result of a construction process by the teller in the course of his or her storytelling and are intended to make sense for the subject as a 'gestalt'. These narratives are fragmented into individual pieces of an experience and then constructed (or recomposed) to a new 'gestalt'—a 'sample' to cover a complete cosmos of patient experiences that should ensure a sort of objectivity or completeness.

This could be a prerequisite for informed choices made on evidence-based information. However, another scenario is also rather likely, if just the reported preliminary results are taken into consideration. There, patients may look for other patients' experiences—as 'companion stories'—to make sense of their own illness and to construct their own narrative. When a patient visits these DIPEx websites or listens to this type of material, a generic illness story may evolve in his or her mind that is a composite of different patient experiences. Additionally, the patient may use experiences of others to complete his or her own illness narrative, to give it a 'gestalt'.

To date, very little is known about what patients expect from patient-orientated websites, and how they select the information and what they do with the information presented. Of course, visitors may use **patient experiences** for their own purposes, but it is important to know more about patients' expectations, their handling, and the outcome. If patients use DIPEx websites mainly to minimize cognitive dissonance, this use corresponds to one of the aims of DIPEx and similar websites, e.g., to support those dealing with illness. However, it would not correspond to other important aims, e.g., to present both evidence-based and experiential information and thus to promote informed decisions (Health Experience Research Group, 2017).

Since evidence is still missing on why and how narratives influence decision-making (Winterbottom et al., 2008), further research is necessary to discover more about what patients seek when listening to other patients' experiences and about the mechanisms of the mental representation of the patient experiences. Methods of evaluation are needed that go beyond surveys of consumer satisfaction and that shed more light on the black box of construction when listening to patient stories and illness experiences: a 'construction' that goes beyond the construction of the teller and the researchers.

In the era of the expert patient, DIPEx websites that support informed decision-making are needed and they may help patients to become more self-confident. In the process of selecting patients, interviewing them about their illness experiences, preparing this subjective material, and presenting parts of it on websites, it is vital to be aware that patient narratives are embedded in a collective process that includes the persons who tell stories, those who arrange them for other sufferers, and those who listen to them. This process should receive more attention in the future to better meet patient needs and expectations.

References

Boothe, B., 2010. *The Narrative: Biographic Storytelling in the Psychotherapeutic Process* [in German]. Stuttgart: Schattauer.

Collie, K. and Long, B.C., 2005. Considering 'meaning' in the context of breast cancer. *Journal of Health Psychology*, **10**, 843–853.

Donaldson, L., 2003. Expert patients usher in a new era of opportunity for the NHS. *British Medical Journal*, **326**, 1279–1280.

Easton, G., 2017. Stories in the consultation. In: C. Robertson and G. Clegg, eds. *Storytelling in medicine: how narrative can improve practice*. Boca Raton, FL: Taylor and Francis. pp. 19–40.

Elliott, J., 2006. I wanted to hear positive stories. *BBC News* [online] (Last updated 11:35 PM on 26 March 2006). Available at: <http://news.bbc.co.uk/1/hi/health/4836464.stm> (Accessed 12 June 2018).

Engler, J., Adami, S., Adam, Y., Keller, B., Repke, T., Fügemann, H., Lucius-Hoene, G., Müller-Nordhorn, J., and Holmberg, C., 2016. Using others' experiences. Cancer patients' expectations and navigation of a website providing narratives on prostate, breast and colorectal cancer. *Patient Education and Counseling*, **99**, 1325–1332.

Festinger, L., 1957. *A theory of cognitive dissonance*. Stanford, CA: Stanford University Press.

Frank, A.W., 2013. *The wounded storyteller: body, illness, and ethics*. 2nd rev. ed. Chicago: University of Chicago Press.

Greenhalgh, T., 1998. *Narrative based medicine.* London, BMJ Books.

Greenhalgh, T., 1999. Narrative based medicine in an evidence based world. *British Medical Journal,* **318,** 323–325.

Health Experiences Research Group, 2014. *Researcher's handbook: Healthtalkonline modules.* Oxford: Nuffield Department of Primary Health Care Sciences, University of Oxford.

Health Experience Research Group, n.d. *The research.* Available at <http://www.healthtalk.org/research/about-herg > (Accessed 12 June 2018).

Hsu, M.Y. and McCormack, B., 2012. Using narrative inquiry with older people to inform practice and service developments. *Journal of Clinical Nursing,* **21**(5–6), 841–849.

Irvine, C. and Charon, R., 2017. Deliver us from certainty: training for narrative ethics. In: R. Charon, S. DasGupta, N. Hermann, C. Irvine, E.R. Marcus, E. Rivera Colon, D. Spencer, and M. Spiegel, eds. *The principles and practice of narrative medicine.* Oxford: Oxford University Press. pp. 110–133.

Kahneman, D., 2003. A perspective on judgment and choice: mapping bounded rationality. *American Psychologist,* **58,** 697–720.

Koschack, J., Weibezahl, L., Friede, T., Himmel, W., Makedonski, P., and Grabowski, J., 2015. Scientific versus experiential evidence: discourse analysis of the chronic cerebrospinal venous insufficiency debate in a multiple sclerosis forum. *Journal of Medical Internet Research,* **17,** e159.

Lucius-Hoene, G., 2010. Narrative analysis. In: G. May and K. Mruck, eds. *The Handbook of Qualitative Research in Psychology.* Wiesbaden: Springer. pp. 584–600.

Mansel, J.K., 2014. The diagnostic and healing qualities of story: goals of care. *JAMA Internal Medicine,* **174**(7), 1037. doi:10.1001/jamainternmed.2014.1800.

Mazanderani, F., Locock, L., and Powell J., 2012. Being differently the same: the mediation of identity tensions in the sharing of illness experiences. *Social Science & MedicineI,* **74,** 546–553.

Overcash, J.A., 2003. Narrative research: a review of methodology and relevance to clinical practice. *Critical Reviews in Oncology/Hematology,* **48**(2), 179–184.

Read, S.J., Vanman, E.J., and Miller, L.C., 1997. Connectionism, parallel constraint satisfaction processes, and gestalt principles: (re)introducing cognitive dynamics to social psychology. *Personality and Social Psychology Review,* **1,** 26–53.

Ricœur, P., 1979. The human experience of time and narrative. *Research in Phenomenology,* **9,** 17–34.

Romanoff, B.D. and Thompson, B.E., 2006. Meaning construction in palliative care: the use of narrative, ritual, and the expressive arts. *American Journal of Hospital Palliative Care,* **23,** 309–316.

Rosenthal, G., 1993. Reconstruction of life stories: principles of selection in generating stories for narrative biographical interviews. *The Narrative Study of Lives,* **1**(1): 59–91 [online] Available at: <http://www.ssoar.info/ssoar/bitstream/handle/document/5929/ssoar-tnsl-1993-1-rosenthal-reconstruction_of_life_stories.pdf?sequence=1> (Accessed 12 June 2018).

Rosenthal, G., 2002. Conducting a conversation in a narrative-biographical style: On the conditions of curative storytelling in the context of research and counselling [in German]. *Psychotherapie und Sozialwissenschaften,* **4,** 204–227 [online] Available at: <http://www.ssoar.info/ssoar/bitstream/handle/document/5676/ssoar-2002-3-rosenthal-biographisch-narrative_gesprachsfuhrung.pdf?sequence=1> (Accessed 12 June 2018).

Sandelowski, M., 1995. Sample size in qualitative research. *Research in Nursing & Health,* **18**(2), 179–183.

Schierholz, H.M., 2016. *Online health experiences as a tool for information and support—Evaluation of the website www.krankheitserfahrungen.de* [in German]. PhD. Georg-August-Universität Göttingen. Available at: <https://ediss.uni-goettingen.de/handle/11858/00-1735-0000-002B-7C41-2>. (Accessed 12 June 2018).

Schreier, M., 2012. *Qualitative content analysis in practice.* Thousands Oaks, CA: Sage.

Schütze, F., 2014. Autobiographical accounts of war experiences. An outline for the analysis of topically focused autobiographical texts—using the example of the 'Robert Rasmus' account in Studs Terkel's book, 'The Good War'. *Qualitative Sociology Review*, 10, 224–283

Smith, J.A., 2015. *Qualitative psychology. A practical guide to research methods*. London: Sage.

Straub, J., 2010. Narrative Theory/Narration [in German]. In: **G. Mey** and **K. Mruck**, eds. *Handbook of Qualitative Research in Psychology*. Wiesbaden: VS Verlag für Sozialwissenschaften. pp. 136–150.

Tuck, M., 2010. *Gestalt Principles Applied in Design*. Available at: <https://www.webpagefx.com/blog/web-design/gestalt-principles-applied-in-design/>(Accessed 12 June 2018).

Ubel, P.A. and **Loewenstein, G.**, 1997. The role of decision analysis in informed consent: choosing between intuition and systematicity. *Social Science & Medicine*, **44**(5), 647–656.

Ville, I. and **Khlat, M.**, 2007. Meaning and coherence of self and health: an approach based on narratives of life events. *Social Science & Medicine*, **64**(4), 1001–1014.

von Müller, M. and **Wermeling, M.**, 2016. Never-ending stories. Strategies to present illness narratives [in German]. *DIEGESIS Interdisciplinary E-Journal for Narrative Research*, 5, 35–62.

Winterbottom, A., **Bekker, H.L., Conner, M.,** and **Mooney, A.**, 2008. Does narrative information bias individual's decision making? A systematic review. *Social Science & Medicine*, 67, 2079–2088.

Ziebland, S. and **McPherson, A.**, 2006. Making sense of qualitative data analysis: an introduction with illustrations from DIPEx (personal experiences of health and illness). *Medical Education*, **40**, 405–414.

Ziebland, S. and **Herxheimer, A.**, 2008. How patients' experiences contribute to decision making: illustrations from DIPEx (personal experiences of health and illness). *Journal of Nursing Management*, **16**, 433–439.

Chapter 4

Stories, illness, and narrative norms

Lars-Christer Hydén

Introduction

Collecting and using illness narratives has become an established practice among social sciences researchers in the medical field to explore illness experiences. One problem in research on illness narratives is that the role of narrative norms—that is, notions of how a story is organized—is rarely discussed, but rather taken for granted by many researchers. Because many people, especially those with neurocognitive disorders, have difficulties living up to and adhering to these narrative norms, there is a risk that their voices and experiences will be excluded from discussions about the consequences of these and other disorders.

Many social scientific researchers have tended to conceive and analyse stories told in interviews or identified in observational data as if they were written. Hence, the focus is often on the *discursive organization* of the narrative in terms of temporal coherence, plot, and so on. Generally, it implies that the *meaning* of the narrative can be found *in* the narrative text and that the narrative primarily is a *representation* of events in the past. Consequently, illness narratives told in interviews are often analysed in relation to norms for written text production, as if they are *written* autobiographical texts. A consequence of—implicitly or explicitly—adhering to literary narrative norms is that social scien-tific researchers often expect and hope to elicit and collect stories that conform to these literary norms.

These types of theoretical conceptions and assumptions—the implicit narrative norms—thus increase the risk of excluding those who cannot live up to the literary narrative norms from studies on illness narratives. The reason often given is that these persons have some kind of 'communicative', 'speech', or 'cognitive' problem, thus meeting exclusion criteria. Their exclusion from projects also means that their voices and experiences are excluded as well. Further, analysing stories that do not comply with the established narrative norms might give the impression that the storyteller is an 'unreliable narrator'—an identity defined by his or her narrative incompetence (cf. Hydén, 2017).

This chapter discusses the role of narrative norms with an emphasis on the notion of temporal coherence.

Narrative norms

The literary scholar Suzanne Fleischman wrote that narrative norms are 'a set of shared conventions and assumptions about what constitutes a well-formed story' that are internalized by speakers (1990, p. 263). These narrative norms guide the storyteller in how to produce a story so that it will be recognized by audiences as a *certain kind* of story. The normative expectations help the listener to build an interpretation of the emerging story: how to understand events up to the present. As the narratologist Wolfgang Iser once pointed out, understanding and interpreting a story is a hypothesis-testing process where the listener tests, revises, and checks interpretations of the story (1978, pp. 107ff). These norms help the storyteller to tell the story in such a way that the listener will understand what is said, and thus understand the emerging story.

These narrative norms are learned by the participants from early age and will result in most people becoming not only very versatile storytellers, but also able to appreciate a wide variety of stories, told by different people, in different contexts. In various social and cultural contexts, most children and adults become familiar with certain shared narrative norms. Research shows that narrative norms are less universal than we might think: they differ between socioeconomic groups, and various social and cultural groups develop these norms even further, thus creating quite specialized stories and understanding of stories (Heath, 1983).

One set of narrative norms are the literary norms that have developed around producing and understanding written stories. Central to the literary, textual narrative norms is the defining of stories as a unit, with a beginning, middle, and end. Integral to the story is also the temporal progression of story events, as well as the expectation of a clear plot, and some kind of moral or lesson. Researchers into illness narratives deal with a subset of the literary norms, i.e., narrative norms having to do with autobiographical storytelling.

Some of the basic aspects of these literary narrative norms are assumed when planning and executing research. There are certain expectations about what kind of stories will be collected through interviews, the way these stories should be told and organized, and their content. There are also certain tools that can be applied in analysing these stories, and later, in reporting them, e.g., in journal articles. In particular, stories are often approached as representations of a set of events leading up to an illness, through the diagnosis, and to the present.

What is problematic here is that the expectation and hope of eliciting, finding, and collecting stories that conform to the literary norms are confounded when storytellers with communicative disabilities, and their stories, do not adhere to these norms. These disabilities are often connected to cognitive and linguistic challenges resulting from neurocognitive disorders or acquired brain injuries. Rather than telling well-organized stories in interviews or in clinical or everyday settings, those with communicative disabilities quite often tend to upset the narrative norms that researchers assume as implicit.

This text-based conception of narrative has been widely—and maybe unintentionally—adopted and used by researchers working on illness narratives, although models for analysis of oral stories have been around for many years (Labov and Waletzky, 1967, 1997; Ochs and Capps, 2001). Consequently, the tendency among social scientific researchers is to conceive and analyse stories told in interviews in the same way as written stories.

A good and influential early example of this approach is *The Wounded Storyteller* (1995, 2015) by sociologist Arthur Frank, whose book maintains a wide influence in the field of illness narratives. Frank introduced the illness narrative as a wider social scientific and medical concern. When looking at the narratives examples he uses to support his arguments and theoretical suggestions, it is clear that all of them are based on written and published stories by patients; none are orally based. A more recent but equally influential example is Rita Charon's 2006 *Narrative Medicine: Honoring the Stories of Illness*. In several of her publications, Charon has argued for what she calls narrative medicine; however, most of her theoretical arguments and examples are based on excerpts from novels and written stories—again, less from interviews or recordings of clinical encounters.

Both Frank's and Charon's work has been widely influential and has worked as a model for what illness narratives look like and how they can be approached. Their work has helped to sustain and spread the notion of illness narratives as well-formed and self-contained units. It has thus geared researchers' attention to finding the meaning in the text, rather than, for example, in the function of the story, or the embodied performance of the story.

As mentioned, treating interview narratives as if they are written texts is problematic, especially in relation to people with neurocognitive disorders but also for many other storytellers with other kinds of disorders. The primary concern is the risk of excluding people, as well as voices and experiences, from research on illness experience.

Temporal coherence

One set of narrative norms that is especially salient in research on illness narratives is the notion of *temporal coherence*; that is, the expectation that the story reflects a set of temporally progressive events which being at the first event and often conclude in the present (Labov, 1972). Temporal coherence can be identified on at least two levels in a story: an event has a microtemporal coherence that results in a temporal organization of the central actions; autobiographical stories often consist of several events that are combined following a macrotemporal order (Gee, 1991; Kintsch and van Dijk, 1978).

Some storytellers have problems with the temporal organization of autobiographical stories for various reasons. Anthropological and other researchers have suggested that stories can be organized along other dimensions, e.g., using space or place as the fundamental organizing principle. In a famous example, Michelle Rosaldo showed how everyday hunting stories among the Ilongot were organized around the physical hunting path, while time was of less importance (Rosaldo, 1980). Other storytellers, like those with neurocognitive disorders (e.g., Alzheimer's disease, acquired brain injuries) often do not tell temporally organized stories because of executive and memory function problems (working memory, episodic memory), which can result in tales about specific events, but where these events have no temporal structure across a whole story.

Researchers usually want to study and analyse the temporal dimensions of interview stories in a linear fashion, e.g., from the present to the future, or how the present can be understood in the light of the past. As there is often an interest in patient experience directly after the diagnosis of an illness, it is not uncommon for researchers to start an interview with questions that relate to just such an experience. In analysing the interviews, the thematic content of the interview is then ordered in such a way that it fits with a preconceived idea of temporal order; that is, the illness process starts with discovery and then progresses from that point. Thus, the medical diagnosis of the illness often achieves the status of something that divides life up into a 'before' and an 'after', which for the individual leads to a 'disrupted life' in which falling ill is a sort of 'turning point'. Thus, illness is described as based on a linear time axis, with the illness as a turning point and a disruption in a temporal flow.

Interview transcripts often show that most storytellers do not tell stories in the temporally ordered way as researchers often would prefer, even if prompted to do so. Instead, storytellers seem to consider the temporal organization of the story as a *device for meaning making*. That is, by re-organizing the order of the events, they can add some new meaning to the story beyond that found in the thematic content often connected to linear organization. Some interviewees tell their illness stories by *backshadowing* and *foreshadowing* events; that is, by indicating that they had a premonition of events to come, thus casting a shadow over future events (Bernstein, 1994; Morson, 1994).

Backshadowing is quite common in interviews, often in the form of small comments about specific events. Many years ago, interviews were done with people diagnosed with chronic fatigue syndrome (CFS) (Bülow and Hydén, 2003). In an interview, 'Tina' described her life situation as she remembered it from the time she began to experience symptoms. Her narrative developed successively from the interviewer's questions. In discussing her work and work situation, she described negative changes in the organization of her work, about her ambition to do a good job, and about the feeling of responsibility that partly stopped her from 'getting out of there'. She talked about how her working situation, in combination with what she called her 'personality', affected her. Tina evaluated the events that led to her eventual CFS diagnosis, saying 'because I should have seen it coming much earlier and left [my job]'.

In Tina's reflections about the time before and during her illness, she anticipates her illness and diagnosis in the stress that eventually led to her illness. The illness thus becomes a given result of her life as she has lived it. It is also a premonition that she 'should have seen'. In Tina's interview, as well as in interviews with others, premonitions of illness consist not only of early signs of the disease in the form of symptoms, but also in images of traumas, life crises, or periods of intense burdens that, in retrospect, may be understood as 'omens' of illness and suffering. However, since the illness could not be anticipated, it could not be prevented, and is instead something that happens as a part of the illness process. Most importantly, in her interview Tina uses time to deliberate on and negotiate her own responsibility for her illness: could she have adapted and changed her lifestyle, and thus, by acting in a 'responsible' way, prevented her illness?

Tina's example highlights the importance of taking the storyteller's temporal organization of their story into consideration when analysing illness narratives. Temporal organization is a way of creating meaning by using formal properties of a story, rather than thematic ones (Bülow and Hydén, 2003).

The next two sections discuss cases in which the basic temporal relation between events in the story has become highly problematic. In both cases the challenged temporal organization of the autobiographical stories result in 'broken' or 'entangled' stories (Hydén and Brockmeier, 2008; Hyden, 2017), i.e., stories where beginnings and endings are twisted together, interwoven with repetitions of the same event that result in shared states of narrative perplexity. In the first case, the entangled story is related to memory challenges resulting from Alzheimer's disease. In the second case, the broken story is connected to a deep despair originating from the consequences of a severe spinal cord injury.

Event organization

Individuals living with Alzheimer's disease are often severely challenged when it comes to the temporal dimension of stories, especially in trying to fit various events or episodes into a general, narrative, temporal organization. Small story parts—episodes or singular events—are often well organized, but it is unclear how these episodes fit together. Often, the same story episode can be told several times during the same storytelling event, thus violating the narrative norm story elements are not repeated if nothing new takes place.

The lack of a temporal macro-organization of a story together with repetitions of the same sequence is often considered as evidence of the person lacking storytelling abilities. Seen from a slightly different point of view, it can be argued that sequences told repeatedly are most likely quite significant for the teller. A recording captures two women, both diagnosed with Alzheimer's disease, telling autobioautobiographical stories. During a 45-minute period, one of the women—here called Martha—tells about getting a driver's license and then buying a car and going on vacation with her family. However, Martha's 'story' does not take a linear form; rather, it consists of roughly 16 small episodes that are repeated and joined together in various ways (Hydén and Örulv 2010; see Box 4.1).

During the 45 minutes, Martha tells—and repeats—some of these smaller episodes between three and six times each; she also joins these episodes together in several ways (Hyden and Örulv, 2009, 2010). Box 4.2 shows how different themes are nested together. Telling the story, Martha is sitting together with her friend Catherine, who is mostly a silent but interested listener. The story starts when Martha visits her sister, driving her new VW car.

At closer inspection, Box 4.2 is divided into at least two thematic sections. The first nine lines are organized around one theme—visiting the sister (see line 3:3 in Box 4.2). Lines 10–15 are organized around a different theme—buying a car (akin to Part 2 in Box 4.1). From a temporal point of view, the events belonging to Part 2 happened before the events in Part 3. In telling the story, Martha does not indicate these thematic and temporal shifts in any way. Still, it is possible to observe an associative connection between two themes in

Box 4.1 The units of Martha's story

Part 1: The son's and/or Martha's getting a driver's licence

(1:1) The local driving instructor encourages the young Martha to learn how to drive.

(1:2) Martha's son gets his driver's licence.

(1:3) A fragmented phrase (used several times).

Part 2: Buying a car

(2:1) Martha decides to buy a car (a VW).

(2:2) Martha's husband questions her ability to save up for a car.

(2:2b) Martha reasserts herself.

(2:3) The look of the car (a VW).

(2:4) Getting help buying a car.

(2:5) Martha plans how to pay for the car.

(2:6) Making a down payment to get the car right away.

(2:7) Martha buys a car.

(2:8) Getting the car.

Part 3: Driving for a vacation and meeting the family

(3:1) Practising before going away.

(3:2) Making a detour.

(3:3) Surprising her sister (later, her mother); the absent husband/driver.

(3:4) Advising her sister about learning to drive; never drive with one's husband.

lines 9, 10, and 11. Line 9 belongs thematically to the preceding strophe, 'Martha's sister and the absent husband/driver'. Line 10 seems to function as a bridge to another part of the story organized around a different theme, namely 'Martha decides to buy a car'. This strophe has already been told previously as it belongs to Part II of the story. It is apparently the words/theme 'driver's license' that functions as an associative connection between the two themes since 'driver's license' belongs to both these themes.

Thus, in this small excerpt, Martha does what is generally considered to be typical for persons with dementia: they repeat stories told the minute before. Generally, those suffering from Alzheimer's disease experience a loss of the short-term and episodic memory (Morris and Becker, 2004).

In analysing Martha's storytelling, the frequent telling and retelling of stories or story fragments was often used to make sense of the current situation or to contribute to an ongoing conversation by the person with dementia. This could be seen as a natural

Box 4.2 Thematic sections in Martha's story

1   'But he's ((Saul—Martha's husband)) not here with us', I said

2   'Saul he's not here now'.

3   'Isn't he here? And who drives the car then?'

4   'Well I guess I do', I said

5   'ARE YOU DRIVING?' she said

6   'Yeah?' //Catherine: She thought you were not all there//

7   no that's what she thought ((laughing))

8   then (I) said ·hh

9   'Well, shouldn't I dr-- shouldn't I', I said

10   'If I have a driver's licence', I said then

11   'I guess I will buy myself a car', I said

12   because I saved up some money

13   but I went to have a look at a car then

14   a VW

15   a new one

(Reported speech is marked by change in tone and prosody.)

strategy considering that dementia, as well as other brain disorders, implies that the person has limited access to cognitive and linguistic resources. Instead, they must make use a smaller set of resources and use these in creative ways. People with dementia generally have a limited access to their previous array of narrative themes and fragments, and often use these repeatedly in different contexts and for different purposes– sometimes in ways that can be quite confusing for other participants (for examples, see Örulv and Hydén, 2006).

In her 1997 book, Vai Ramanathan indicates that repetition of the same story or story fragment can have a further function, specifically, relating certain events by telling a story can be a way to present important aspects of the Self. In Martha's story, fragments appear that establish her as an independently minded person—although others, like her husband and sister, had objected. When Martha tells and retells those story fragments, she is close to 90 years old and lives in a residential care unit with a dementia diagnosis. But by repeating the story fragments, listeners are reminded that she was also a woman who was independent and autonomous.

Thus, although severe problems with the temporal organization of story might result in broken stories, a closer look at these stories may simultaneously reveal subtle meaning-making strategies that are used by storytellers who have limited linguistic and cognitive resources.

Chaos narratives

For some suffering from illness or injury, the linear aspect of time has disappeared, and these types of stories told are called 'chaos narratives' (Frank, 1995). These narratives are characterized by the the storyteller always seeming to be in the present; there is no future horizon that helps to establish hope. The sufferer tells a disjointed story:

> Stories are chaotic in their absence of narrative order. Events are told as the storyteller experiences life: without sequence or discernable causality. (Frank, 1995, p. 97)

A visit to the storyworld of a chaos narrative is a visit to a world beyond the moral norms and standards of everyday life. It is a non-sequential story that tries to describe a world that is difficult to imagine and to inhabit, that is about the physically and morally broken body, and that is told from the immediacy of the actual body. The story often creates strong emotional responses in the listener, not the least because any possibilities for change in any direction or any hope are totally absent.

In a study of athletes who have suffered severe physical traumas, the British sociologists Brett Smith and Andrew Sparkes interviewed several rugby players that became disabled because of their rugby playing (Smith and Sparkes, 2008; cf. Smith and Sparkes, 2011). One of their interviewees was a 35-year-old man who suffered an upper spinal cord injury resulting in paraplegia. In a life-history orientated research interview, 'Jamie' tells about the accident and its consequences on his life. The story declares that the accident was not a turning point. Rather, his life as he had known it stopped with the accident, and nothing happened after the injury, except for a faint wish to walk again. Later, he divorced his wife and only saw his children occasionally.

In the interview, the interviewer tries to enter Jamie's experiences and feelings related to the consequences of his spinal injury (Box 4.3).

The answer to the initial interview question is interspersed by four very long silences (in an interview five to ten seconds silences are extremely long and marked pauses). In their way these pauses underline the patient's belief that there is nothing more to say—the silences are equal to speech. Silence or words—it does not matter. Jamie not only tells the interviewer (and thus other listeners and readers) that his life is over, but also that there is no way forward after the accident; there is no future and nothing will happen that changes his situation. For Jamie's chaos narrative, there is no progression of narrative events—beginning, middle and end—only an eternal now.

The interviewer is drawn into this chaos storyworld, and after the two first silences is obviously immersed in Jamie's feelings of hopelessness and demoralization, and offers 'I'm not sure what to say'. This empathy of hopelessness again appears when the interviewer asks, 'You've gone?' in response to Jamie's use of the word 'gone'; Jamie's words reflect his former life.

When Jamie tells his story, there is no separation between his actual body and the body projected into the storyworld. This identity between the actual and the narrative bodies makes it difficult, almost impossible, for both storyteller and listener to view, understand, describe, or experience the body in any other way. For Jamie, the body in the real world and the story world are the same; time has stopped for both.

Box 4.3 Jamie tells his story

Jamie: I feel nothing. Feel, it's shattering, shattering.

(ten second silence)

The whole thing, just completely shattering. Life has been, it's been beaten, life's been beaten out of me.

(eight second silence)

Interviewer: I'm, I'm not sure what to say.

Jamie: What is there to say? My life is a mess now. I can't remember when I was happy last. I feel, I feel, dead now. Since the accident, it's like this all the time. Life was good before it. I was happy. Then, then, I, I don't know. My life is over. It is over. Over. I've gone.

(five second silence)

Interviewer: You've gone?

Jamie: Yes. I am no one now. I may as well be dead. The accident has left me with nothing. No one. Life is a mess. The neck is broke, and, and, and it was awful. Last night I couldn't sleep. I can't sleep at the moment. I lie there. My life has ended.

(five second silence)

My life ended when, when. I don't know how to say it. It's difficult. I sit here. What do I have? Nothing. It's, it's, it's over. Nothing to live for. I don't know how else to say it. What can I say? I'm gone. The accident took everything from me. Now what? And then, then, then, I don't know. I don't know why I live. Nothing has changed since the accident. The body has had it. Life has, has, stopped. I have no life left in me now. Just darkness. Darkness. I'm worthless. And then, then, life has ended. No cure. Life ended the day I broke this neck.

(From Smith and Sparkes, 2008; transcription slightly changed by adding new lines when there is a pause in order to clarify the structure of the told story.)

Discussion

When researchers encounter patients who tell stories that seem to lack temporal coherence or dimension, one possible response is to in some way attempt to amend the interview and the story. This can be done by compiling a narrative out of the story fragments and creating a temporally coherent narrative, i.e., a story that adheres to the norms of written text narratives. It is also possible to use stories *about* the person with dementia told by others (relatives, carers, professionals) and use this material to compile a story.

This procedure has, in fact, profound consequences both for the conception of what a narrative is and for the ways narratives are analysed. However, the question then emerges of *whose story* it is that is being told and presented in research, and *whose voice* is heard in the storytelling. Is the researcher's attempt at the story the patient's true story, or is it the story that the researcher *believes* that the patient wanted to tell? Additionally, people with communicative disabilities tend to appear less competent as storytellers than they actually are. Telling stories that do not comply with the established narrative norms often results in the conclusion that if the story is somehow defective or incompetent, so, too, is the storyteller.

At the same time, people telling illness stories are often quite creative storytellers—especially if they have communicative disabilities. Often, they try to find new semiotic resources to overcome the effects of their brain disorder in order to be able to continue as participants in storytelling activities (as in interviews) and thus sustain both their personhood and their sense of self and identity. However, this can create complications for the other participants, expecially the interviewer.

A problem is that literary narrative norms often tend to exclude creative use of communicative resources. Stories told by people with brain disorders often defy ordinary ways of listening to and understanding stories. As such, this lack of an ordinary storytelling relationship easily can result in a situation that often is described in the literature as a 'communicative breakdown'. That is, the participants cannot establish a shared understanding and meaning, resulting in one or both of the participants wanting to withdraw from the ongoing activity. This could increase the risk of what Paula Freed (2002) calls another 'disencounter'. One way around such a relational defeat would be for the participants, and especially the healthy participants, to engage in the meaning-making process in a way that is open to new possibilities of meaning. Metaphors used in psychoanalysis could help conceptualize this possibility.

In 1948, the Austrian-American psychoanalyst Theodor Reik published *Listening with a Third Ear*, which in part described his ideas on how clinical psychoanalysts should listen to their patients. He argued that the established idea about how to listen to patient was to focus on what today is called the verbal utterances of the patients; that is, the words. Reik pointed out that the 'verbal message' only constituted a minor part of the resources the analyst uses in constructing an understanding of the meaning of the patient's stories. Other extremely important resources were found in embodied communication—the way the patients made use of their bodies, voices, gestures (the rhythm and prosody)—as well as the timing in telling a story. Thus, in constructing meaning, the 'conjecturing analyst'

> does not concern himself first and foremost with the logical proof of his idea, and often pursues contradictory trains of thought. He has an open mind and does not shrink from yielding himself, by way of experiment, to a train of thought that seems senseless and absurd. (...) He must learn to listen 'with the third ear.' (Reik, 1949, pp. 223, 144)

According to Reik, it is thus less important to adhere to the traditional communicative norms having to do with coherence and truth than 'to a train of thought that seems senseless and absurd'. The 'senseless and absurd' could even perhaps be poetic rather than just imply meaning. In other words, it is important sometimes to engage in mutual meaning-making through listening and understanding in new and often surprising ways, especially to find out what could be salvaged beyond the pure verbal utterance. Although people engaging in storytelling with persons with dementia rarely are psychoanalysts, Reik's advice is still worth considering.

Reseachers above all must be aware of the often implicit narrative norms that guide not only the analysis of interviews, but also the interview design and the way studies are reported.

References

Bernstein, M. A., 1994. *Foregone Conclusions: Against Apocalyptic History*. Berkeley, CA: University of California Press.

Bülow, P and Hydén, L-C., 2003. In dialogue with time: Identity and illness in narratives about chronic fatigue. *Narrative Inquiry*, 13, 71–97.

Charon, R., 2006. *Narrative Medicine: Honoring the Stories of Illness*. New York: Oxford University Press.

Frank, A. W., 1995. *The Wounded Storyteller. Body, Illness, and Ethics*. Chicago: The University of Chicago Press.

Fleischman, S., 1990. *Tense and Narrativity: From Medieval Performance to Modern Fiction*. Austin: University of Texas Press.

Freed, P., 2002. Meeting of the minds: ego reintegration after traumatic brain injury. *Bulletin of the Menninger Clinic*, 66, 61–78.

Gee, J. P., 1991. A linguistic approach to narrative. *Journal of Narrative and Life History*, 1, 15–39.

Heath, S. B., 1983. *Ways With Words. Language, Life, and Work in Communities and Classrooms*. New York: Cambridge University Press.

Hydén, L-C., 2017. *Entangled Narratives. Collaborative Storytelling and the Re-Imagining of Dementia*. New York: Oxford University Press.

Hydén, L-C. and Brockmeier, J., eds., 2008. *Health, culture and illness: broken narratives*. New York: Routledge.

Hydén, L-C. and Örulv, L., 2009. Narrative and identity in Alzheimer's disease: a case study. *Journal of Aging Studies*, 23, 205–214.

Hydén L-C & Örulv, L., 2010. Interaction and narrative in dementia. In: D. Schiffrin, A. De Fina and A. Nylund, eds. *Telling stories: language, narrative, and social life*. Washington, DC: Georgetown University Press. pp. 149–160.

Iser, W., 1978. *The Act of Reading. A Theory of Aesthetic Response*. Baltimore: Johns Hopkins University Press.

Kintsch, W. and van Dijk, T., 1978. Toward a model of text comprehension and production. *Psychological Review*, 85, 363–394.

Labov, W., 1972. The transformation of experience in narrative syntax. In: W. Labov, ed., *Language in the Inner City*. Philadelphia: University of Pennsylvania Press. pp. 354–405.

Labov, W. and Waletzky, J., 1967/1997. Narrative analysis: oral versions of personal experience. *Journal of Narrative and Life History*, 7, 3–38.

Morris, R. and Becker, J., eds., 2004. *Cognitive Neuropsychology of Alzheimer's Disease* 2nd ed. Oxford: Oxford University Press.

Morson, G. S., 1994. *Narrative and Freedom. The Shadows of Time*. New Haven, CT: Yale University Press.

Ochs, E & Capps, L., 2001. *Living Narrative. Creating Lives in Everyday Storytelling*. Cambridge, MA: Harvard University Press.

Ramanathan, V., 1997. *Alzheimer Discourse. Some Sociolinguistic Dimensions*. Mahwah, NJ: Lawrence Erlbaum Associates.

Reik, T., 1949. *Listening with the Third Ear. The inner experience of a psychoanalyst*. London: George Allen & Unwin Ltd.

Rosaldo, M. Z., 1980. *Knowledge and passion. Ilongot notions of self and social life.* Cambridge: Cambridge University Press.

Smith, B. and Sparkes, A. C., 2008. Changing bodies, changing narratives and the consequences of tellability: a case study of becoming disabled through sport. *Sociology of Health and Illness*, **30**, 1–20.

Smith, B. and Sparkes, A. C., 2011. Exploring multiple responses to a chaos narrative. *Health*, **15**, 38–53.

Örulv, L. and Hydén, L-C., 2006. Confabulation: sense-making, self-making and world-making in dementia. *Discourse Studies*, **8**, 647–673.

Chapter 5

Choices of illness narratives in practice

Applying ideas of sampling and generalizability

Thorsten Meyer and Margret Xyländer

Patients' stories in practice

Illness narratives have found their way into the daily lives of thousands of people. For example, the association of German medical schools has recently set up an exhibition based on patients' reports about their illness and care. This exhibition has been shown at different medical schools in Germany, and it is available to view on the association's homepage[1]. The exhibition, 'Hinter den Kulissen: Patienten erzählen' (Behind the Scenery: Patients Report), compiles 33 different patient stories that focus on the unique supporting role of highly specialized university medical centres. There are stories from different fields, including oncology, hearing loss, transplantation, perinatal medicine, neurology, and surgery. In the exhibition's introduction, the president of the association points out that these stories provide a very private insight into the lives of the patients; at the same time, they illustrate the importance of university-based medical care for the German health system and how much the staff accomplished each and every day. The patients' stories drew a very personal picture of these accomplishments, which expressed the significance of this highly specialized medical care.

Increasingly, these kinds of patient accounts appear regularly in the daily lives of millions of people. However, the exhibition mentioned is special because it comes from a university background. It is clear that, while the exhibition shows very comprehensive and realistic insights into patients' experiences, its main purpose is to show that these stories support a predefined and politically important message—that medical schools play an important and specific part in the health care of the German population, and that they should be acknowledged accordingly. From this perspective, patients' stories are being used to convey a political message. This chapter is not an appropriate forum for an ethical discussion regarding the part politics can play in medical care provision. However, this example is similar to many others in that patients' stories often provide a persuasive approach to convey a pre-defined message.

Sampling illness narratives in practice

This chapter takes the perspective of qualitative researchers on how to select illness narratives for a specific use in practice, and which part of these narratives should be chosen. From a pragmatic perspective, it is easy to argue that this issue is not of great importance. Perhaps those cases from a study that fit our purpose(s) best are those that are selected. And, in the same vein, so are those citations within the case that fit the purpose(s) best. However, in doing so, the credibility of the work can be jeopardized as this approach is commonly used in journalism, politics, or marketing, which are fields that deal with disseminating messages that are pre-defined and simple.

Why, then, should there be a bother about issues of sampling illness narratives in practice? Firstly, there is the important—or even central—issue of sampling or choosing cases as a prerequisite for drawing generalizations. In this context, sampling or choosing cases is not only related to the process of selecting cases for research, but also to further aspects of the research process. This includes how to deal with conflicting results, or which results should be reported in a research paper, and how. Secondly, it should sensitize researchers to the different political roles they might play when working in practice-related fields, such as health research. The medical school example shows that the selection of cases and of the information provided within each case is predetermined by the message they are intended to convey: one based on persuasion and motivated by marketing or advocacy. Researchers might find themselves sometimes in a similar position—qualitative research is inherently value-driven and can adhere to an advocacy framework. How then do researchers deal with these issues of sampling in these situations?

By looking at the issue of selecting cases or citations of illness narratives for use in practice from the perspective of qualitative researchers, awareness is needed when determining approaches or criteria that guide the selections. This chapter asserts that the selection of illness narratives for use in practice should likewise be guided by those used in sampling, representativeness, and generalizability in qualitative research in the planning and active research phases. Therefore, this chapter reviews these concepts and considers their relevance for case or information selection in illness narratives for use in practice.

To begin, the chapter discusses issues of sampling in qualitative research. Next, it reflects on the different roles researchers play in using illness narratives. Finally, it attempts to distil these issues to sensitize for matters of scientific probity in using illness narratives in practice and concludes by suggesting alternative ways that patients' stories might increase understanding of patient care provided in medical schools.

Qualitative research: sampling strategies and generalization

A great weakness, even danger, of qualitative research lies in its potential to 'prove' almost anything. If there are strong assumptions about a topic and a personal agenda about what results should lead to, then there is a strong risk that the research renders poor quality results (Meyer, 2015). A major challenge in qualitative research is how to deal with assumptions and presuppositions, which, if unchecked, may determine the research process and forego innovative conclusions and result in assumptions getting proven because the research process was set up not to be open to alternatives. There is a common temptation to look especially for citations, cases, or situations that prove the original question, but this is poor qualitative research.

One central strategy to counteract this tendency is related to what Patton called 'purposeful sampling', or the sampling of information-rich cases (2002, p. 230). Sampling should not be based on randomness, nor on convenience. Instead, a strategy should be applied that allows researchers to learn the most in relation to the research question. Patton has compiled 15 different sampling strategies (14 + 1 to represent all useful triangulation options) that could serve this purpose (2002; for a discussion see also Emmel, 2013). These strategies include *maximum variation sampling*, i.e., selecting a wide range of cases on dimensions of interest; *extreme or deviant case sampling*, i.e., the selection of unusual cases to provide a special way of learning about a phenomena; *sampling confirming and disconfirming cases*, which is especially valuable for facilitating analytical generalizations; and *critical case sampling*, which allows for logical generalizations in the sense that if an assumption holds in the case sampled, it also should hold in other cases (Patton, 2002, pp. 230–242). Theoretical sampling, as has been elaborated on within the framework of grounded theory (Corbin and Strauss, 1990), is also one of these sampling strategies. Here, the process of data acquisition and data analysis are interdependent and build on each other. Therefore, theoretical sampling is deeply integrated in the research process and the development of empirically based theoretical assumptions. Along with the technique of constant comparison, this strategy helps to continuously challenge researchers' thinking against the data and emerging theory. In this vein, sampling represents an important building block in the generalizability of study results (cf. Mayring, 2007).

In general, research techniques should be reflective and explicit about the rationale behind case selection, which should be conceptually driven (by a predetermined theoretical framework or by evolving theory), and sampling should be designed to make analytical generalizations possible, where samples should not usually be wholly pre-specified, but rather selected sequentially. Sample size should be small enough to accomplish 'the deep, case-oriented analysis that is a hallmark of all qualitative inquiry', and large enough to ensure 'a new and richly textured understanding of experience' (Sandelowski, 1995, p. 183).

There should be such an emphasis on sampling because it helps researchers to remain alert to a lack of openness or selective construction of their results. Additionally, sampling represents the silver bullet to making generalizations from qualitative research. This chapter makes the strong assumption at this point that research should strive for generalizable results (cf. Daly et al., 2007). In reference to Polit and Beck's work on generalization in qualitative research, this chapter considers purposeful sampling to be a prerequisite of analytical generalization. By doing so it prioritizes the concept of analytical generalization over the concept of transferability (including reader generalizability or case-to-case translation, see Polit and Beck, 2010, p. 1453). In the latter, the task of providing a statement of generalization is understood as a collaborative effort between researcher and reader, with both parties having responsibilities (e.g., for the research to provide detailed descriptions, and for the reader to evaluate the extent to which the findings apply to situations familiar to them in terms of proximal similarities). Sampling understood in this way offers a way to accomplish *findings* that are representative—not samples as 'a sub-set that is a miniature of the population' (Gobo, 2004, p. 439). Ideally, analytical generalization should be based on a dynamic research process in which sampling is done in continuous dialogue with field incidents, contingencies, theoretical developments (Gobo, 2004; Polit and Beck, 2010), and integrating inductive and confirmatory strategies.

Choosing cases for research is, however, only one aspect of sampling. When presenting results, researchers are again confronted with tough selection decisions: selecting cases for the report, and selecting appropriate citations or other parts of the original data. This problem relates to what Jeanne Daly once called 'the curse [of] the illustrative quotation' (2009, p. 405). Should those cases be selected that are most suitable to convey the main message? Should those citations be used that best convey the main (or favourite) findings? Or, as an alternative, should the strategy for case and citation selection be developed and put forward transparently, using the same method that should be employed in sampling? This chapter argues that presentation of qualitative research results should allow the audience to reconstruct the interpretation and should therefore be as transparent as possible in the interpretation (Kruse, 2014, p. 638). Therefore, the claim of generalizability is intricately related to intersubjective comprehension. It could be, for example, appropriate to provide an insight into the spectrum of different—more or less convincing—cases, or to provide an additional insight into those quotations that might contradict possible results of the study (and to explain why they do not). As Sandelowksi notes, one way of acknowledging and taking seriously the diverse views and stances of the persons and stories that pique researchers' interest is not to try to reduce results to one representative voice, but instead to respect their polyvocal characteristic (Sandelowski, 1998). The audience has to be sure that researchers have acknowledged all of the available data, or as Luborsky and Rubinstein put it:

> '… the entire corpus of materials and observations with informants needs to be examined in the discovery and interpretative process aimed at describing relevant units for analyses and dimensions of meanings. This is in contrast to reading the texts to describe and confirm a finding without then systematically rereading the texts for sections that may provide alternative or contradictory interpretations' (1995, p. 103–104).

While this statement refers explicitly to qualitative analysis, it can also be read as a call to sensitize the selection of citations for the presentation of results.

Another important ethical issue related to citing a personal account is to assure that the person's account has been respected in its entirety. Researchers often see their work referenced by another colleague and feel misunderstood or supporting conclusions they do not support. If a certain citation of a patient is used, it is vital to ensure it is not reframed or put in a context that it was not meant for. Researchers must always ask if the participant read her citations, would she feel understood and respected? There is no claim that participants should have the last word about whether an interpretation is correct, as suggested by some quality-improvement approaches to qualitative research (i.e., a 'member check' or 'responded validation'; see Meyer, 2007), which has been criticized by different authors (see e.g., Britten, 2001). Instead, perhaps the role of the participant in this process should be related to the type of enquiry, as expressed by Lucius-Hoene, Breuning, and Helfferich in Chapter 2, i.e., whether we deal with experiential, naturalistic, or performative approaches to narrations. In any case, it is imperative to confirm that all relevant context information and personal understandings are acknowledged in order to properly interpret the patients' reports.

Before discussing these considerations on sampling and generalization to the selection of cases or citations of illness narratives, the next section first reflects on the different roles qualitative researchers might take or find themselves in when using illness narratives in practice.

Roles of qualitative researchers

Who has an interest in using illness narratives in practice? What is the professional role—if any—to which individuals interested in using illness narratives in practice adhere? This book suggests that there are myriad motivations for or interest in using illness narratives. On one side of a continuum may be societal groups or institutions with special interests in pushing a topic or message of their primary concern, e.g., those opposed to immunization (Meyer and Reiter, 2004) or the exhibition of the German medical school association mentioned earlier. Cases, and information within these cases, are selected to best fit the purposes of the person who selects the cases, taking up different social roles. The selection of cases and of information is determined by the respective political or marketing goals of the stakeholders. There is a danger of misusing or abusing the stories or experiences of the patients involved (assuming they are true, and not fabricated). In the middle of the continuum is the role of the journalist, who is trained to write 'stories'. In this instance, personal accounts are a powerful way to add authenticity to a story, and depending on the professional self-concept of the journalists, as well as their available resources and competencies, journalists might use illness narratives to support and steer readers towards accepting a pre-determined message. That is, original stories are searched and excerpts harvested in order to convey a specific message. The media may also have a 'story' to tell, and people's experiences may sway their views. In the end, patients' original accounts or narratives may 'prove' their story. It should also be acknowledged that journalists must juggle the commercial interests of the media organization they work for with their professional obligation to report the truth (Deyo and Patrick, 2005).

At the other side of the continuum are qualitative researchers, who are trained to recognize the fallacies of selective information processing and the importance of striving for a research stance that allows for empathy and distance as well as the integration of different perspectives onto the phenomenon under study. Still, there are barriers that might result in findings that are much more restricted than originally anticipated, being a rough outline, or overly 'to the point' (suggesting that researchers should strive for or be able to reduce the different facets of their results into a single point).[2] A long research report must be condensed into the frame of a journal paper format, leaving space for only a small number of citations. Not only might important results in terms of case illustrations or citations be excluded, but so also might important methodological reflections, due to space limitation. Another source of restriction might be represented by the audience addressed. Considering the limited time spent reading journal papers, there is a temptation to overemphasize certain aspects of results in order to reach the audience. Another strong source of possible distortion of the presentation of results might be the degree of advocacy which researchers are obliged to maintain. If the project is responsible for setting up an intervention or programme for some disadvantaged people—will the results reflect the whole picture, including unwanted effects or failures?

How should we select illness narratives in practice?

Sampling or selecting cases of illness narratives for use in practice should be guided by the same criteria used for sampling and generalizability in qualitative research. Grob and Schlesinger support this view (see Chapter 23 this volume) and suggest that 'when narratives evolve from informal stories to qualitative data put to use in the public domain, that use must be guided by standards of practice just as rigorous as those employed for quantitative data'. Additionally, those decisions should be guided by the rigour developed in the conduct of a qualitative study.

This section now looks at the well-known DIPEx programme on illness narratives, and reflects on the way how illness narratives should be used for public presentation. In 2003, Herxheimer and Ziebland stated that the ' ... primary aim of DIPEx is to describe the widest practicable range of individual experiences from the patients' points of view and to provide a rich information resource for patients affected by the diseases and for those who look after them' (p. 209). Accordingly, the

> ' ... sampling method used should ensure a wide range of patients' experiences because factors expected to be associated with different experiences (such as age, sex, social class, and stage of illness and condition-specific factors) will guide the selection of interviewees.... The intention is to represent the fullest possible range of experiences irrespective of frequency of occurrence' (Herxheimer et al., 2000, p. 1542).

The format of websites such as www.healthtalk.org carries huge potential in its sampling idea. However, these formats are not always possible (and arguably) suitable for the different audiences and purposes for which we illness narratives are used in practice. Still, it is important to consider the creative ways illness narratives can be used in practice with the same rigour used in qualitative research. At the least, researchers' awareness of case-selection strategy, transparency, and stance to make the audience aware of the richness of different perspectives must be front of mind.

Discussion

It is tempting to grab the audience's attention by using the most intense or compelling illness stories. However, qualitative researchers should be aware that this is but one strategy among many. This chapter suggests that researchers strive to be transparent in the approach of how cases or information from these cases in practice are selected, make explicit the strategy and criteria, and indicate that there is much more to a phenomenon that cannot be easily distilled 'to a point'. Instead, perhaps the 'point' is rather a point of departure.

Returning to the introductory example: medical schools experience tension similar to journalists. On the one hand are tangible economic interests, but on the other is the strongest obligation to truth (in its different connotations). An approach that harvests illness narratives for public-relations purposes does not necessarily support truthful reporting, and is in conflict with what a university, and a medical school, as an institution stands for.

Notes

1. http://www.deutsche-uniklinika.de/themen-die-bewegen/hinter-den-kulissen-patienten-erzaehlen (Accessed 31 October 2017).
2. We are grateful to Professor Maren Stamer, Berlin, for introducing us to this metaphor.

References

Britten, R., 2001. Checklists for improving rigour in qualitative research: a case of the tail wagging the dog? *British Medical Journal*, **322**, 1115.

Corbin, J. and Strauss, A., 1990. Grounded theory research: procedures, canons and evaluative criteria. *Qualitative Sociology*, **13**, 3–21.

Daly, J., 2009. Qualitative methods and the curse the illustrative quotation. *Australian and New Zealand Journal of Public Health*, **33**, 405–406.

Daly, J., Willis, K., Small, R., Green, J., Welch, N., Kealy, M., and Hughes, E., 2007. A hierarchy of evidence for assessing qualitative research. *Journal of Clinical Epidemiology*, **60**, 43–49.

Deyo, R. A. and Patrick, D. L., 2005. *Hope or hype: the obsession with medical advances and the high cost of false promises*. New York: Amacom.

Emmel, N., 2013. *Sampling and choosing cases in qualitative research. A realist approach*. London: Sage.

Gobo, G., 2004. Sampling, representativeness and generalizability. In: C. Seale, G. Gobo, J. F. Gubrium, and D. Silverman, eds. *Qualitative research in practice*. London: Sage. pp. 435–456.

Grob, R. and Schlesinger, M., 2018. When public and private narratives diverge: media, policy advocacy, and the paradoxes of newborn screening policy. In: G. Lucius-Hoene, C. Holmberg, and T. Meyer, eds. *Illness narratives in practice*. Oxford: OUP. pp. 286–298.

Herxheimer, A., McPherson, A., Miller, R., Shepperd, S., Yaphe, J., and Ziebland, S., 2000. Database of patients' experiences (DIPEx): a multi-media approach to sharing experiences and information. *Lancet*, **355**, 1540–43.

Herxheimer, A. and Ziebland, S., 2003. DIPEx: fresh insights for medical practice. *Journal of the Royal Society of Medicine*, **96**, 209–210.

Kruse, J., 2014. *Qualitative Interviewforschung. Ein integrativer Ansatz*. Weinheim: Beltz Juventa.

Luborsky, M. R. and **Rubinstein, R. L.**, 1995. Sampling in qualitative research. *Research on Aging*, **17**, 89–113.

Lucius-Hoene, G., **Helfferich, C., Breuning, M.**, 2018. Illness narratives in practice: which questions do we have to face when collecting and using them? In: **G. Lucius-Hoene, C. Holmberg**, and **T. Meyer**, eds. *Illness narratives in practice*. Oxford, OUP: pp. 13–26.

Mayring, P., 2007. On Generalization in Qualitatively Oriented Research. *Forum: Qualitative Social Research/Sozialforschung*, [e-journal] 8(3): Art. 26. Available from http://nbn-resolving.de/urn:nbn:de:0114-fqs0703262.

Meyer, C. and **Reiter, S.**, 2004. Impfgegner und Impfskeptiker. Geschichte, Hintergründe, Thesen, Umgang. *Bundesgesundheitsbl Gesundheitsforsch Gesundheitsschutz*, **47**(12), 1182–1188.

Meyer, T., 2007. Kritische Bewertung von Qualitativen Studien. In: **R. Kunz, G. Ollenschläger, H. Raspe, G. Jonitz**, and **F-W. Kolkmann**, eds. *Lehrbuch evidenzbasierte Medizin in Klinik und Praxis*. (**2. Auflage**). Köln: Deutscher Ärzte-Verlag. 159–176.

Meyer, T., 2015. Health Research, Qualitative. In: **J. D. Wright**., ed, International Encyclopedia of the Social & Behavioral Sciences, 2nd edition, Vol **10**. Oxford: Elsevier. pp. 692–697.

Patton, M. Q., 2002. *Qualitative Research & Evaluation Methods*. 3rd ed. Thousand Oaks: Sage.

Polit, D. F. and **Beck, C. T.**, 2010. Generalization in quantitative and qualitative research: myths and strategies. *International Journal of Nursing Studies*, **47**, 1451–1458.

Sandelowski, M., 1995. Sample size in qualitative research. *Research in Nursing & Health*, **18**, 179–183.

Sandelowski, M., 1998. Writing a good read. Strategies for re-presenting qualitative data. *Research in Nursing & Health*, **21**, 375–382.

Ethical and communicational aspects of using narratives in medicine

Chapter 6

Illness narratives in counselling—narrative medicine and narrative ethics

Hille Haker

The narrative turn in medicine

Since the 1970s, criticism of a 'reductionist' approach within medicine has resulted in a return to narratives and the review of the role of narratives in medical practice. Hence, narrative medicine is part of a broader epistemological shift—medicine must complement its science-based method with hermeneutics that understand medicine as social praxis (Gadamer, 1996)—and a cultural shift that mirrors the turn to postmodern pluralism (and sometimes to relativism). Both shifts result in a new attention to experiential stories and a critique of the exclusive reign of evidence-based empirical knowledge to determine a person's health status. Ronald Schleifer and Jerry Vannatta follow Marshall Marinter's definition:

> Disease then [...] is the pathological process, deviation from a biological norm. Illness is the patient's experience of ill health, sometimes when no disease can be found. Sickness is the role negotiated with society (Schleifer and Vannatta, 2013).

In the context of this chapter, I add a fourth category, namely 'disability', a specific 'deviation from the norm'.

Medical doctor and literature scholar Rita Charon who coined the term 'narrative medicine' is one prominent representative of this turn to experiential competency, but given the long history of medicine and literature, for example, she is hardly exceptional in the shift to narratives (Charon and Montello, 2002; Charon, 2006). Charon aims to return the power of storytelling to the patient, shifting the emphasis to collaborative meaning-making and interpretation. This chapter argues that counsellors indeed co-construct stories and engage in storytelling, too. Charon, however, misinterprets the communicative structure of the encounter because in professional contexts, expertise, knowledge, and power are distributed differently among the partners. In a more recent work, Charon stresses the role of recognition and reciprocity (Charon, 2012). She recalls encounters with a patient she has seen over an extended period of time and argues that the patient comes to know much about the doctor's life, too—but it is a misconception of professional relations to assume that this fact creates a *reciprocal recognition*. In my view, Charon overstates her argument: while the understanding of disease and disability, illness, and sickness overlap in both counsellor and client/patient understanding, the very term 'counselling' constitutes their positional asymmetry regarding the knowledge about the empirical dimension of health, i.e., the 'disease' or 'disability' as medical terms. As I show at the end of this chapter, Charon is correct that doctors and/or counsellors cannot but 'reveal' something about their own selves, interpretation, and meaning-making in the encounter with their patients or clients. But this does not mean that patients or clients are interested (or should be interested) in a *reciprocal relationship* that resembles more a friendship than a professional relationship.

The relationship between counsellor and client to which I here constrain my reflections requires specific norms that ensure the respect and avoid the exploitation of a dependent's vulnerability. *Recognition* is indeed an appropriate concept for this relationship, but in its ethical dimension, it is much more complex than Charon has it. Recognition entails, first, the *identification* of the partners *as* counsellor and client; it entails the *acknowledgment* that both the client's and counsellor's perspective is meaningful and counts in the counselling; and it entails the *respect* for each other's rights and obligations, including the scope and limits of actions. While the counsellor has more initial agential power in the constellation, the patient or client, vulnerable because of her dependency on help, must be supported as much as possible in her agency. Narrative is one element among several others to achieve this goal; and recognition in the above-mentioned threefold understanding replaces a paternalistic and sometimes authoritarian understanding of the professional role of counsellors.

Narrative medicine has its critics, too. In his critique of the postmodern shift to narratives within the medical humanities, Seamus Mahony, for example, criticizes Charon in particular for promoting a 'dangerous' concept of empathy and understanding (Mahony, 2013). He claims that the discourse in narrative medicine is clouded in impenetrable jargon, strongly influenced by postmodernist literary theory. And much of the language employed, he argues, has a religious flavour that is uncalled for within medical communication: 'witnessing', 'professing', and 'honouring' are activities, Mahony argues, that do not belong in the doctor-patient communication (Mahony, 2013, p. 614). I echo a caution about the status of narrative medicine, but Mahony and others misplace their critique: it is due to the insufficient theory, not the concept as such, that narrative medicine is often merely used as an appeal to be more 'humane' in the context of a highly bureaucratic, technocratic, and automated medical practice.

This chapter focuses on ethics in genetic counselling and explores the role of narratives in this context. Counselling practices have been submitted to professional ethical standards over the last few decades. These are often tied to codes of conduct that professional societies developed as their ethical guidelines beyond the legal requirements. They are meant to orientate the counselling profession in their encounters with clients, colleagues, and society.

The practice of counselling—standards and competencies

The mission statement of the American Counseling Association (ACA) states the following:

- The mission of the American Counseling Association is to enhance the quality of life in society by promoting the development of professional counselors, advancing the counseling profession, and using the profession and practice of counseling to promote respect for human dignity and diversity (ACA, 2014, p. 2), and

- Counseling is a professional relationship that empowers diverse individuals, families, and groups to accomplish mental health, wellness, education, and career goals (ACA, 2014, p. 3).

The ACA's *Code of Ethics* entails not only the broad goal of promoting and enhancing the quality of life in different social spheres, but also explicitly draws on the ethical principles of respect for human dignity and diversity. The principles echo the main bioethical principles that have been developed over the last decades, especially by James Childress and Tom Beauchamp (2012).

The National Society of Genetic Counselors (NSGC) adopted an ethics code in 1992 (with the last revision in 2006), which is more specific to genetic counselling. In relation to their clients, it spells out that counsellors are to respect their clients' 'beliefs, inclinations, circumstances, feelings, family relationships and cultural traditions' (NSGC, 2006, Section II, Nr. 3), and enable them 'to make informed decisions, free of coercion, by providing or illuminating the necessary facts, and clarifying the alternatives and anticipated consequences' (NSGC, 2006, Section II, Nr. 4). Because of the specific sensitivity of genetic information, the NSGC opposes 'the use of genetic information as the basis for discrimination' and supports 'policies that assure ethically responsible research' (NSGC, 2006, Section IV, Nr. 7).

Ethical values, norms, and principles are professional standards; they are norms that constitute 'good' and 'right' counselling. They link counselling to the overall framework of medical ethics. Comparing it to the narrative turn in medicine, the ethical standards do *not* reflect the so-called postmodern trend that has often been labelled antinormative; rather, both codes represent an ethics that is abstract, decontextualized, and faced with multiple difficulties in its application (Page, 2012). Following the mainstream Anglo-American medical ethics approaches, the ACA and the NSGC embrace the medical-ethical principles without attending to discourses that question the normative framework to which they apply; this, I argue, creates a tension for the implementation of narratives. In contrast, postmodern theorists consider the abstract normative frameworks as an obstacle to respect diversity and the multiplicities of identities. Postmodern theories of ethics, though plural themselves, emphasize instead difference, multiplicity, and the interrelation of science and society (Bauman, 1993; Harding, 2009; Reuter and Wieser, 2006). In the following, I suggest that the approach of *narrative ethics*, albeit not an approach that covers all ethical issues, can bridge the two sides: the dimension of (illness) narratives in counselling on the one side, and the normative framework of ethics that defines the standard of a good practice on the other.

Narratives in counselling

The question is not *whether* narratives matter in the encounters between counsellors and clients, but rather *how* they matter. Counsellors necessarily listen to clients' personal narratives to understand what matters to clients. There is an ongoing debate, however, about the status of narratives regarding its potency (or claim) to *re*present (Aristotle's term of *mimesis*) a person's 'real' life and identity. More specifically, narrative theory analyses the different ways of narration or *presentation* (Atkins, 2004). Over the last two decades, I have worked on the literary forms within the genre of (fictional) biographies and auto-biographies within narrative ethics (Haker, 2006; Haker, 1999; Haker, 2009), arguing that a critical hermeneutics is required as part of narrative theory; life-stories entail *formal* structures of narratives, including life stories as a quest or journey, conversion narratives, healing narratives, or any teleological narrative of a 'good life'. These forms owe much to literary traditions of oral and written nature, and as such they must be scrutinized in their aesthetic (and social) function. Arthur Frank, for example, identifies several genres in patients' stories of illness: narratives of restitution, narratives of chaos, narratives of quest, life reviews, and trauma narratives (Frank, 1995). Interestingly, life reviews have become most prominent in hospice care (Flanagan, 2017)—their *narrative* function is dominated by their *ethical* (and *spiritual*) function, often conveyed in spiritual care concepts, to bring closure, peace, and forgiveness. It is this practice of narrative ethics that sparked Mahony's criticism of the (often unaccounted) appeal to particular forms of the 'good life' within narrative medicine. In contrast to such 'big stories' of a person's life, metaphors and 'small stories' (Bamberg, 2006; Georgakopoulou, 2007), i.e., fragments of stories that require unfolding, may be much more important *ethically*, because values, particular interpretations, and judgments entailed in them often remain un(dis)covered and hence undiscussed:

> [T]he smallness of talk, where fleeting moments of narrative orientation to the world can be easily missed out by an analytical lens that only takes fully fledged ('big') stories as the prototype from where the analytic vocabulary is supposed to emerge. (Bamberg & Georgakopoulou, 2008).

Narratives are necessarily addressed, and they are necessarily mediated by the public language and public concepts of reasoning (Korsgaard, 2009). I agree with Bamberg that there is no necessity to speak of 'narrative exceptionalism' when it comes to identity (Bamberg, 2012); but it is certainly fair to say that in counselling and personal decision making, narratives and storytelling play a more important role than, for example, argumentation and democratic public reasoning. Both forms of 'communicative action' complement each other and overlap considerably: narrative and argumentative reasoning intertwine and overlap, and the practice of genetic counselling has as much affinity to narratives as it has affinities to scientific empirical knowledge. Both, however, are linked to 'sickness', i.e., the social interpretations of illness, disease, and disability. Unfortunately, narrative theories often tend to ignore the social—and that means, among other things, the *social-normative*—contexts of personal narratives. Postmodern, poststructural, feminist, and postcolonial studies are right to criticize the lack of social analyses and the socially mediated epistemological frames of the health discourse. I would therefore caution against an uncritical reception of narratives, taking them merely as representations, rather than presentations of reality, and, likewise, caution against an uncritical reception of narrative ethics.

Against the critics of narrative medicine, however, I believe there cannot be any doubt that narrative competency helps counsellors to understand, to recognize and respect, and to empathize with clients. These required competencies call for special attention to *oral* narratives told in the counselling sessions, which function differently from written stories: oral stories can guide the understanding and interpretation through gestures, body language, spaces between sentences, emphasis, etc. (Arduser, 2014).

The 'meaning-making' and interpretation is never value-neutral. In their effort to render the evaluation as reflective as possible, Schleifer and Vandatta point to the shared enterprise of practical reasoning, including the reasoning of ethical issues, which they identify as the Aristotelian practice of phronesis:

> The job is to listen carefully (listening for what is said and for what is not said), to facilitate the parts of the story that are not there, and to join with the patient in articulating what is important, the patient's chief concern. But the physician does not have to drive the train; the patient drives the train, and the burden for doing all the work is lifted from the doctor (Schleifer and Vannatta, 2013, p. 169).

The following setion takes a closer look at ways of practical reasoning in the decision-making processes of genetic counselling.

Genetic counselling and decision-making in ethical conflicts

Genetic counselling not only provides information but also supports a client in the deliberation of decisions in view of a genetic information. The models of decision-making must reflect the normative standards of the profession and hence realize, for example, the respect of dignity and diversity stated as core principles in the above-mentioned codes. Furthermore, counselling concerns *procedural* issues of decision making, such as transparency and the respect for the noncoerced choice by the clients. Counselling necessarily entails the conversation about *substantial* ethical issues, and hence the ethical values that inform the clients' choices. Since the counselling ethics standards call for an abstract and vague respect of the client's decisions, counsellors often merely apply the *procedural* guidelines and pay far less attention to the substantive ethical issues their clients are facing.

The ACA emphasizes the role of counsellors in the decision-making process:

> When counselors are faced with ethical dilemmas that are difficult to resolve, they are expected to engage in a carefully considered ethical decision-making process, consulting available resources as needed.... ethical reasoning includes consideration of professional values, professional ethical principles, and ethical standards (ACA, 2014, p. 19).

Non-directive counselling rests upon this framing of moral pluralism that often translates into a liberal understanding of autonomy as choice that owes more to the Anglo-American tradition than to the Kantian understanding of autonomy as moral agency and responsibility (O'Neill, 2002). As long as the counsellor complies with the procedural rules of respect, transparency, and non-coercion, the professional standards seem to be met. Nevertheless, the ACA puts considerable weight on the counsellor to guide the process; it proposes to follow common models of decision making. It recommends the following steps, although they are not meant to be exhaustive:

1. Identify the problem.
2. Consider the standards of the ACA, principles, and laws.
3. Generate the course of action.
4. Consider the consequences.
5. Deliberate the risks and benefits.
6. Select the objective course of action based on the circumstances and welfare of all involved (cf. p. 19).

It is clear that it is the counsellor who is in the driver's seat of the process. This observation underscores the power differential or asymmetry between counsellor and client, because *how* a problem is described, for example, will determine in good part the options and choices. Clearly, the counsellor is supposed to steer the conversation. She should follow the principle-based approach of medical ethics, but there is no indication how the different principles relate to each other, how they are to be prioritized, and how one may define a 'dilemma'. Most likely, the description of the problem will be oriented by the medical epistemology: the 'problem' will then be described in terms of genetic risks. Hence, the connection between the different semantics of disease and disability, illness, and sickness is lost, and most likely, only one semantic is favoured. Narrative ethics offers at least two important corrections. First, it will reflect on *different* understandings of health and its counterparts: counsellors must attend to the personal, experiential notion of *illness* as well as to the role of social mediations in the construction, for example, of disability. Second, narrative ethics will operate with a model of shared decision making that secures the client's position as the centre of the conversation and the counsellor's role as a resource of expert knowledge, which the client does not have. In other words, narrative ethics will attend to the 'ethical dimensions' not merely as the normative principles of generalized *respect*, but also as personalized, relational *recognition* of the other who is faced with choices that are, in part, pre-structured by social norms and the genre of genetic counselling.

Already in 1986, Albrecht Wellmer stated that most ethical controversies may rest upon different analyses of situations; he therefore called for paying more attention to contextual analyses (Wellmer, 1986). In an effort to connect the hermeneutical and the normative dimension of ethical reflection, in 2002 Dietmar Mieth proposed a method, originally developed for bioethics deliberations, which he called 'conductive'—it complements an inductive, contextual approach with a deductive, normative approach. It is possible to rephrase the steps in this way:

1. Determine the pre-understanding and context of action.
2. Identify what the situation is about (facts).
3. Identify possible ethical orientations.
4. Determine alternative actions.
5. Assess the ethical priorities.
6. Implement the action.

Since Mieth developed this sequence mainly for political/social deliberations, it is only applicable with modifications. Nevertheless, it is possible to see that it would require the counsellor to attend much more to the social analysis and interpretation, instead of defining risks and benefits that are dependent on probabilistic projections and subject to plural interpretations of risk-taking. While I have previously proposed a general model for gen-ethical counselling that also attends to the evaluative and normative dimensions of ethics (Haker, 2002), here I will focus more on the role of small stories in the configuration of narratives. Paul Ricoeur's concept of a threefold mimesis, which aims to address the above-mentioned question of presentation and representation, or, in other words, the relationship between narrative and reality, stories and life, considers stories neither as a realist representation of a person's life nor as merely imagined construction that has no root in the experienced life of the narrator. Rather, the *configuration* has a *pre-figured* background in the praxis and a person's lifeworld, for example her pre-judgment of disabilities. Likewise, the story told in the counselling will *re-figure* or shape a person's understanding in the future (Ricoeur, 1988; Ricoeur, 1992). With these insights, the following steps could serve as a practical guide for counsellors:

1. Determine the context (narrative *prefiguration* of praxis).
2. Analyse the relational constellation relevant for the decision—narrative *configuration I.*
3. Identify the ethical conflict and the underlying norms (principles, standards, laws) of action in relation to the situation in question (*configuration II*).
4. Identify potential conflicts between personal values and normative principles.
5. Explore the consequences of all options together with the client (*configuration III*), support the client to determine priorities and make a decision.
6. Determine the steps of action, based upon the decision.
7. Explore with the client how to implement the course of action (*refiguration*).

This model needs to be elaborated further, and the terminology of 'sequence' must be adjusted in the real-life communications. The model is neither 'directive' nor 'non-directive' in the traditional sense, but *correlative*. It leaves room for narrative enactment and interpretation, but it has the advantage over other narrative medicine models in that it does not jump from stories to ethical assessments and decision. Rather, it correlates the descriptive and the normative dimension of ethics, with narratives functioning as a *bridge* between description and prescription (Haker, 2010; Ricoeur, 1992). Counsellors need to attend to signals that are inherent to narratives, however 'small' they are, and take them as occasions to begin the 'meaning-making' process.

Narratives in gen-ethical counselling

Susan Markens conducted interviews with genetic counsellors to better understand their role in decision making and to explore the publicly raised concern that counsellors implicitly or explicitly encourage couples to terminate pregnancies. The question concerns the *prefiguration* of prenatal genetic counselling:

> [B]y implicating their role in the normalization process, much research seems to suggest that genetic counsellors explicitly and implicitly encourage women to undergo prenatal testing and to terminate pregnancies with abnormalities (Markens, 2013, p. 434).

Her interviews demonstrate that counsellors take the medical information as guide for action—following the communicative norms of *information,* which demand 'description' without 'prescription'. I have said that narratives are bridges between description and prescription, and this may often happen through 'small stories'. Counsellors must understand, however, that it is not only their clients who step on this 'bridge'—in entering a conversation beyond the 'transmission' of facts (though their communication can never be *entirely* value-neutral), they step on it, too. The counsellors' ethical neutrality ('be descriptive, not prescriptive') may be especially challenged when the clients' assessments of an ethical conflict departs from the counsellor's own assessment. Narrative ethics, I argue, helps to better understand that the position of the counsellor as objective 'reporter' of medical facts is as misleading as its opposite. Yet, 'morality' is in fact often understood as taking a prescriptive position, rendering counsellors as 'moral police'. In contrast to both positions, narrative ethics reflects on the encounters on the 'narrative bridge' exactly between description and prescription. The narrative analysis enables the ethical reflection, understood as practical reason in the above-mentioned sense. The counsellor's concern for narrative will not *appeal* to a client's life-story but rather attend to the 'small stories' that require analysis and unfolding. Markens documents the following encounter, told by a genetic counsellor:

> There was one case that I remember that was—so when they measure fetal bones... so these percentiles are averages. They're norms.... Well, I had a couple whose measurements were consistently below normal, consistently below 10%.... But not all over, and really it was just a femur and a humerus.... Otherwise the baby seemed to be growing—progressing normally, was a normal amniocentesis. There [were] no birth defects. (Markens, 2013, p. 444)

The counsellor recalls the medical diagnosis. Yet, there are two terms that entail 'small stories': the counsellor calls the foetus (the medical terminology) a 'baby' and refers to the lack of 'birth defects'. The language of 'birth defects' is often used in medical information, but it nevertheless is a non-neutral, value-laden term, because it interprets particular genetic features as 'defects'—something that disabilities studies would strongly oppose because it employs a biological concept of disability. This is how the counsellor recalls the couples' response:

> And they were really worried about having a baby who was going to be a dwarf. Even though there was really nothing to indicate.... There was a lot more leaning towards normal than there was leaning towards dwarf, and they terminated that pregnancy.

Again, the 'small story' is entailed in one word: the prospective parents identify their future child as a 'dwarf'. Identification is *one* aspect of recognition, as I have argued earlier—in this case a stigmatizing *misrecognition* that distances the prospective parents from their future child, now called the 'foetus', 'baby', or 'dwarf'. The counsellor repeats this term uncritically, merely pointing out that s/he could not convey to the clients that their evaluation does not match the *facts* of the medical diagnosis. The tension the counsellor recalls seems to entirely rest on the wrong application of a valid concept ('dwarfness') to the actual case, not on the concept itself:

> And I—I didn't say 'I think you're wrong,' but I spent a lot of time being, like, 'Are you sure? Because this is a really big decision, and most likely there's really only a tiny chance that this baby ... '—and I was trying to ... and they were, like, 'Nope, nope, nope. We just can't. We can't. We're too scared.'... And they terminated this pregnancy, and they sent the baby off for a skeleton review for skeletal dysplasia, there was nothing wrong with this baby. They couldn't find anything. So they most likely terminated a very normal pregnancy.... I had a really hard time with that one because... I don't know. It was just so hard because there most likely was nothing going to be wrong with this kid, but how do I know.... But it's those, like, sort of soft calls where you're, like, come on (Markens, 2013, p. 445).

The counsellor disagrees with the couple's ethical assessment and subsequent course of action, the termination of pregnancy, expressed in the repeated use of the term 'baby'; but s/he also feels bound by the ethical principle of non-directive counselling that prohibited counsellors from becoming prescriptive. Yet, his/her retrospective attitude is clearly disrespectful of the clients: 'But it's those, like, sort of soft calls where you're, like, come on'.

My proposed model of ethical decision making would start with the one-word small story: it would require the counsellor to unpack the term 'dwarf' (Step 1) and its underlying social imagery. S/he could explore how the prospective parents imagine their child, giving them the opportunity to speak of their own desires, imaginations, and anxieties. The counsellor could emphasize the different layers of non-health, i.e., disease and disability, illness, and sickness—including the tension between the medical and the social concept of disability. S/he could address the tension between what they assumed to be an existential threat and the medical findings (Step 2). S/he could ask questions and interpret the (small) story, thereby co-constructing a narrative that addresses the moral emotions relevant to the conflict (Step 3). Potentially, even the concept of parenthood and the concept of recognition—as acknowledgment and respect as process in addition to a static identification—could become part of the conversation (Step 4), making the tension of the ethical assessment a part of the conversation, rather than evading it. Step 5 could allow for more imagining of the future—inquiring how the clients envision their life with their future child, or after losing it under the given circumstances. Step 6 would follow the ACA, assuring the clients that it is up to them to make the best possible decision within the legal constraints.

My model creates both more space for the narrative and hermeneutical work of meaning-making and space for the ethical deliberation. This does not mean that the counsellor uses his or her power to *judge* the values or tries to convince the clients of his or her own ethical values; rather, it means that counsellors understand that ethical deliberation is part of the interpretation and co-construction of narratives. Learning to identify and analyse such 'small stories' must be part of the education and ongoing training of counsellors.

The model does not depart from a non-directive approach. But it would not suppress the conversation about moral judgments (including the prejudgment of the prefiguration of narratives in the lifeworld) and explicate them in order to reason about them. It would enable counsellors to concretize their professional ethical standards, in reflecting upon the medical terminology, their own pre-judgments that they necessarily enact in conversations, and potentially in correcting (denigrating) imageries or attitudes they may hear from their clients. Narrative ethics examines all stories critically, considering medical information *and* ethical concepts that the counsellor must have available. While narrative ethics cannot *resolve* the tensions, it may clarify the role of counsellors in the ethical decision making, attending especially to the theory of oral narratives and the theory of 'small stories' that accompany oral narratives.

Conclusion

This chapter argued that narratives play a role in counselling, 'no matter what'. Counsellors must acquire the competence to understand how stories entail moral understandings. At times, these may be in tension with the ethical principles counsellors stand for as a profession, namely to respect the dignity and diversity, well-being, and social justice of all people. I am not following postmodern ethics approaches, but I echo the critique of 'principles' when they are merely used as a normative fig leaf with no practical impact. Narratives, I have argued, are the bridge between descriptions and prescriptions; their function is hermeneutic, i.e., to discern the (necessarily) evaluative understanding of reality, experiences, and social contexts. Narrative ethics defends an ethics approach that takes narratives and principles as complementary, i.e., correlative, corrective, and constructive resources in ethical decision making—but it also upholds the obligation to respect and recognize the concrete 'other'.

Acquiring competence in narrative ethics involves much training in narrative theory as well as in ethics. The model proposed here needs to be tested and further developed in the professional education and training forum. But in my experience, the 'gen-ethical' model is better than the one implemented by most genetic counsellors. The standard models leave little room for either narrative competency or ethical deliberation as a collaborative endeavour between counsellors and their clients, and therefore remain abstract and often purely rhetorical. Recognition, spelled out as *respect*, obliges the counsellor to take seriously the client's agency, capability, right, and responsibility to make decisions (Ricoeur, 2006). Recognition, spelled out as *acknowledgment*, however, requires that the counsellor attends to the concreteness of the 'other'. It requires a critical listening and 'unpacking' of the 'small stories' that are rooted as much in the social lifeworld as in the personal lives of the clients. After the process of having 'all things considered' collaboratively, counsellors will be better able to leave it to the clients to make their decisions.

References

American Counseling Association. (2014). *ACA Code of Ethics*. Available at: <http://www.counseling. org/docs/ethics/2014-aca-code-of-ethics.pdf?sfvrsn=4> (Accessed 17 January 2017).

Arduser, L., 2014. Agency in illness narratives. A pluralistic analysis. *Narrative Inquiry*, 24, 1–27.

Atkins, K., 2004. Narrative identity, practical identity and ethical subjectivity. *Continental Philosophy Review*, 37, 341–366.

Bamberg, M., 2006. Stories, Big or small, Why do we care? *Narrative Inquiry*, 16, 139–147.

Bamberg, M., 2012. Why Narrative? *Narrative Inquiry*, 22, 202–210.

Bamberg, M. and **Georgakopoulou A** (2008). Small stories as a new perspective in narrative and identity analysis. *Text & Talk*, 28, 377–396.

Bauman Z (1993). *Postmodern Ethics*. London: Wiley Blackwell.

Beauchamp, T. L. and **Childress, J. F.,** eds., 2012. *Principles of biomedical ethics*. 7th ed. New York: Oxford University Press.

Charon, R., 2006. *Narrative medicine. Honoring the stories of illness.* Oxford: Oxford University Press.

Charon, R., 2012. The reciprocity of recognition—what medicine exposes about self and other. *The New England Journal of Medicine*, 367, 1878–1881.

Charon, R. and **Montello, M. M.,** 2002. *Stories matter: the role of narrative in medical ethics.* New York: Routledge.

Flanagan, T. E., 2017. Narrative medicine and health care ethics: religious and literary approaches to patient identity and clinical practice. Chicago: Dissertation Manuscript, Loyola University Chicago.

Frank, A. W., 1995. *The wounded storyteller, body, illness, and the human condition.* Chicago: University of Chicago Press.

Gadamer, H. G., 1996. *The enigma of health* (originally published as *Über die Verborgenheit der Gesundheit*, 1993). Stanford: Stanford University Press.

Georgakopoulou, A., 2007. *Small stories, interaction and identities.* Amsterdam: John Benjamin Publishing Company.

Haker, H., 1999. *Moralische Identität. Literarische Lebensgeschichten als Medium ethischer Reflexion. Mit einer Interpretation der 'Jahrestage' von Uwe Johnson.* Tübingen: Francke.

Haker, H., 2002. *Ethik der genetischen Frühdiagnostik. Sozialethische Reflexionen zur Verantwortung am menschlichen Lebensbeginn.* Paderborn: Mentis.

Haker, H., 2006. Narrative bioethics. In: C. **Rehmann-Sutter** and D. **Mieth,** eds. *Bioethics in cultural contexts: reflections on methods and finitude.* Berlin, Springer. pp. 353–376.

Haker, H., 2009. Narrative ethics in health care chaplaincy. In W. **Moczynski, H. Haker,** and **K. Bentele,** eds. *Medical ethics in health care chaplaincy.* Essay. Münster, LIT Verlag. pp.143–174.

Haker, H., 2010. Narrative ethik. *Zeitschrift für Didaktik der Philosophie und Ethik*, 2, 74–83.

Harding, S., 2009. Postcolonial and feminist philosophies of science and technology, convergences and dissonances. *Postcolonial Studies*, 12, 401–421.

Korsgaard, C., 2009. *Self-constitution. Agency, identity, and integrity.* Oxford: Oxford University Press.

Mahony, S., 2013. Against narrative medicine. *Perspectives in Biology and Medicine*, 56, 611–619.

Markens, S., 2013. Is this something you want? Genetic counselors' accounts of their role in prenatal decision making. *Sociological Forum*, 28, 431–451.

Mieth, D., 2002. *Was wollen wir können? Ethik im Zeitalter der Biotechnik.* Freiburg: Herder.

National Society of Genetic Counselors, 2006. *NSGC Code of Ethics.* Available at: <https://www.nsgc. org/p/cm/ld/fid=12> (Accessed 17 January 2017).

O'Neill, O., 2002. *Autonomy and trust in bioethics.* Cambridge: Cambridge University Press.

Page, K., 2012. The four principles. Can they be measured and do they predict ethical decision making? *BMC Medical Ethics*, **13**, 10. doi: 10.1186/1472-6939-13-10

Reuter, J. and **Wieser, M.**, 2006. Postcolonial, gender und science studies als Herausforderung der Soziologie. *Soziale Welt*, **57**, 177–191.

Ricoeur, P., 1988. *Time and Narrative, Vol. 3*. Chicago: Chicago University Press.

Ricoeur, P., 1992. *Oneself as another.* Chicago: University of Chicago Press.

Ricoeur, P., 2006. *The Course of Recognition.* Cambridge, MA: Harvard University Press.

Schleifer, R. and **Vannatta, J.**, 2013. *The chief concern of medicine. The integration of the medical humanities and narrative knowledge into medical practices.* Ann Arbor: University of Michigan Press.

Wellmer, A., 1986. *Ethik und Dialog—Elemente des moralischen Urteils bei Kant und in der Diskursethik.* Frankfurt: Suhrkamp.

Chapter 7

An illness narrative or a social injustice narrative?

Maya Lavie-Ajayi and Ora Nakash

Introduction

In narrative research, stories are considered subjective representations of the world, formed within a specific socio-cultural and relational context (Spector-Mersel, 2010). Actors construct narratives by choosing a beginning and an end-point by selecting the appropriate events, actions, and characters to be included in the narrative, and by attributing value to these selections. Hence, it is only within specific discursive circumstances that a narrative and its specific 'valued goal' can be told and heard, i.e., can be made intelligible (Gergen, 2005).

Within a specific context, narratives serve to both reflect and create cultural values. When analysing a narrative, it is important to focus on its performative aspects in generating, sustaining, and disrupting cultural traditions (Gergen, 2005) or 'master narratives' (Hyvärinen, 2008). Taking into account the range of narratives available at any given time means it is necessary to explore who is entitled to tell a narrative and when, how narratives are received, and how they work in the social world (Hyvärinen, 2008). This chapter explores these questions within the context of mental health facility intake procedures (hereafter referred to as 'mental health intake' or 'intake'). The mental health intake is usually the first point of contact between clients and therapists (mostly psychologists or social workers). The primary goal of intake is to gather information about the presented problem and psycho-social history of the client in order to make a first diagnosis and a treatment plan.

Many different kinds of narratives can be told during intake, and these narratives, told by either client or therapist, can generate, sustain, and disrupt contemporary psychotherapeutic discourse. This chapter first considers a critique of contemporary psychotherapeutic discourse. It then explores in detail a single intake session in which the client relates a narrative of social injustice, reconfigured by the therapist as a mental illness narrative. The last section argues that social injustice narratives disrupt the master narrative of contemporary psychotherapeutic discourse, and consequently cannot be accepted.

Current criticism on mainstream psychotherapeutic discourse

A rich theoretical critique of current mainstream psychotherapy discourse and practice has gathered momentum over the last three decades (Parker, 1999; Avissar, 2009).
The hegemonic psychotherapeutic discourse has been criticized for emphasizing intra-
personal processes while ignoring—or at best, underestimating—the social, economic, and cultural context in which the individual lives, and through which suffering
emerges (Avissar, 2009; Cushman, 1990; Masson, 2012; Nakash et al., 2009; Parker, 1999;
Prilleltensky, Prilleltensky, and Voorhees, 2008). This discourse exists despite the accu-
mulation of research attesting to the impact of the social determinants of mental health
inequities (Alegría et al., 2009; Braveman, Egerter, and Williams, 2011; Nakash, Levav,
and Gal, 2013; Nakash, Saguy, and Levav, 2012; Nakash, Nagar, Danilovich et al., 2014).

A number of scholars have argued that regardless of their different practices, all dominant psychotherapy discourses share a profound disinterest in social injustice and a
complete acceptance of the existing political status quo (Clark, 2002; Masson, 2012).
For example, Cushman (1990) argues that most psychotherapy discourses use the dominant ideology of individualism, ignoring the political and economic arrangements that
may be responsible for a client's suffering. Advocating a more contextualized psychotherapy discourse stems from the understanding that psychotherapists can be more
effective if they integrate an understanding of how power influences oppression and
liberation—and ultimately, wellbeing—into their practice (Prilleltensky, Prilleltensky,
and Voorhees, 2008).

From a critical perspective, psychotherapy can no longer be viewed as politically neutral if we understand 'political' as relating to the distribution of societal power and resources (Sucharov, 2013). On the contrary, psychotherapy is 'a field of political action, a
place where power is exercised and contested, as therapists try to affect clients' lives and
clients acquiesce, resist or do both at the same time' (Totton, 2006).

This critique of current mainstream psychotherapeutic discourse tends to be theoretical, and the actual analyses of psychotherapy sessions—and specifically, intake sessions—
published to date are few (Georgaca, 2014). This chapter presents a detailed, qualitative
analysis of a single mental health intake session from a critical perspective.

The research context

The intake and interviews that underpin this chapter were conducted and recorded as
part of a larger study on mental health disparities (Nakash, Nakar, and Levav, 2014;
Nakash, Nagar, Danilovich et al., 2014), and took place in a community mental health
centre in a major Israeli city. The clinic offers free services to a diverse, socio-economically
disadvantaged adult client population, under the provisions of the extant health care
law. Therapist participants in the study were recruited at the clinic through introductory
informational meetings. Client participant recruitment was conducted through direct
person-to-person solicitation at the time of presentation for intake. The appropriate

Institutional Ethics Committees at the participating clinics approved all aspects of the study and ensured that data collection complied with all human subject protocols. These protocols included a detailed informed consent process (which included an assessment of the client's capacity to consent) and assurances of patient care and confidentiality throughout participation in the study. After consent was obtained, both clients and therapists participated in the three separate components of the study: 1) audiotaping the intake; 2) participation in a post-intake, semi-structured interview; and 3) completion of a demographic questionnaire. Post-intake interviews with the therapist and client occurred immediately following the intake, and each was interviewed alone. The interviews focused on the evaluation of the clinical encounter. Questions included the presenting issue, nature of the client–therapist rapport, and the role of socio-cultural factors during the meeting. The post-session interviews included in this chapter were conducted by two graduate students in clinical psychology. The intake session and subsequent interviews were transcribed in full.

Following Parker's (1999) call for critical research to focus on particularity, this chapter focuses on one of the 129 intakes that were recorded. Detailed analyses of language using qualitative methods often examine only a small number of texts due to the intensive nature of the process (Lamb, 2013). This intake is not intended to be representative of intakes in general, or of the intakes in this particular study. Rather, the intake was selected because it contained explicit disagreement. The explicit nature of the disagreement between therapist and client, and the client's open criticism of the hegemonic psychotherapy discourse, presented an opportunity to highlight the limits of current mainstream psychotherapeutic discourse.

Intake participants and structure

The intake participants were Rivka[1], the therapist, a 54-year-old *Ashkenazi* (Jews of European/American origin, considered an advantaged ethnic group in Israel) senior clinical psychologist, and Sima, the client, a 53-year-old *Mizrahi* (Jews of Middle Eastern/ North African/Asian origin, considered a disadvantaged ethnic group in Israel) woman. Sima presented herself at the intake in a state of crisis, following the downgrading of her employment status, which occurred at a period during which her family circumstances changed dramatically. According to her, the changes at work and in her family circumstances had left her feeling lonely and isolated.

The intake session lasted 55 minutes. Throughout the session, Sima mostly spoke in a clear and strong voice; from time to time, her voice broke and she cried. Rivka, the therapist, moved from mostly nodding and asking a few open questions, to progressively employing a mixture of open and closed questions during the latter part of the intake.

The following sections present Sima's and Rivka's narratives on the basis of what they said during the intake and the post-intake, semi-structured interviews. The narratives were analysed holistically, focusing on content (what was said), structure (how it was said), and underlying motives (Rosenthal, 1993).

Sima's social injustice narrative

Sima presented herself at the intake in the throes of a legal battle with her employer. Sima had worked for the Post Office, in a range of clerical and managerial positions, for 34 years, ever since graduating from high school. Ten months before the intake session Sima was removed from her position as a registration clerk and placed in the more junior position of cashier. She perceived this change as a major demotion that had caused her depression. Sima believed that her position was taken from her as the result of false allegations:

> It was planned and it was very obvious, it was planned. They brought someone who had been suspended and at home for two years, following suspicions of financial fraud. He was acquitted in the trial; they were forced to find him a position without a cash register, and he obviously did not want the kind of physical jobs that I also did not want. So they had to give him my unique position, they had to ... find him the most appropriate role, and so they created problems for me, and this was obvious (Intake, lines 465–468).

Sima diagnosed herself as suffering from depression; she defined this depression as resulting from the injustice she had experienced in her work. Yet she contextualized her mental state within the wider context of her life as a whole:

Sima (S): I came [to the mental health clinic] following a depression that was caused by a problem I have at work.

Interviewer: Yes ...

S: Now the depression was caused mainly by the problem at work, but ... it is particularly severe because of other reasons, and the timing of its occurrence. (Sima's interview, lines 83–86).

At the intake itself, Sima discussed the internal and external reasons for her suffering more fully, connecting her depression not only to work, but also to her divorce eight months earlier, to the onset of her menopause, and to a feeling of 'empty nest' syndrome. Sima explained that she felt unable, both physically and emotionally, to work as a cashier twenty years after leaving her previous position. For a long period, she tried to fight against this change, but could not find any allies for her fight. Sima told that she singlehandedly continued to struggle against the changes via different health and legal committees within the workplace. During this period, she visited a psychiatrist in order to establish the negative implications of the change foisted upon her on her mental health, i.e., her depression. She said that the psychiatrist issued a letter with four recommendations: 1) to do more physical activity; 2) psychoactive medication; 3) psychological treatment; and 4) recommendation to change her role. Sima presented the psychiatrist's medical opinion and recommendations to the health committee. She also said that this letter was not sufficient in itself, as the workplace presented a letter from a different psychiatrist to the committee, without the recommendation that Sima be given back her position. The committee refused her request, and backed the Post Office's decision.

As a last resort, Sima turned to an appeal committee. Its final session was due to take place a week after the intake interview. Sima reports that she was very worried about her chances with the appeal committee. She believed that she only had a very slim chance of winning her case against the Post Office. She had decided to book an appointment with a mental health clinic, in order to boost her chances with the appeal committee, as she explains in the post-intake interview:

S: I have obtained a psychiatric recommendation to change my position at work but still they insist, so I thought that here I could receive help in obtaining a medical opinion from a psychologist with a specific recommendation, with a specific opinion that might determine my fate.

Interviewer: The external fate of your work.

S: The external fate. Because I am going to an appeal committee. Now, in the appeal committee, they will bring their own doctor: my work place will bring, among others, a psychiatrist. Because I have obtained a recommendation from a psychiatrist, they will bring the appropriate medical profession in accordance with the disciplines I turn to. They will bring their own psychiatrist, and it is important to me that he will see that indeed I have looked for psychological treatment, as my psychiatrist recommended. (Sima's interview, line 156–163).

Sima's narrative highlights the political power of psychotherapy as a social institution. In the narrative she explained that both she and her work place were using mental health professionals in a legal struggle to define reality: she and the Post Office had brought a psychiatric recommendation to back their legal claims and their opposing narratives. Sima described how, in order to secure her rights at work, she needed to use the political power of psychotherapy in two ways: first, to use the psychological diagnosis to prove that she had suffered as a result of the Post Office's decision; and second, to prove that she was a 'good patient'—i.e., one who followed the psychiatrist's orders. She hoped that both methods would help to support her account of reality.

Hence, Sima turned to the community mental health centre to ask for help with her depression. She did not want therapy and most of all she did not want psychoactive medication, but rather she wanted a professional letter with a diagnosis of her as suffering from depression because of the crisis at work. In her post-intake interview Sima shows she understood that her request did not fit the hegemonic therapeutic discourse:

I assume that I am an unusual case ... I feel that I am probably an unusual case here, that the psychologist does not really understand my expectations from you. And I think that in a place like this, maybe there is a need to designate a person for special cases like mine (...). I think that instead of insisting and, as they say, get locked on psychiatric medication, one could think beyond that, even though this may be unacceptable in this kind of setting. To consider some, some different things from what they have learned so far. To consider, for example in my specific case, what is needed is a medical evaluation [to the committee] so maybe ... now, if she had helped me to solve the problem at my workplace, she would have cured me! (Sima's interview, lines 123–180).

Sima's advice echoes contemporary scholarship on context-sensitive and politically sensitive therapy (Avissar, 2009; Prilleltensky, Prilleltensky, and Voorhees, 2008; Sucharov, 2013). This line of thinking urges therapists to think critically and to expand the context of their work to embrace social, cultural, and political issues. This therapeutic position is based on the ecological discourse that sees the person as part of the socio-cultural systems that largely shape people's identity and lives. The basic assumption of this ecological position is that it is not possible to properly understand and address well-being and suffering without looking at the context of the power relationships within which suffering occurs (Totton, 2006).

The next section returns to Rivka's post-intake interview and explores her account of Sima's narrative.

Rivka's narrative of mental illness

Based on the interview with Rivka, it seems that she tried her best to be empathetic; she tried not to ask too many questions about Sima's past, so as not to put Sima in an uncomfortable position:

> Look, I think it is difficult to ask a person in a very difficult crisis ... ahh ... to expand about the background and ... to collect more information, like I said to you, about the personality aspect that is the basis of the issues, because she is very riled up and this ... and right now the emotional flooding ... there is something not empathetic if you start asking too many questions (Rivka's post-intake interview, lines 58–60).

Rivka realized that it was the first time that Sima had consulted a psychologist and wanted Sima to have a positive experience so she would feel comfortable enough to return. Hence, it was very important for Rivka 'to be attuned' toward Sima. However, she found it hard to feel positively toward her:

> On the one hand, it really hurts what she is going through; on the other hand, I felt that there was something tough in her, like she has her own position and she is not open to hear others (...) like pain, together with something that ... it is not easy to connect to. (Rivka's interview, lines 93–97).

Rivka took into account the possibility that Sima's story, about the injustice of the workplace, was true. She did not ignore the external explanations Sima gave for her depression, but she positioned the external factors as almost irrelevant to the psychiatric diagnosis and therapy that would follow. Rivka believed that Sima's reaction was inappropriate to the circumstances. In the post-intake interview she said that Sima's reaction to the crisis and the depression that followed '*sit on something else*':

> Look, I have all kinds of diagnostic thoughts about her beyond the crisis, I mean like a personality that is more ... maybe schizoid or something more rigid (Rivka's interview, line 127–129).

By focusing on Sima's reaction as mainly stemming from her '*personality*', the external factors were discussed only through an interpretative lens, i.e., using external reality to explore internal patterns. Through this focus, the political nature of the external factors was rejected. The external factors were appended into an essentialist discourse and an inherent personality-based explanation. Rivka's final diagnosis was Personality Disorder Not Otherwise Specified, alongside an adjustment disorder with prolonged depressive reaction. A diagnosis of depression could have helped Sima, without taking explicit sides. A personality-based diagnosis means that not only did Rivka's recommendation not support Sima's narrative, but also, in fact, actively challenged her narrative by offering a personality-based explanation for her difficulties. Rivka may have been unable to recognize that her diagnosis strengthened the position of Sima's workplace in the legal battle against her.

It is possible to assume that Rivka's inability to accept Sima's social injustice narrative relates, at least in part, to her inability to see the implications of her diagnosis in the legal battle, as well as to the current hegemonic psychotherapeutic discourse. This discourse framed and directed Rivka's thoughts and actions from the beginning of the intake interview. For example, when asked during the interview about her aims for this meeting, Rivka said:

R: First of all, I wanted to get to know her and check what is the problem. Ah … to try and reach a diagnosis, to see what she would like to get from us, from the clinic … and to think if we are the right place for her, what might be the optimal treatment to offer her.

Interviewer: Ok, so you have said four things, how would you grade these in terms of priorities, what was most important?

R: Everything. (Rivka's interview, lines 30–36).

Rivka insisted that she saw all four aims as inseparable. She could not see her diagnosis as differing from learning about the problem. This extract highlights the basic assumption in mainstream therapeutic discourse—one that conceptualizes emotional difficulties as located 'inside' the individual (Avdi, 2005); thus, an inseparable connection between problem, diagnosis, and treatment. In this discourse, the context is understood only as background to the problem, and is not given any importance. This conceptualization limited Rivka's ability to accept Sima's social injustice narrative and also to recognize the political aspect of her diagnoses. Since contemporary psychotherapeutic discourse disregards the political aspect of this profession, Rivka's attempt not to take sides in this power struggle made her incapable of seeing that her diagnosis actually sides with the workplace and blames Sima for her crisis.

Narratological disagreement

Though most of the discussion during the intake was very pleasant—as both Sima and Rivka acknowledged in their post-intake interviews—by the end of the intake, the two narratives—social injustice and mental illness—clashed around the mandate of the intake and the matter of psychoactive medication. The following is a short extract from the final ten minutes of their discussion:

R: Is there anything else that you think is important that I should know about you, about the past, the present?

S: No in my past there were no … I told you, in general I had no special events in my life. That's it. I never thought that I will be thrown into this situation (starts crying). I just looked for help because I see that nothing helps my position at work. Undoubtedly not, I think that if I go back to work, this will change my life in a significant way and if not, my life will deteriorate and I will go downhill. I say it honestly, and no I am not coming to pretend or act and I am not coming to do, ah, nothing. There are no games here. I am a very honest person, I don't play any games, I don't do any shows. This is the situation now.

R: So let's ... let's stop for a moment here. In terms of work, I have no way and cap-ability to help you because, you know, we have no mandate.

S: I understand.

R: More personally to you, first of all I really recommend that you start somewhere. There is no doubt that I see the depression. The deep sadness, as you said, there have been many changes in the last year, everything happened at the same time. The ad-justment to a new way of living is not easy in all respects. I am very much in favour of starting medication, very, because you have no idea how much this medication will influence, the influence of the Cipramil or Cipralex that they gave you, it takes three to four weeks before it starts to have an influence on you, and to accumulate some basic energy to help you help yourself. You see?

(Two-minute discussion about the other medications Sima takes).

R: Now I really think that you should start [psychiatric medications], and that's it for me. I return the question to you again, and because we already need to stop, let's do it briefly: What would you like from us? What are you asking from us?

S: I repeat myself again, I think that if my problem at work had been solved ...

R: Ok, this, let's ...

S: I know that you cannot help ...

R: Assuming that this is not solved, or assuming that ...

S: This is not solved, I don't know, right now I really do not want to use medication (Intake, lines 502–533).

This extract presents a juxtaposition of the two narratives. While Sima clearly reiterated that she came to ask for help in her battle with her workplace, Rivka limited the bound-aries of her practice, focusing on what she could offer—psychoactive medication. Two minutes later, they were repeating almost the same dialogue. Their discussion became immobilized in a clash between the two narratives, which highlights the limits of the mental health profession in general, and psychology in particular, through the exclusion of the political context, and limiting—even objecting to—the role of therapists as social advocates, particularly for socially and culturally oppressed populations. The discussion between Sima and Rivka shed light on Rivka's inability to help her as long as Rivka was not ready to face the last taboo of psychotherapy—its political power (Altman et al., 2004). As long as Rivka did not acknowledge the political blindness of her practice, Sima's narrative could not be validated.

Conclusion

This chapter's analysis of an intake session illustrates how the hegemonic psychotherapeutic discourse in regular mental health practice is characterized and shaped by an individualistic view (Cushman, 1990), and a profound disinterest in social injustice (Clark, 2002; Masson, 2012). This psychotherapeutic discourse emphasizes personal pathology, while underestimating the socio-cultural context within which the individual lives and through which suffering emerges. In contrast, it also argues that Sima offers a 'counternarrative'. Counternarratives are stories told 'against' dominant cultural narratives, often by placing marginalization in the context of oppression and economic, social and cultural inequality (Fine and Harris, 2001). Counternarrative demands the ability to perceive and interrogate the various forms of oppression that shape a life, and to take action against the status quo (Lavie-Ajayi and Krumer-Nevo, 2013). Sima tried to offer a counternarrative to the hegemonic psychotherapy narrative, which is essentialist and individualistic and defines psychopathology as a set of symptoms and internal personality structures. Sima's counternarrative defines her depression as related to inequality, rather than her personality. The context of inequality can cause pain and demoralization, as well as psychological damage by challenging the sense of worth, dignity, and an appreciation of one's own place in the world (Prilleltensky, Prilleltensky, and Voorhees, 2008). This chapter suggests that Rivka could have supported Sima's counternarrative without ignoring the aspects of Sima's behaviour, which might have contributed to this situation. Rivka could rather have tried and incorporated these in a complex story using a contextualized perspective (Lavie-Ajayi and Krumer-Nevo, 2013).

Moreover, Sima's request for help disrupted the view of psychotherapy as politically neutral. Sima needed Rivka to be aware of psychotherapy as 'a field of political action'—a socio-cultural institution where power is exercised and contested, as therapists try to influence the lives of their clients and to construct knowledge through the establishment of psychiatric nosology (Totton, 2006). Rivka did not want to take sides in a power battle between Sima and her workplace. However, in her attempt to be politically neutral, she increased the (unintentional) impact of her own actions, i.e., of a personality-based diagnosis. As argued by other researchers—and as suggested by this chapter—in ignoring the power they possess as well as the political aspects of their practice, therapists may be oblivious to their own role in perpetuating the status quo, and the suffering that derives from it (Altman et al., 2004; Samuels, 2004; Totton, 2006).

The role of unequal power relations in the clinical encounter becomes even more pronounced when the client comes from a disadvantaged social group. Gender, ethnicity, class, and other social identifiers often translate to asymmetrical power relations in society, and this imbalance can seep into the therapeutic encounter. Therapists must acknowledge this power discrepancy, and find ways to diminish its effect; clinical empathy is not enough. What is needed is political empathy. In the exchange between Sima and Rivka, Rivka did her best to be empathetic—to be aware of the thoughts and feelings of her client, and to understand her state of mind. However, Rivka failed to demonstrate an understanding of social marginalization as an everyday process that is embedded in un-equal power relations in society (Prilleltensky, Prilleltensky, and Voorhees, 2008), as well as an awareness of the unquestioned psychological, social, and cultural discourses and the structural features of bureaucratic hierarchies (Deutsch, 2011). Political empathy urges practitioners to constantly reach for the inclusion of the other by taking into account the whole person as an ecological system within a specific, often unequal, socio-political-economical context (Samuels, 2004).

Note

1. Pseudonyms are used in this paper, to preserve the anonymity of the participants.

References

Alegría, M., Sribney, W., Perez, D., Laderman, M. and Keefe, K., 2009. The role of patient activation on patient–provider communication and quality of care for US and foreign born Latino patients. *Journal of General Internal Medicine*, **24**(3), 534–541.

Altman, N., Benjamin, J., Jacobs, T., Wachtel, P., and Geffner, A. H., 2004. Is politics the last taboo in psychoanalysis? *Psychoanalytic Perspectives*, **2**(1), 5–37.

Avdi, E., 2005. Negotiating a pathological identity in the clinical dialogue: discourse analysis of a family therapy. *Psychology and Psychotherapy: Theory, Research and Practice*, **78**(4), 493–511.

Avissar, N., 2009. Clinical psychologists do politics: attitudes and reactions of Israeli psychologists toward the political. *Psychotherapy and Politics International*, **7**(3), 174–189.

Braveman, P., Egerter, S., and Williams, D. R., 2011. The social determinants of health: coming of age. *Annual Review of Public Health*, **32**, 381–398.

Clark, C., 2002. Identity, individual rights and social justice. In: R. Adams, L. Dominelli, and M. Payne, eds. *Critical Practice in Social Work*. London: Palgrave. pp. 38–45.

Cushman, P., 1990. Why the self is empty: toward a historically situated psychology. *American Psychologist* **45**(5), 599.

Deutsch, M., 2011. Justice and conflict. In: P. T. Coleman, ed. *Conflict, Interdependence, and Justice: The Intellectual Legacy of Morton Deutsch*. New York: Springer. pp. 95–118.

Fine, M. and Harris, A., 2001. Under the covers: theorizing the politics of counter stories. *International Journal of Critical Psychology*, **4**, 183–99.

Georgaca, E., 2014. Discourse analytic research on mental distress: a critical overview. *Journal of Mental Health*, **23**(2), 55–61.

Gergen, K. J., 2005. Narrative, moral identity, and historical consciousness. In: J. Straub, ed. *Narration, Identity and Historical Consciousness*. New York: Berghan Books. pp. 99–119.

Hyvärinen, M., 2008. Analyzing narratives and story-telling. In: P. Alasuutari, L. Bickman, and J. Brannen, eds. Sage Handbook of Social Science Research Methods. London: Sage. pp. 447–460.

Lamb, E. C., 2013. Power and resistance: new methods for analysis across genres in critical discourse analysis. *Discourse & Society*, **24**(3), 334–360.

Lavie-Ajayi, M. and Krumer-Nevo, M., 2013. In a different mindset: critical, accessible youth work with marginalized youth. *Children and Youth Services Review*, **35**, 1698–1704.

Masson, J. M., 2012. *Against Therapy, Emotional Tyranny and the Myth of Psychological Healing*. San Francisco: Untreed Reads.

Nakash, O., Levav, I., and **Gal, G.**, 2013. Ethnic-based intra-and inter-generational disparities in mental health, results from the Israel-World Mental Health Survey. *International Journal of Social Psychiatry*, 59, 508–515.

Nakash, O., **Dargouth, S.**, **Oddo, V.**, Gao, S., and **Alegría, M.**, 2009. Patient initiation of information: exploring its role during the mental health intake visit. *Patient Education and Counseling*, 75(2), 220–226.

Nakash, O., **Nagar, M.**, and **Levav, I.**, 2014. Presenting problems and treatment expectations among service users accessing psychiatric outpatient care: are there gender differences? *The Israel Journal of Psychiatry and Related Sciences*, 51(3), 212–217.

Nakash, O., **Saguy, T.**, and **Levav, I.**, 2012. The effect of social identities of service-users and clinicians on mental health disparities, A review of theory and facts. *The Israel Journal of Psychiatry and Related Sciences*, 49(3), 202–210.

Nakash, O., **Nagar, M.**, **Danilovich, E.**, **Bentov-Gofrit, D.**, **Lurie, I.**, **Steiner, E.**, **Sadeh-Sharvit, S**, **Szor, H**, and **Levav, I.**, 2014. Ethnic disparities in mental health treatment gap in a community-based survey and in access to care in psychiatric clinics. *The International Journal of Social Psychiatry*, 60(6), 575–583.

Parker, I., 1999. *Deconstructing Psychotherapy*. London, Sage.

Prilleltensky, I., **Prilleltensky, O.**, and **Voorhees, C.**, 2008. Psychopolitical validity in the helping professions: applications to research, interventions, case conceptualization, and therapy. In: C. I. **Cohen** and S. **Timimi**, eds. *Liberatory psychiatry: philosophy, politics, and mental health*, 105–130.

Rosenthal, G., 1993. Reconstruction of life stories: principles of selection in generating stories for narrative biographical interviews. In: R. **Josselson** and A. **Lieblich**, eds. *The narrative study of lives*. London: Sage. pp. 59–91.

Samuels, A., 2004. Politics on the couch? Psychotherapy and society—some possibilities and some limitations. *Psychoanalytic Dialogues*, 14(6), 817–834.

Spector-Mersel, G., 2010. Narrative research—time for a paradigm. *Narrative Inquiry* 20(1), 204–224.

Sucharov, M., 2013. Politics, race, and class in the analytic space, The healing power of therapeutic advocacy. *International Journal of Psychoanalytic Self Psychology* 8(1), 29–45.

Totton, N., 2006. Power in the therapeutic relationship. In: N. **Totton**, ed. *The politics of psychotherapy: new perspectives*. Maidenhead: Open University Press. pp. 83–96.

Narratives in psychotherapy, rehabilitation, and vocational training

Chapter 8

Retelling one's life story—how narratives improve quality of life in chronic language impairment

Sabine Corsten and Friedericke Hardering

Introduction

There is an increasing interest among health professionals regarding the emotional problems, and their psychosocial consequences, faced by people with chronic diseases. The growing awareness that neurogenic communication problems caused by aphasia can have a devastating effect on family and social life has led to a shift of focus in speech and language therapy (e.g., Hilari et al., 2015; Hinckley, 2016). While earlier interventions primarily addressed the language deficit, more recent socio-pragmatic approaches have concentrated on communicative resources and social consequences of aphasia (Duchan and Byng, 2013), which follows the model of functioning of the International Classification of Functioning, Disability and Health (ICF) of the World Health Organization (2001). The ICF model especially focuses on restriction in participation related to impairments in body functions as well as to personal and environmental factors. The approaches are based on supporting coping processes and helping patients to rediscover meaningful roles. They aim at improving quality of life (QoL) by developing strategies that assist individuals in managing their lives after experiencing aphasia.

This chapter presents an interdisciplinary multimodal approach called *narraktiv*, an acronym for 'Narrative Kompetenzen Aktivieren', i.e., activation of narrative competencies. The intervention was developed in the research project *Improving Quality of Life in Aphasia: Activation of Narrative Competencies by Biographic-Narrative Intervention*[1] at the Catholic University of Applied Sciences Mainz, and is a biographic-narrative approach to improve QoL for people with aphasia. The key idea is that self-perception changes considerably when people are diagnosed with aphasia. They lose key aspects of their premorbid self-image, e.g., perceiving themselves as incompetent, which is the primary reason for their diminished QoL (Le Dorze et al., 2014). Shadden (2005) even talks about 'identity theft' in a case of aphasia. Therefore, the aim of this biographic–narrative approach was to support patients in renegotiating their own identity.

The chapter[2] provides an overview of the psychosocial situation in case of aphasia, and explores the concept of identity, particularly the concept of narrative identity (Bauer, McAdams, and Pals, 2008; McAdams, 2008), as well as approaches to identity work. In conclusion, it presents a biographic-narrative concept including biographic-narrative interviews and group interventions developed specifically for people with aphasia. It also discusses evidence of psychosocial benefits of the approach.

Aphasia and quality of life

Aphasia, a neurologically based language disorder, occurs in about 30% of stroke patients (Engelter et al., 2006), impairing their language skills, including verbal expression, auditory comprehension, reading, and writing. Aphasia is associated with significant life-altering psychosocial consequences, including changes in relationships and social isolation, along with deficits in communication (Le Dorze et al., 2014). The incidence of depression is estimated to be as high as 62%—higher than in stroke survivors not suffering from aphasia (Kauhanen et al., 2000; Hackett et al., 2005). Aphasia reduces health-related QoL even more substantially than cancer or Alzheimer's disease, and this reduction in QoL has also been associated with changes in physical activity (Lam and Wodchis, 2010). Even improved language skills do not necessarily lead to a comparable improvement in QoL (e.g., Franzén-Dahlin et al., 2010).

The great and lasting losses in QoL are due to the strong impact of aphasia on self-perception (Shadden, 2005). As a disruptive life event it affects everyday routines, expectations, and aims (Bury, 1982; Lucius-Hoene, 2002). It changes the individual's sense of self, their roles, and their relationships (Musser et al., 2015). In their 2012 review, Hilari and colleagues found that social aspects, emotional distress, and changes in perception reduce QoL in people with aphasia. Brown and colleagues (2012), in a qualitative meta-analysis, show that having a sense of purpose and usefulness is crucial to living successfully with aphasia. As the sense of self is always framed within the social exchange, and powerfully influenced by social relationships, aphasia can lead to devastating consequences. Failed exchanges due to the language deficit can cause feelings of inferiority and devaluation, which then can lead to a permanent sense of incompetence. Shadden's 2005 study introduces a man with aphasia who declares, 'I don't have aphasia when I'm alone' (p. 215). In aphasia, the required reframing of self-perception when in relationships with others cannot take place to a sufficient and appropriate extent.

Given their failure in social exchanges, people with aphasia need specific support in creating a new story for themselves in order to cope with the changed situation. For example, narrative therapy uses life-storytelling as a process of reconstructing identity (White and Epston, 1990). Life narratives facilitate the process of making sense of the illness experience by reconstructing the meaning and purpose of life and reviewing patients' own strengths and resources that might help overcome personal and environmental challenges. Disruptive life events can be integrated into the life story, generating a new perspective on the self (Brody, 1994). The extent to which people restore their sense of identity and bring renewed meaning to their lives is in turn related to improved QoL (Bauer, McAdams, and Pals, 2008). In case of aphasia, such a narrative-based approach needs to be modified.

Identity work and the concept of narrative identity

Identity and identity work are central concepts in various research trends in the social sciences. Many definitions commonly conceive of identity work as integrative and connective, which produces continuity and coherence based on narration (Keupp et al., 2006; McAdams, 2008). Identity work thus is the central mechanism to produce a sense of identity (Keupp et al., 2006). There are four crucial aspects of identity work:

1) Identity work is an ongoing process. Where some older identity theories assume that identity evolves in the process of growing up and becoming stable at some point (Erikson, 1973), modern identity theories stress that identity has to be worked on throughout life. Identity is never complete but must be continually negotiated, and these negotiations happen constantly. Therefore, social theorists speak of everyday identity work (Keupp et al., 2006). Identity work takes place not only when individuals focus on their own personality, but also on their actions. Nor is the *result* of identity work fixed. Keupp and colleagues (2006) assume that identity constructions are always fragile.

2) Identity work creates connections between different areas of life. Everyday connecting and structuring involves several aspects of organizing experiences. Keupp and colleagues (2006) identify temporal connections, which link past, present, and future, and interactive connections, which link different roles and areas of life (work, leisure time, family). Additionally, they introduce 'content-based' connections, which link past experiences to similar new experiences.

3) Narration is an important medium of identity work. Several identity theories postulate that identity work takes place mainly based on narration (McAdams, 2008). The term narration stresses the linguistic aspect, and some theoretical approaches in narrative psychology also assume that all of human experience has a narrative quality. The concept of narration implies a narrative scheme with a beginning, middle, and end. It connects the past to the future. This highlights the temporal aspect of connection. The concept of 'narrative identity' (Bauer, McAdams, and Pals, 2008) combines these considerations and focuses on the part of identity that becomes accessible when people talk about themselves or tell stories about their own lives.

4) The aim of identity work is to create coherence, continuity, and agency (Lucius-Hoene and Nerb, 2010). This means that people recognize themselves as the same person despite changes in life (coherence), and perceive different phases of life as connected with and related to each other (continuity). A central goal of identity work is to create a positive sense of identity, making it possible for people to perceive themselves as being able to act (agency). While the sense of identity influences narrations of the self, changed narrations of the self in turn affect the sense of identity (Keupp et al., 2006).

Successful identity work results in a meaningful experience of the self and has, therefore, a major effect on QoL.

This chapter stresses the procedural, connecting, and narrative character of the identity concept based on the different aspects of the definition. The chapter uses the terms 'narrative identity' and 'identity' as synonyms, assuming that narration is fundamentally constitutive of identity.

Narrating and coping with illness

Identity work is an everyday process that depends on many preconditions and draws on specific resources. Narrative identity constitutes itself based on references to the self (Keupp et al., 2006), which mainly take place in intersubjective contexts. People negotiate the image they have of themselves and their own histories in conversations with other people in which they then re-interpret events and images together. Because of communicative limitations, people with aphasia are often faced with the challenge of having fewer opportunities to narrate and talk about themselves. They often withdraw or are excluded from situations of social exchange. This removal changes both the frequency and the intensity of narrations of the self. As a consequence of the decrease in narrations of the self, the relevant identity-work mechanisms that help in coping with the biographical disruption cannot take place. Furthermore, in case of communicative failure due to the language deficit, failures in social exchanges strengthen the feelings of stigmatization and incompetence. Thus, there is a lack of successful and appreciative exchanges, which usually foster identity work.

Scholarly work in *narrative-based medicine* has pointed out that talking about an illness can be helpful for the individual experiencing it. Both 'narrative therapy' and 'narrative coping' take this view as a starting point and presume that the telling of a life story has a 'healing' effect on the person telling the story (Brody, 1994). The aim of these therapeutic interventions is to cope with biographical breaches caused by aphasia using techniques of biographical revision. The basic assumption of these concepts is that people repeatedly tell certain stories about their own life (retelling, re-authoring; see Parry and Doan, 1994). Telling others repeatedly about stressful experiences enables people to find a kind of narrative that helps them integrate the stressful event better into their own life story (Brody, 1994). Their strengths and resources become visible again, such as having coped successfully with a crisis earlier in their life. This memory of successful coping may make persons with aphasia feel more confident of their own ability to approach challenges actively and competently. Supporting processes of identity work seems to be a promising way forward in view of the special situation of people with aphasia and the insights gained from narrative-based medicine and biographical work. It facilitates coming to terms with biographical breaches and creates a sense of continuity and coherence. People develop a sense of identity that helps them see themselves as creators of their own life stories (see Figure 8.1). The next section shows how adapting these narrative methods to suit people with aphasia is particularly challenging.

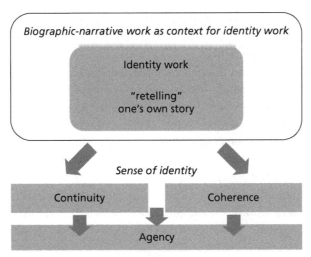

Figure 8.1 Biographic-narrative work as context for identity work.
Adapted with permission from Corsten, S et al. Biographisch-narrative Intervention bei Aphasie. Sprachtherapie aktuell 2. Copyright 2015 © Deutschen Bundesverbandes für akademische Sprachtherapie und Logopädie. Available at: http://sprachtherapie-aktuell.de/files/e2015-07_Corsten_Hardering.pdf

Biographic-narrative approach

Educational and nursing approaches use biography work to work on identity and enhance QoL (e.g., Korte, Westerhof, and Bohlmeijer, 2012), resulting in guides on developing biographical work with individuals and groups (e.g., Kaiser and Eley, 2016). Approaches focusing on activities are used alongside approaches focusing on narratives. Ruhe (1998) differentiates between unstructured and structured biography work.

Projects for people with aphasia mainly use group approaches focusing on participation to improve QoL. This is based on the idea that facilitating meaningful activities might improve the perception of gaining mastery, which then should lead to a more positive sense of self (Attard et al., 2015). There are already some large-scale projects in the Anglo-American world, such as the *Life Participation Approach to Aphasia* (LPAA Project Group, 2008) and *Connect—the communication disability network* (Duchan and Byng, 2013), that was unfortunately recently abandoned. In such projects, people with aphasia take part in group programmes on biographical writing, discussing daily politics, hobbies, and many other things. They are supported by speech therapists in all these activities. It is also possible to participate in book clubs or online activities such as chat rooms. Several early studies have shown that these methods result in improved participation and QoL (e.g., Pound, 2011; van der Gaag et al., 2005). However, a minority of people with aphasia, as van der Gaag and colleagues' 2005 study showed, experienced no changes in QoL. These individuals did not like the group setting and did not feel comfortable being with other people with aphasia. There were not enough people in the study to determine which type of participants would benefit most from such an approach. However, the conclusion is that each individual's ability to handle interactions with other people who experience similar constraints influences the benefit of the approach. Finally, the described projects do not include systematic biography work as they rather focus on encouraging activity.

Only two qualitative studies to date have focused on purely narrative-based biographical work for people with aphasia. Shadden and Hagstrom (2007) showed that a patient with chronic mild aphasia benefited from telling his life story in a self-help group and developed a more positive view of himself. The procedure was recently further elaborated by Strong, Lagerwey, and Shadden (2018). In their 2012 single-case study, Bronken and colleagues worked on biographical themes individually with a patient suffering from aphasia. As the individual conversations lasted for a year after the onset of aphasia, the recovery process, including useful experiences and strategies, was framed as a kind of 'journey of recovery'. Worksheets and graphical illustrations were used to support the expression of feelings and experiences of the changing self-image. The findings were comparable with the ones from Shadden and Hagstrom (2007). In both studies, the biography work was not structured systematically and both studies focused on illness narratives by asking questions specifically about the experience with aphasia. In a new, more recent approach, Worrall and colleagues (2016) evaluate an early intervention for both the person with aphasia after stroke and their family members. Among other interventions, narratives in groups are expected to lead to better mood and QoL outcomes for people with aphasia and their caregivers. However, evidence has not yet been put forward to suggest that the approach is successful.

The *narraktiv* intervention presented here is a structured narrative approach that was especially conceptualized for people with aphasia. In the course of three years, the approach was evaluated as part of a mixed-method design including pre- and post-tests and follow-up testing after an intervention-free phase of three months (see Corsten et al. 2015). Semi-structured interviews were conducted for the qualitative evaluation. The following description refers to the observations during the intervention and the post-intervention interview data of the 27 participants in order to focus on the individual perspective of the people with aphasia.

The approach consisted of five biographic-narrative interviews and seven group sessions of 90 minutes each. The aim of the intervention was to use autobiographical narration in the sense of identity work to motivate participants to address their own situation in life. They were encouraged to recognize their own resources and abilities to cope with their illness and everyday life. The personal history was used as a pool of resources that participants could draw on to remind themselves of their own strengths and abilities. The approach aimed to enable them to further develop their own identity by perceiving life as meaningful and feeling more confident. Another aim was to support them in interacting with others. People with a severe impairment to speech production feel particularly isolated and have few opportunities to talk, as they were able to take part in individual interviews and group meetings, they were included in the intervention (see e.g., van der Gaag et al., 2005). However, a medium level of speech comprehension was required.

Biographic–narrative interview

The in-depth interviews that have been conducted as part of the *narraktiv* approach are based on the narrative interview, which is primarily a sociological research tool (Schütze, 1983; Wengraf, 2001). This kind of unstructured interview can be used as a biographic–narrative method as it facilitates renegotiating identity (Lucius-Hoene, 2002). In this approach, participants are specifically invited to talk about their personal history.

The biographic–narrative interview consists of two phases (see Rosenthal, 2005). The first phase includes the invitation to biographical self-portrayal and to tell one's own life story. Moderators ask the participants to tell as much as they want about their personal history. The aim is that participants tell a detailed coherent story, deciding which parts they want to focus on.

In the second phase of the interview moderators can ask questions in order to generate new narratives after the end of the story. These questions might include aspects mentioned only briefly in the main story, e.g., a phase of life that the speaker referred to only briefly. Questions may also go beyond the story. It is useful to address successful coping strategies and important areas of life to focus on patients' own resources. Asking resource-oriented questions draws attention to the patient's strengths and to challenges the patient has mastered. As part of the *narraktiv* intervention, participants were asked what they were particularly proud of. The questions can also relate to specific phases of life, e.g., youth, for example, 'How did you make friends?'. It is also possible to address challenging situations, e.g., 'How did you cope with changing your job?'. Questions with negative connotations about situations of failure should be avoided if possible (for more on resource-oriented questions, see Flückiger and Wüsten, 2010). However, it is not possible to foresee all the questions which might evoke negative emotions in an individual participant. On the one hand, when this occurs it might be useful to get the discussion back to topics associated with more positive emotions. On the other hand, initially negative experiences can eventually engender feelings of strength, which could be emphasized in the further course of the conversation.

According to the people with aphasia who took part in the *narraktiv* intervention, openly sharing one's life story requires an atmosphere of trust. This trust was linked to the experience of having sufficient time to create narrations as well as to the interviewers' patience during communication difficulties. The interviews showed that reflecting on the past triggered mostly positive reactions. Most participants were glad about remembering almost forgotten times or situations. They reflected on successful life events or periods. For example, one participant mentioned memories of his great professional life. However, a few participants related less pleasant memories. For example, one participant was confronted with a difficult family event represented by the death of her father: 'My father, he died in war … I did not have a childhood at all …'. In most cases, participants managed to recover from such an emotional outburst by continuing their storytelling, and finally discussing more positive life events. Furthermore, the impact of negative experiences may be reduced in a social exchange. Based on a controlled reconstruction of the events a sense of control could be developed (Lucius-Hoene, 2002). Finally, the memory of mastering challenging situations and the experience of successful communication during the narrative interviews strengthened patients' belief in their competencies. As one participant pointed out, '[…] I lost my fear of being unable to speak. And this restored my confidence in communicating longer without difficulties'.

Biographical group work

Biographical work in a group of people sharing the experience of suffering from a chronic illness may contribute to stabilize identity (cf. Kaiser and Eley, 2016). The group environment is particularly conducive to intersubjective aspects, which play a crucial role in the process of telling or recounting personal life stories, and are therefore of central importance for producing identity (Keupp et al., 2006; Shadden, 2005). The group can be an accepting environment where people are not alone with their illness. Therefore, the group setting has the potential to facilitate the openness required in order to share personal histories with each other. This enables persons with aphasia to become aware of their own coping skills. Listening to other participants' stories may result in changing someone's perspective, making personal impairments seem less severe. Participants are also able to 'learn from each other', as they can adopt other people's strategies for coping with the illness (for a further discussion of characteristics and mechanisms of groups for people with aphasia that may mediate psychological well-being, see Attard et al., 2015).

The research literature includes varying recommendations on the size of the groups (see e.g., Brown and Knox, 2010). The *narraktiv* groups demonstrated that working in groups with five to seven participants provided a setting in which everyone was able to contribute to the group conversation. It seems useful for the group to be heterogeneous, as the work does not involve functional practising (Simmons-Mackie and Elman, 2011). People with more severe impairments will be able to learn or receive support from others, while participants with less severe impairments will learn to assess their own abilities better.

There is a wide range of different methods for the group work. The *narraktiv* intervention used a guide and focused on a separate biographical topic in every session. Given that the topics for each session were selected beforehand, people with severe speech impairments were able to prepare for the session and bring along support materials, e.g., photos. The topics were set to allow a specific focus on identity. Subjects such as family life inspire participants to think about challenging situations and the ways these were mastered. The guiding principle of identity work is to focus on topics relating to the past and the present, as well as to look at future perspectives. Participants were first asked for their own definitions of the topic at the beginning of the *narraktiv* group sessions, and then encouraged to tell situational stories. This approach is inspired by episodic interviews (Flick, 2011).

Furthermore, it is advisable to draw up a schedule for every session (see Brown and Knox, 2010). Important phases include introducing the topic, working on the topic, and concluding the work. The group should also agree on certain rules of communication, to which participants can refer at all subsequent meetings. One possible rule might be that group members give the group immediate feedback whenever they have not understood something (for other rules, see Brown and Knox, 2010).

Group moderators do not take on a leading role in the biographic-narrative groups, but instead act as 'communication brokers' (Beeson and Holland, 2006, p. 148). They guide the discussion methodologically, creating space for communication and helping individual participants take part in the discussion, but neither contributing their own opinion nor offering any advice. The *narraktiv* groups discussed in this chapter were led by two moderators in order to be able to integrate people with severe speech impairments and adequately respond to non-verbal communication attempts. One of the facilitators moderated the discussion, helping participants communicate, while the other observed the group, reacting to non-verbal communication attempts. The *narraktiv* team consisted of a speech therapist and a pedagogue due to the interdisciplinary focus of the project. It is worth noting that expertise in speech therapy is indispensable, as it is important to give people with aphasia, who have difficulty expressing themselves, the help they require.

Similarly to the biographic-narrative interviews, *narraktiv* participants reported appreciating the trusting atmosphere during the group sessions. The group moderators' ability to maintain the focus on the participants' messages, rather than on fixing the language impairment, helped participants get the feeling of being capable. Getting to know other people in similar situations led to the exchange between participants of similar experiences and helpful strategies. However, confronting people with serious disabilities was hard to bear for a few participants. One of the participants decided only to take part in the interviews. She said that 'The three people they are aphasic, too ... and that's very hard. I thought a lot about the time I went through at the beginning and could just say "yes" ... '. In contrast, other participants benefited from comparison with other group members with more severe disabilities. Afterwards, they reported a positive change towards their sense of the disease, and a corresponding greater sense of control. Here, control addresses internal processes which help to minimize losses in and expand existing levels of autonomy and activity (Heckhausen, Wrosch, and Schulz, 2010). Internal control processes help to develop compensatory strategies and adaption focusing on protective self-attribution. Social comparison in particular refers to compensatory feelings. Furthermore, having the chance to support others also made people feel more competent. However, for one participant, comparison to others who were perceived as better off led to diminished self-respect. For others, this kind of upward comparison was an inspiration to work on further improvement. One participant, for example, stated: 'Because of realizing that Mr. XX is better off than me I want to get there as well.' Despite some divergent opinions, biographic-narrative work in a group led most participants to a more positive self-attribution and increased feelings of control and agency.

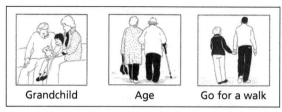

Figure 8.2 Pictograms including important persons, life stages, and activities.
Adapted with permission from Corsten, S et al. Biographisch-narrative Intervention bei Aphasie. Sprachtherapie aktuell 2. Copyright 2015 © Deutschen Bundesverbandes für akademische Sprachtherapie und Logopädie. Available at: http://sprachtherapie-aktuell.de/files/e2015-07_Corsten_Hardering.pdf

Interviewing tools to support people with aphasia

Moderators can offer communicative assistance, e.g., eye contact, active listening, inviting participants to use other means of communication, both in individual and group interviews. They can also use tools specific to speech, such as phonological or semantic assistance (e.g., initial sounds or asking to paraphrase something; see also Luck and Rose, 2007). These tools should be used sparingly, particularly in the biographic-narrative interview, to avoid influencing the narration too much.

The *narraktiv* approach used writing and visualising tools known from biography work such as 'trees of life' for depicting important events (see Kaiser and Eley, 2016). It also used pictograms allowing participants to present their personal history as they would in a diary (Schimpf and Corsten, 2016). Pictograms included important persons, phases of life, important places, and activities, such as going for a walk (see Figure 8.2).

People with severe apraxia of speech, a neurologically based articulation disorder leading to the near-inability to initiate speech, were especially able to use the pictograms in the interviews to reconstruct their personal history. Although the pictograms encouraged telling a chronological story, individuals could make their own choices about what they wanted to stress. Additionally, visualizations can also be used to inspire discussions outside the individual interview, for instance, in the groups. These tools, in particular the visualizations, allowed people with aphasia access to biographical narrative work specifically adapted to their needs.

Conclusion

People with aphasia experience severe losses of QoL, which are associated with a changed sense of identity (Shadden, 2005). Sociocultural theories assume that the so-called narrative identity is constantly transformed as part of intersubjective exchange. This process requires narrative skills. It is particularly important to talk about critical life events and integrate them into one's personal history to guarantee an optimal development of identity. Biographic-narrative interventions facilitate processes of developing identity (Korte, Westerhof, and Bohlmeijer, 2012). These language-based methods have to be modified for people with speech impairments. Qualitative studies provide preliminary evidence that the approach can be used with people with aphasia (Bronken et al., 2012; Shadden and Hagstrom, 2007).

Narraktiv is the first intervention involving a systematically structured process consisting of individual biographic-narrative interviews and group sessions for persons with aphasia. In this approach a multimodal method was used to adapt the approach for them. Observations during the intervention as well as in the reports of the participants in the semi-standardized interviews conducted after the intervention showed that a vast majority of participants valued both kinds of intervention, in individual as well as group sessions.

Three main topics have been identified that relate to processes of identity renegotiating: 'increased confidence with regard to patients' own agency', 'changed, resource-oriented concept of the illness', and 'increased sense of control' (see Corsten et al., 2015 for a differentiated description of the results), which resulted in an enlarged scope of action as well. For example, one participant reported that 'before being part of the project I didn't care about other people anymore. But I learned that I should write an email. And then I did so (...) and then I visited someone. And now I will go on like this'. The quote also illustrates the striving for activity in already known fields despite having a chronic illness.

The study outlined here confirms that participants with aphasia are able to benefit from the biographic-narrative intervention, despite their speech difficulties, if they receive adequate support. However, speech and language therapists and group facilitators must be aware that biographic–narrative work can evoke negative emotions, e.g., when someone remembered negative life events. As Lucius-Hoene (2002) points out, a structured reconstruction of such events can also support the development of a sense of control, which again might help to integrate negative memories in one's own life story. Strategies used to master a challenging situation can thus promote feelings of strength. Furthermore, the group setting allows the exchange of feelings and strategies for social comparisons, which might be stimulating but could also provoke feelings of incompetence (Heckhausen, Wrosch, and Schulz, 2010), although the latter was true only for one participant. Considering the specific target group, it is important to remember that people with aphasia have very few possibilities for social exchange, and that traditional speech and language therapy concentrates on patients' deficits (Kovarsky, Shaw, and Adingono-Smith, 2007), and not patients' strengths. Therefore, people with aphasia especially appreciate social interactions with an anticipated focus on the content of the conversation that may outweigh a feeling of incompetence, which might result from upward comparisons. Narrative interventions therefore must take into account factors such as the setting, the characteristics of the target group, and the skills of the facilitators. The facilitators need to ask questions that promote problem-solving reminiscence in order to help reframing the meaning of past events.

Finally, it is important to consider that the biographic-narrative approach presented here is *not* a kind of psychotherapy. Therefore, people with suspected depression were excluded from the intervention, which means there was less danger of evoking negative emotions that could not be resolved. A current review about aphasia and depression suggests making use of biographic-narrative work in order to prevent manifest depression (Baker et al., 2017). Considering the results of this evaluation and the current state of research, aphasic people with mild psychological distress might also benefit from the approach (see also Webster, Bohlmeijer, and Westerhof, 2010). Thus, the presented narrative approach might be a form of prevention that assists people in coping with transitions in their life. Furthermore, a close exchange with psychotherapists might be advisable, as there are almost no appropriate interventions for aphasic people with signs of depression, and the preventive possibilities of speech therapy are largely unclear (Northcott et al., 2017). This issue needs further research.

In conclusion, the biographic–narrative approach supports identity work and increases successful adapting processes in people with aphasia. This study shows that participants were still aware of their disabilities, but were able to integrate them in a first step towards improving their self-concept.

Notes

1. The current work is supported by a grant of the German Federal Ministry of Education and Research (FKZ 17S10X11).

2. This contribution is based in parts on Corsten & Hardering (2015). Translation and linguistic improvement were done by Andrea von Kameke and Mary Beth Volker.

References

Attard, M., Lanyon, L., Togher, L., and Rose, M., 2015. Consumer perspectives on community aphasia groups: a narrative literature review in the context of psychological well-being. *Aphasiology*, **29**(8), 983–1019.

Baker, C., Worrall, L., Rose, M., Hudson, K., Ryan, B., & O'Byrne, L., 2017. A systematic review of rehabilitation interventions to prevent and treat depression in post-stroke aphasia. *Disability and Rehabilitation*, 40(16), 1870–1892.

Bauer, J., McAdams, D., and Pals, J., 2008. Narrative identity and eudaimonic well-being. *Journal of Happiness Studies*, **9**(1), 81–104.

Beeson, P. M. and Holland, A. L., 2006. Aphasia groups in a university setting. In: R. Elman, ed. *Group treatment of neurogenic communication disorders: the expert clinician's approach*. San Diego: Plural Publishing, Inc. pp. 145–158.

Brody, H., 1994. My story is broken, can you help me fix it? Medical ethics and the joint construction of narrative. *Literature and Medicine*, **13**(1), 79–92.

Bronken, B. A., Kirkevold, M., Martinsen, R., and Kvigne, K., 2012. The aphasic storyteller: coconstructing stories to promote psychosocial well-being after stroke. *Qualitative Health Research*, **22**(10), 1303–1316.

Brown, D. and Knox, M., 2010. Group Therapy—An Interprofessional Approach, In: S. Brumfitt, ed. *Psychological Well-Being in Acquired Communication Impairments*. Chichester: John Wiley and Sons, Ltd. pp. 175–196.

Brown, K., Worrall, L., Davidson, B., and Howe, T., 2012. Living successfully with aphasia: a qualitative meta-analysis of the perspectives of individuals with aphasia, family members, and speech-language pathologists. *International Journal of Speech-Language Pathology*, **14**(2), 141–155

Bury, M., 1982. Chronic illness as biographical disruption. *Sociology of Health & Illness*, **4**(2), 167–182.

Corsten, S. and Hardering, F., 2015. Biographisch-narrative Intervention bei Aphasie. *Sprachtherapie aktuell: Schwerpunktthema: Aus der Praxis für die Praxis2*, e2015-07. doi: 10.14620/stadbsstadbs150907.

Corsten, S., Schimpf, E. J., Konradi, J., Keilmann, A., and Hardering, F. 2015. The participants' perspective: how biographic-narrative intervention influences identity negotiation and quality of life in aphasia. *International Journal of Language & Communication Disorders*, 50(6), 788–800.

Duchan, J. F. and Byng, S., 2013. *Challenging aphasia therapies: broadening the discourse and extending the boundaries*. Hove, NY: Psychology Press.

Engelter, S. T., Gostynski, M., Papa, S., Frei, M., Born, C., Ajdacic-Gross, V., Gutzwiller, F., and Lyrer, P. A., 2006. Epidemiology of aphasia attributable to first ischemic stroke: incidence, severity, fluency, etiology, and thrombolysis. *Stroke*, 37(6), 1379–1384.

Erikson, E. H., 1973. *Identität und Lebenszyklus*. Frankfurt: Suhrkamp.

Flick, U., 2011. Das episodische Interview. In: G. Oelerich and H. U. Otto, eds. *Empirische Forschung und soziale Arbeit*. Wiesbaden: Verlag. pp. 273–280.

Flückiger C., Wüsten, G., Zinbarg, R. E., and Wampold, B. E., 2010. *Resource activation: using clients' own strengths in psychotherapy and counseling*. Göttingen: Hogrefe.

Franzén-Dahlin, A., Karlsson, M. R., Mejhert, M., and Laska, A. C., 2010. QoL in chronic disease: a comparison between patients with heart failure and patients with aphasia after stroke. *Journal of Clinical Nursing*, 19(13–14), 1855–1860.

Hackett, M. L., Yapa, C., Parag, V., and Anderson, C. S., 2005. Frequency of depression after stroke. *Stroke*, 36(6), 1330–1340.

Heckhausen, J., Wrosch, C., and Schulz, R., 2010. A motivational theory of life-span development. *Psychological Review*, 117(1), 32–60.

Hilari, K., Needle, J. J., and Harrison, K. L., 2012. What are the important factors in health-related quality of life for people with aphasia? A systematic review. *Archives of Physical Medicine and Rehabilitation*, 93(1), 86–95.

Hilari, K., Cruice, M., Sorin-Peters, R., and Worrall, L., 2015. Quality of life in aphasia: state of the art. *Folia Phoniatrica et Logopaedica*, 67(3), 114–118.

Hinckley, J. J., 2016. Aphasia practice in the year 2026. *Seminars in Speech and Language*, 37(3), 166–172.

Kaiser, P. and Eley, R., 2016. *Life story work with people with dementia: ordinary lives, extraordinary people*. London: Jessica Kingsley Publishers.

Kauhanen, M. L., Korpelainen, J. T., Hiltunen, P., Määttä, R., Mononen, H., Brusin, E., Sotaniemi, K. A., and Myllylä, V. V., 2000. Aphasia, depression and non-verbal cognitive impairment in ischaemic stroke. *Cerebrovascular Disease*, 10(6), 455–461.

Keupp, H., Ahbe, T., Gmür, W., Höfer, R., Mitzscherlich, B., Kraus W., and Straus F,. 2006. *Identitätskonstruktionen. Das Patchwork der Identitäten in der Spätmoderne*. Reinbek bei Hamburg: Rowohlt-Taschenbuch-Verlag.

Korte, J., Westerhof, G. J., and Bohlmeijer, E. T., 2012. Mediating processes in an effective life-review intervention. *Psychol Aging*, 27(4), 1172–1181.

Kovarsky, D., Shaw, A., and Adingono-Smith, M., 2007. The construction of identity during group therapy among adults with traumatic brain injury. *Communication & Medicine*, 4(1), 53–66.

Lam, J. M. and Wodchis, W. P., 2010. The relationship of 60 disease diagnoses and 15 conditions to preference-based health-related quality of life in Ontario hospital-based long-term care residents. *Medical Care*, 48(4), 380–387.

Le Dorze, G., Salois-Bellerose, É., Alepins, M., Croteau, C., and Hallé, C., 2014. A description of the personal and environmental determinants of participation several years post-stroke according to the views of people who have aphasia. *Aphasiology*, 28(4), 421–439.

LPAA Project Group, 2008. Life participation approaches to aphasia. In: **R. Chapey**, ed. *Language Intervention strategies in aphasia and related neurogenic communication disorders.* Philadelphia: Lippicott, Williams & Williams. pp. 235–245.

Lucius-Hoene, G., 2002. Narrative Bewältigung von Krankheit und Coping-Forschung. In: **J. Bergmann**, ed. *Die heilende Kraft des Erzählens. Psychotherapie und Sozialwissenschaft. Zeitschrift für Qualitative Forschung. 3. Band 4.* Göttingen: Vandenhoeck & Ruprecht. pp. 166–203.

Lucius-Hoene, G. and **Nerb, N.**, 2010. Hirnschädigung, Identität und Biographie. In: **P. Frommelt** and **H. Lösslein**, eds. *Neurorehabilitation.* Heidelberg: Springer. pp. 93–106.

Luck, A. and **Rose, M.**, 2007. Interviewing people with *aphasia*. Insights into methods adjustments from a pilot study. *Aphasiology*, **21**(2), 208–224.

McAdams PD (2008) Personal narratives and the life story. In **O. John, R. Robins**, and l> **A. Pervin**, eds. *Handbook of personality: theory and research.* New York: Guilford Press. pp. 241–261.

Musser, B., Wilkinson, J., Gilbert, T., and **Bokhour, B. G.**, 2015. Changes in identity after aphasic stroke: implications for primary care. *International Journal of Family Medicine*, Article ID 970345, 8 pages. Available at: <http://dx.doi.org/10.1155/2015/970345>.

Northcott, S., Simpson, A., Moss, B., Ahmed, N., and **Hilari, K.**, 2017. How do speech and language therapists address the psychosocial well-being of people with aphasia? Results of a UK on-line survey. *International Journal of Language & Communication Disorders*, **52**(3), 356–373.

Parry, A. and **Doan, R. E.**, 1994. *Story re-visions: Narrative therapy in the postmodern world.* New York: Guilford Press.

Pound, C., 2011. Reciprocity, resources, and relationships: new discourses in healthcare personal, and social relationships. *International Journal of Speech-Language Pathology*, **13**(3), 197–206.

Rosenthal, G., 2005. *Interpretative Sozialforschung. Eine Einführung.* Munich: Weinheim und Juventa.

Ruhe, H. G., 1998. *Methoden der Biographiearbeit, Lebensgeschichten und Lebensbilanz in Therapie, Altenhilfe und Erwachsenenbildung.* Weinheim: Beltz.

Schimpf, E. and **Corsten. S.**, 2016. Der Einsatz von Piktogrammen zur Ermöglichung biographischer und alltäglicher Selbstthematisierungen. In: **G. Burkart** and **N. Meyer**, eds. *'Die Welt anhalten' Von Bildern, Fotografie und Wissenschaft.* Weinheim: Beltz Verlag. pp. 222–238.

Schütze, F., 1983. Biografieforschung und narratives interview. *Neue Praxis*, **1**(3), 283–293.

Shadden, B. B., 2005. Aphasia as identify theft: theory and practice. *Aphasiology*, **19**(3–5), 211–223.

Shadden, B. B. and **Hagstrom, F.**, 2007. The role of narrative in the life participation approach to aphasia. *Topics in Language Disorders*, **27**(4), 324–338

Simmons-Mackie, N. and **Elman, R. J.**, 2011. Negotiation of identity in group therapy for aphasia: the Aphasia Café. *International Journal of Language & Communication Disorders*, **46**(3), 312–323.

Strong, K. A., Lagerwey, M. D., Shadden, B. B., 2018. More than a story: my life came back to life. *American Journal of Speech and Language Pathology*, **1**(27), 464–476.

van der Gaag, A., Smith, L., Davis, S., Moss, B., Cornelius, V., Laing, S., and **Mowles, C.**, 2005. Therapy and support services for people with long-term stroke and aphasia and their relatives: a six-month follow-up study. *Clinical Rehabilitation*, **19**(4), 372–380.

Webster, J. D., Bohlmeijer, E. T., and **Westerhof, G. J.**, 2010. Mapping the future of reminiscence: a conceptual guide for research and practice. *Research on Aging*, **32**(4), 527–564.

Wengraf, T., 2001. *Qualitative research interviewing: biographic narrative and semi-structured methods.* London: Sage.

White, M. and **Epston, D.**, 1990. *Narrative means to therapeutic ends.* New York: W.W. Norton.

World Health Organization, 2001. *International classification of functioning, disability and health.* Geneva: World Health Organization.

Worrall, L., Ryan, B., Hudson, K., Kneebone, I., Simmons-Mackie, N., Khan, A., Hoffmann, T., Power, E., Togher, L., and Rose, M., 2016. Reducing the psychosocial impact of aphasia on mood and quality of life in people with aphasia and the impact of caregiving in family members through the Aphasia Action Success Knowledge (Aphasia ASK) program: study protocol for a randomized controlled trial. *Trials*, **17**(153), 1–7.

Chapter 9

Narrative practice, neurotrauma, and rehabilitation

Peter Frommelt, Maria I. Medved,
and Jens Brockmeier

Narrative practices as practices of meaning-making

Over the last decades, the significance of narrative practices has become recognized in a broad spectrum of medical and clinical specialties. Narrative practices have been identified to play an important role within scientific research and its overarching conceptual and philosophical framing; they are intertwined with the clinical activities of examining, healing, and caring; they are integral to the teaching and training of novices in the field; and they are crucial to the ways people reflect on and cope with the extraordinary challenges and experiences of illness and suffering (Jones and Tansey, 2015). Whether these are experiences of persons who are directly affected in their bodily and mental life or of individuals who care for them as professionals, family members, and friends, at stake are experiences that often have an existential dimension. They touch human life as a whole, and they are fundamental to a person's sense of self and identity.

Why do these experiences tend to take the form of narrative? One reason has to do with their complexity, another with their potentially all-encompassing scope. Narrative is not only omnipresent, but it also is the most complex form of linguistic discourse. It offers a synthesis of all registers of language, that is, it can involve many other forms and practices of communication and reflection. Because of its linguistic and dialogical richness, we argue that narrative is the most differentiated venue of human meaning formation, especially if things get messy and complicated. And this is almost always the case under conditions of illness, injury, and suffering. Whenever a person's 'being' in the world is at stake—with all its concerns and troubles, anxieties and hopes, the hurly-burly of life—people use narrative to understand and to communicate about their situation. Medical and healthcare scholars therefore have pointed out that what needs to be included in all clinical areas and practices (and in many cases what is missing) is narrative competence. Narrative abilities are seen as pivotal for the manifold interactions among patients, their families, doctors and other health practitioners, and the public. All these encounters require an advanced ability to tell, listen, understand, and interpret stories—stories of oneself and others, stories that struggle with the challenges of illness and injury, and stories of how to come to terms with them. In this chapter, we draw attention to a specific area of narrative meaning-making that in the research literature on narrative medicine and, more broadly, on narrative, health, and illness has been neglected: rehabilitation after neurotrauma (which includes stroke, traumatic brain injury, or encephalitis). We highlight the nature and need of narrative competence in this field and outline some particularities of the narrative formation and negotiation of meaning in the context of rehabilitative interactions after brain trauma. Individuals who take part in these interactions are continuously engaged in acts of understanding, interpreting, explaining, convincing, and motivating—rather than simply dealing with medical or biological 'facts'.

In the literature, there are two different strategies to advance narrative competence in medicine. Both consider the present state of health care as highly problematic—more specifically, the dominance of biomedical- and technology-based approaches, the influence of the medical and pharmaceutical industrial complex, and the excessive commodification of health care in the wake of neoliberal policies. In view of this situation, one line of argument offers an alternative option of better healthcare by implementing more humane (or humanistic or person-centred) and ethically responsible principles of medicine, including narrative medicine. The other line is committed to the same mission but chooses to bring to the fore how much even the present clinical system, indeed, every kind of health system, is already undergirded by narrative practices of understanding and care, with the implication that providers should become further aware of them and develop them proactively (e.g., Charon, 2008; Charon et al., 2017). In taking a closer look at various practices of narrative meaning-making in neurorehabilitation we consider these lines as informing two different but interrelated perspectives.

A new narrative for neurotrauma rehabilitation

Considering the current clinical realities of neurotrauma rehabilitation, we first must emphasize, however, that conscious attention to narrative practice is by far the exception rather than the rule (Frommelt and Lösslein, 2010). What dominates is a biomedical model of function repair, often called restorative neurology. In restorative neurology, assessment results of a single motor, sensory, or cognitive domain form an algorithm for retraining impaired functions and providing compensatory strategies. It is no secret that this compartmentalized approach in which each function is separately dealt with is not particularly effective in the context of everyday life (e.g., Chung et al., 2013; Gillespie et al., 2015; Loetscher and Lincoln, 2013; Pollock et al., 2014).

One aspect we believe is strongly neglected in current rehabilitation is patients' experience of therapy as being meaningful—not only with respect to everyday functioning but also in relation to their biographic and social world and their projects of life (e.g., Bruner, 1990). Conventional therapies focus on decontextualized techniques, but what they typically fail to achieve is to create or rehabilitate a sense of the patient as a whole person with an integrated identity. There is an array of studies demonstrating that it is precisely one of the functions of narrative discourse to evoke such sense of personal (or individual) identity (Brockmeier and Carbaugh, 2001; Hurwitz, 2016, 2017; Medved and Brockmeier, 2004).

This argument does not claim that narrative practices should replace therapies in neurorehabilitation that solely focus on separate impairments; rather it suggests that they complement each other in a way that addresses some of the unmet needs of the 'person' in neurology. Narrative is the hinge that connects the subjective, the phenomenological, and the world of biomedical rehabilitation. Narrative practices realize a transition from a predominantly biomedical model to a model of person-centred medicine and psychology—a model that incorporates (auto-)biographical memory, emotions, and social and cultural dimensions of lived experience (Brockmeier, 2015).

Co-narration

Illness narratives, the stories told by patients about their lived experience of illness, injury, and suffering are, by now, a well-established genre of narrative practices, but they are not the only genre. Especially in neurorehabilitation, a number of other genres of narrative practices are important; in this chapter, we highlight three of them: co-narration, conversational narrative, and performative narrative.

As neurologists Goldstein (1934/1995) and Luria (1973) pointed out, neurological and neuropsychological functioning is intertwined with that of other people, whether health care providers, family, or friends. It is even dependent on others, especially when, as a consequence of brain damage and traumatically caused deficits, these others need to facilitate certain neurocognitive functions such as 'bridging the cognitive gaps' (Goldstein, 1934/1995) and creating new 'functional systems' (Luria, 1973). In many cases, what these 'others' offer is 'narrative care' (Randall, 2009). This care begins by providing the social space—a communicative space and time—in which others can tell and respond to stories. What emerges in this way are acts of co-narration for which the dialogical (or discursive) articulation of the story is pivotal. Storytelling becomes a process of interaction, a time of concentrated cooperation, which, especially after neurotrauma, can be pivotal to bridge cognitive gaps (e.g., Medved and Brockmeier, 2010). These acts of social co-construction even play a crucial role for restoring narrative competency after neurotrauma itself. Jorgensen and Togher illustrated this in their 2009 study in which individuals were asked to create narratives on their own; their stories appeared to lack cohesion, elaboration, and other qualities of language. However, if participants were asked to create narratives with the communicative support of a friend, performance was comparable to controls without neurotrauma.

Conversational narratives

Such interactions, especially if they take place in an everyday setting, are fundamental for the restoration of storytelling capabilities and the rehearsal of stories that help patients, families, and even health professionals. In many cases, these interactions comprise more than two co-narrators; they can be conversational narratives that extend in space and time. The discursive net of everyday communication is of particular importance when people might have forgotten details of their everyday life. There are countless narrative everyday practices that 'fill in' what is missing and compensate for a neurological failure. They work as micro-acts of recognition and reassurance, and thus of rehabilitation. Robert MacKay's (2003) *Tell them who I was* described this scaffolding function of narrative. Along these lines, family members or friends might become 'vicarious voices' (Hydén, 2008) of individuals with neurotrauma. Sometimes they may even turn into 'holders' of the brain injured person's identity (Lindemann, 2014).

Narrative discourse can involve a variety of narrators, at various points in time, and variously involved in the illness or injury process and in activities of healing and rehabilitation (Hydén and Brockmeier, 2008). Mattingly (1998) investigated how health professionals give meaning to patients' behaviour, achievements, and dysfunctions in rehabilitation arrangements, and how both caregivers and patients act on these interpretations. She called these scenarios, ones that typically embrace a few people within a certain time span, 'healing dramas.' The dramatic stories Mattingly examined realized a 'therapeutic emplotment', a term she borrowed from narratology, whereby events or dramas are arranged along a therapeutic plotline.

Performative narratives

Narration in rehabilitation need not be restricted to illness narratives, co-narrations, conversational stories, and narrative networks. It can also include narrative practices that go beyond the obvious linguistic sphere. In fact, many stories are told in and through images, artifacts, and performances that realize narrative sequences without words, or with a very reduced number of words. A narrative, as a narratological definition goes, is everything that tells a story.

In clinical practice, there are various interventions that can utilize and promote performative narrative competencies. Carless and Douglas (2008), for example, had men with neurotrauma engage in sport activities that were designed to promote the development of stories emphasizing agency, self-awareness, and relating to others. Likewise, there are several arts-based interventions, such as drawing or painting, that boost narrative competencies (Weston and Liebmann, 2015). Michel Meinhart (personal communication) from the University Hospital Linz, Austria, reported an experience from his 'Healing Drama Group' about a woman on a stroke unit. In the biographical interview, the patient talked about her fondness for roses, including some autobiographical vignettes about her seeking out the scent of roses. When she was asked about her favorite spot in her apartment she answered the bathtub. Figure 9.1 captures how one of the unit's nurses used these narrative vignettes to arrange a 'rose bath' for this woman, creating a joint narrative performance of a memory.

Within rehabilitation settings, other patients can become effective players in participating in and supporting narrative processes. A key element in such a comprehensive programme is the idea that narrative practices aim at 'a change in both the patient's sense of oneself and their social role in relation to their pre-trauma situation, a change in social identity as much as social participation' (Cicerone, 2013, p. 1421). The recovery

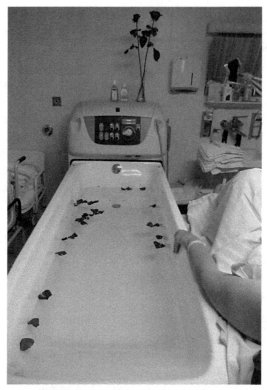

Figure 9.1 A joint narrative performance: *The rose bath*.
Reproduced courtesy of Michael Meinhart, Johannes Kepler University Linz, Austria.

of one's sense of self can be supported by the performance of stories that survivors of neurotrauma proactively tell each other. This can take place as a guided exchange of self-related narratives in peer groups, which might be integral to a holistic neuropsychological rehabilitation programme. It could also be part of a group therapy programme for persons with aphasia that aims to strengthen their narrative competencies and, in this way, their sense of agency (Simmons-Mackie and Elman, 2011; Weatherhead and Todd, 2013). Group therapies that foreground narrative practices engender the development and enactment of agency—which, of course, always has a performative component.

Outside of the hospital or rehabilitation centre the primary responsibility of performatively emploting the individuals' dramas into 'healing narratives' is left to families and wounded or sick persons. As observed by Knechel Johansen (2002), an anthropologist and mother of a severely brain-injured son, it is imperative to include family members' narratives because brain injury impacts every family member. It is therefore necessary to tell the story of this experience from as many angles as possible, creating a multi-voiced family narrative that unavoidably comprises all narrative potentials—including all kinds of performative ones. This multi-voicedness also encompasses narratives from the community at large (e.g., Stewart, 2013).

To sum up thus far, narrative practices in neurorehabilitation reach beyond the classical monological genres of illness stories. Accordingly, we have focused our discussion in this chapter on discursive practices: co-narration, conversational narrative, and performative narrative. What has emerged is a multi-voiced and multi-centred narrative fabric that is not restricted to language, although it binds together the stories and storytelling practices of a wide spectrum of narrators and listeners. Health professionals, family members, friends, colleagues, fellow sufferers, and communities all potentially contribute to the dense narrative reality of neurorehabilitation. The next section turns to one specific phenomenon of this reality that has received particular attention in the research literature: the question of individuals' personal identity and sense of self, and the impact of narrative practices on them.

Self and identity

Learning to live with a brain that has suddenly changed after neurotrauma is a long-term process; it involves developing and perhaps fortifying a new identity. Both immediately and for years after the injury, people experience floods of intensely bewildering emotions—shock, sadness, anger, fear, and downright existential panic. People with acquired brain injury often say that their being in the world has been dramatically altered, that a fundamental threat to their identity has occurred, and that their sense of self has been 'shattered', 'broken', 'stolen', or 'lost' (e.g., Lucius-Hoene, 1997; Luria, 1973, Nochi, 1998; Shadden, 2005). In contrast to other injuries and illnesses, there seems to be a unique developmental trajectory after neurotrauma that challenges people's identity and sense of self. This disorientation can worsen months, even years post-neurotrauma (e.g., Prigatano and Summers, 1997).

In trying to become aware of these changes and, perhaps, sustain a sense of self and identity, individuals almost always turn to narrative practices because, as already noted, narrative is one of the premier venues for making sense of our experiences and dealing with the many puzzling questions of one's identity. It offers an experiential space to weave together personal and medical concerns where individuals try out stories of their lives, to figure out what their injury means for them, and to discern what can and cannot be done about it. These stories are commonly called illness or injury narratives. However, things are not so straightforward for people with neurological lesions. Because brain injury impacts their very ability to narrate, these individuals can be left with reduced narrative competence. In this case, people not only suffer from neurotrauma and the struggles and existential crises that often accompany the injury, but they are also afflicted with the catastrophe of narrative dysfunction, the inability to tell stories, and, sometimes, to use language at all.

Such a radical alteration of narrative competence has profound consequences for one's experience of oneself, in fact, for one's entire identity construction. If identity is not primarily understood as a given entity, but as an ongoing process of self-narration of one's being in the world, then serious restriction and damage to one's narrative competences cannot but result in a challenge to one's identity.

Even though challenges to identity and sense of self after neurotrauma have been reported as psychologically highly dramatic problems, examination of them has begun only recently. One reason for this neglect is that traditional neurology has viewed narrative and the self—and their disorders—as expressions of brain functioning. Although we agree that it is essential to appreciate the role of the brain in rehabilitation settings, we see momentous limitations when self and narrative are conceived in a predominantly neurobiological way. Likewise, we take it to be problematic to define 'disorders' of self and narrative as dependent variables causally linked to brain damage. Localizing narrative exclusively as a function of brain, ultimately as a neural capacity, ignores and excludes the quality of storytelling as a social form of life, and as a way of communicating and reflecting embedded in real-world activities. It also is in these activities that narrative's important role in shaping personal identity becomes manifest. If restricted narrative competence after a neurotrauma is seen as pathological representation of a disturbed biological construct of self and identity, narrative is reduced to a *symptom*. Such a view negates the complexity of narrative competence; it ignores the agentive role of storytelling, even if it might be limited, as well as its rehabilitative function. It also leaves out the rehabilitative role of others, the 'narrative community', in scaffolding and bolstering a person's narrative competence.

In our own work, we found that individuals left primarily with anterograde amnesia after neurotrauma managed to form and tell stories about their everyday lives, because they were able, despite certain restrictions, to draw on readily available linguistic resources (Medved and Brockmeier, 2008a, 2008b). Among the techniques identified were 'memory importation' (transplanting a past memory into the present), 'memory appropriation' (taking another's memory as one's own), and 'memory compensation' (talking about trying to find a memory). All of these techniques are built on remaining forms of narrative competence. Although these resources were not always efficiently used—often the resulting stories were incohesive, vague, inconsistent, and confabulatory, they nevertheless provided a helpful means to sustain a sense of self and a basic form of identity.

For instance, a woman related a small story about going to Kansas when the car she was in got stuck in a ditch—an event she did not really remember, but could 'recollect' because it had been repeatedly told by family members. In telling her story, this woman was able to position herself as someone who can, and does, travel the same way she did before her neurotrauma, thereby ensuring a continuous sense of identity pre-to post-injury. In whatever way possible thus she demonstrated (in fact, performed) a type of narrative agency. But while this agency is necessary, it is important to note that it is not sufficient to sustain a coherent self or tell an identity story. What is also required, as pointed out earlier in this chapter, is a supportive narrative environment—a discursive space in which co-narrators comment on and bridge conversation gaps, helping to give shape to personal experiences, thoughts, and feelings (Hydén, 2014; Hydén, Lindemann, and Brockmeier, 2014).

As discussed, the idea that stories are jointly constructed elaborates on an understanding of narrative as a communicative activity, whether with one or multiple co-narrators. This idea has huge ramifications for patients' identities, as becomes evident in a study on conversational narratives among family members (Medved, 2011). In one of the participating families, family members were grappling with ways to tell and interpret an event that involved the mother (who had suffered a stroke) going to a mall alone without telling anybody. Some family members used the incident as evidence that she had pretty much recovered; they took it as proof of her restored neurological capabilities. This reading asserted that the woman was no longer in need of a 'rehabilitation identity', which implied she did not need additional attention and care. In contrast, other family members used this event as evidence to boost their claim that she continued to suffer serious cognitive impairments (for example, poor judgment). In this reading, the woman was positioned as someone who should have her independence and autonomy curtailed. The patient herself seemed unable to construct a coherent narrative storyline, hence relying on the multi-voiced narrative care provided by her family.

As this example shows, patients' narrative environments encompass extended social networks within which the work of storytelling and story construction about neurotrauma gets done. Often these narrative realities are discussed as if they were a homogeneous entity, but the story is more complex. The voices of family members might vary in terms of their themes, interests, and commitments. The same is the case within formal rehabilitation settings, and even within society. This cacophony of co-narrators can make it very challenging for the person with neurotrauma to find their own injury narrative.

Person-centred neurorehabilitation and the narrative approach

As a reaction to the shortcomings of the traditional biomedical approach already sketched, various authors have advocated a shift to a holistic, person-centred neurorehabilitation (e.g., Ben-Yishay and Diller 2011; Christensen et al., 1992; Prigatano, 1999). Within the 'context-sensitive approach' to neurorehabilitation proposed by Ylsivaker (2003), cognitive functions are regarded not as isolated biological structures and operations but as 'essentially connected to an individual's goal, emotions, contexts of action and domains of content' (2003, p. 1). But what exactly is meant by contexts of action and domains of content? Frommelt and Grötzbach (2010) indicate that there is a prominent place for the inclusion of narrative practices. In the last section of our chapter we discuss results of research on such inclusion.

Based on their experience utilizing and researching narrative interaction, Frommelt and Grötzbach (2010) recommended that therapeutic tasks which cut across the boundaries of single cognitive domains be incorporated into rehabilitation. Designed to be meaningful for the person, these tasks reflect his or her social and cultural context of life; often they are integrated in collaborative actions. The setting of goals is commonly considered crucial for successful outcomes in rehabilitation after neurotrauma (Wade, 2009). In the traditional goal-setting process, health professionals define goals in relation to functional deficits detected in assessments. The narrative approach works differently. The implementation and encouragement of narrative practices (e.g., in therapies) are not primarily focused on functional impairments, but rather on long-term goals and projects in the life of the person. Instead of trying to access these goals through standardized interviews or questionnaires, health professionals need to listen attentively to the stories injured people and their family members tell, paying particular attention to what they hope and expect from life, and what guides their projects and visions. King (2004) observed three fundamental ways in which his participants gave meaning to their lives: through a sense of belonging (relationships), doing (meaningful engagements), and self-understanding (identity).

Frommelt and Grötzbach (2007, 2008) proposed a narrative based 'top-down model' for setting goals. Drawing on the stories of brain-injured persons and their proxies, primary long-term goals are discussed and agreed on in a shared goal-setting meeting. These goals orient interdisciplinary teams and allow therapists to formulate short-term goals related to specific functions and daily activities. Observing rehabilitation therapists, Struhkamp (2004) found that they were more effective when they engaged in narrative exchanges with their patients. Among others, they could modify and adapt goals and therapies in a flexible, empathic, and creative way. However, therapists need to be mindful of imposing their own agenda on individuals' 'raw narratives'. They also need to be aware of the dangers of thickening problematic illness identity narratives.

Conclusion

In this chapter, we put forward various arguments to advance the idea that a narrative approach to neurorehabilitation is a person-centered approach. Arguing that there is no person-centered neurorehabilitation without a central place for narrative practices, we prefer to talk about a 'person-centred' approach over a 'patient-centred' approach because we want to open the perspective toward all domains of human existence, and not only disease-related domains, that is, toward the *person* and his or her being in the world. We view injuries and their consequences from the standpoint of the subject, a subject who is injured but still a subject. Thus, person-centred care is concerned with individuals in their (auto-)biographical, social, and cultural life worlds. The goal of neurorehabilitation is to enable persons with a neurotrauma to regain full agency, autonomy, and subjectivity. The narrative approach, as we have suggested in this chapter, is a powerful way to reach this goal.

References

Ben-Yishay, Y. and Diller, L., 2011. *Handbook of holistic neuropsychological rehabilitation*. Oxford; Oxford University Press.

Bruner, J. S., 1990. *Acts of meaning*. Cambridge, MA: Harvard University Press.

Brockmeier, J., 2015. *Beyond the archive: narrative, memory, and the autobiographical process*. Oxford: Oxford University Press.

Brockmeier, J. and Carbaugh, D., eds., 2001. *Narrative and identity: studies in autobiography, self and culture*. Philadelphia: John Benjamins.

Carless, D. and Douglas, K., 2008. Narrative, identity and mental health: how men with serious mental illness re-story their lives through sport and exercise. *Psychol Sport Exerc*, **9**, 576–594.

Charon, R., 2008. *Narrative medicine: honoring the stories of illness*. Oxford: Oxford University Press.

Charon, R., DasGupta, S., Hermann, N., Irvine, C., Marcus, E. R., Rivera Colón, E., Spencer, D., and Spiegel, M., 2017. *The principles and practice of narrative medicine*. New York: Oxford University Press.

Christensen, A. L., Pinner, E. M., Møller Pedersen, P., and Teasdale, T. W., 1992. Psychosocial outcome following individualized neuropsychological rehabilitation of brain damage. *Acta Neurologica Scandinavica*, **85**, 32–38

Chung, S. Y., Pollock, A., Campbell, T., Durward, B. R., and Hagen, S., 2013. Cognitive rehabilitation for executive dysfunction in adults with stroke or other adult non-progressive acquired brain damage. *Cochrane Database of Systematic Reviews*, **4**. CD008391. doi: 10.1002/14651858.CD008391.pub2.

Cicerone, K. D., 2013. Participation after multidisciplinary rehabilitation for moderate to severe traumatic brain injury adults. *Archives of Physical Medicine and Rehabilitation*, **94**, 1421–1423.

Frommelt, P. and Grötzbach, H., 2007. Zielsetzung in der Schlaganfallrehabilitation. In: C. Dettmer, P. Bülau, and C. Weiller, eds. *Schlaganfallrehabilitation*. Bad Honeff: Hippocampus. pp. 121–133.

Frommelt, P. and Grötzbach, H., 2008. Das Narrative in der Neurorehabilitation. *Neurological Rehabilitation*, **14**, 3–11.

Frommelt, P. and Lösslein, H., eds., 2010. *NeuroRehabilitation*. 3rd ed. Berlin: Springer.

Frommelt, P. and Grötzbach, H., 2010. *Kontextsensitive Neurorehabilitation*: Einführung in die klinische Neurorehabilitation. In: P. Frommelt and H. Lösslein, eds. *Neurorehabilitation*. 3rd ed. Berlin: Springer. pp. 3–22.

Gillespie, D. C., Bowen, A., Chung, C. S., Cockburn, J., Knapp, P., and Pollock, A., 2015. Rehabilitation for post-stroke cognitive impairment: an overview of recommendations arising from systematic reviews of current evidence. *Clin Rehabil* **29**, 120–128.

Goldstein, K., 1934/1995. *The organism: a holistic approach to biology derived from pathological data in man*. New York: Zone Books.

Hurwitz, B., 2016. What Archie Cochrane learnt from a single case. *Lancet*, **389**, 594–595. doi.org/10.1016/j.shpsa.2017.03.004.

Hurwitz, B., 2017. Narrative constructs in modern clinical case reporting. *Studies in the History and Philosophy of Science Part A*.

Hydén, L. C., 2008. Broken and vicarious voices in narrative. In: L. C. Hydén and J. Brockmeier, eds. *Health, illness and culture: broken narratives*. New York: Routledge. pp. 36–54.

Hydén, L. C., 2014. How to do things with others: joint activities in involving persons with Alzheimer's disease. In: L. C. Hydén and J. Brockmeier, eds. *Beyond loss: dementia, identity, and personhood*. New York: Oxford University Press. pp. 137–154.

Hydén, L. C., Lindemann, H., and Brockmeier, J., eds., 2014. *Beyond loss: dementia, identity, and personhood*. New York: Oxford University Press.

Hydén, L. C. and Brockmeier, J (2008). From the retold to the performed story. In: L. C. Hydén and J. Brockmeier, eds. *Health, illness and culture: broken narratives*. New York: Routledge. pp. 1–15.

Jones, E. M. and Tansey, F. M., eds., 2015. *The development of narrative practices in medicine c.1960—c.2000: Wellcome witnesses to contemporary medicine*. Vol. 52. London: Queen Mary University of London.

Jorgensen, M. and Togher, L., 2009. Narrative after traumatic brain injury: a comparison of monologic and jointly-produced discourse. *Brain Injury*, **23**, 727–740.

King, G. A., 2004. The meaning of life experiences: application of a meta-model to rehabilitation sciences and services. *American Journal of Orthopsychiatry*, **74**, 72–88.

Knechel Johansen, R., 2002. *Listening in the silence, seeing in the dark: reconstructing life after brain injury*. Tuscaloosa, AL: University of Alabama Press.

Lindemann, H., 2014. *Holding and letting go: the social practice of personal identities*. New York: Oxford University Press.

Loetscher, T. and Lincoln, N. B., 2013. Cognitive rehabilitation for attention deficits following stroke. *Cochrane Database of Systematic Reviews*, 5. CD002842. doi: 10.1002/14651858.CD002842.pub2.

Lucius-Hoene, G., 1997. *Leben mit dem Hirntrauma: Autobiographische Erzählungen von Kriegshirnverletzten und Ihren Ehefrauen*. Bern: Hans Huber.

Luria, A., 1973. *The working brain*. New York: Basic Books.

Mackay, R., 2003. 'Tell them who I was': the social construction of aphasia. *Disability & Society*, **18**, 811–826.

Mattingly, C., 1998. *Healing dramas and clinical plots: the narrative structure of experience*. New York: Cambridge University Press.

Medved, M. I. and Brockmeier, J., 2004. Making sense of traumatic experiences: telling your life with Fragile X syndrome. *Qualitative Health Research*, **14**, 741–759.

Medved, M. I. and Brockmeier, J., 2008a. Continuity amidst chaos: neurotrauma, loss of memory and sense of self. *Qualitative Health Research*, **18**, 469–479.

Medved M. I. and Brockmeier, J., 2008b. Talking about the unthinkable: brain injuries and the 'catastrophic reaction'. In: L. C. Hydén and J. Brockmeier, eds. *Culture, Health and Illness: Broken Narratives*. New York: Routledge. pp. 54–72.

Medved, M. I. and Brockmeier, J., 2010. Weird stories: brain, mind, and self. In: M. Hyvarinen, L. C. Hydén, and M. Tamboukou, eds. *Beyond narrative coherence*. Philadelphia: John Benjamins. pp. 17–32.

Medved, M. I., 2011. Recovered or recovering: negotiating rehabilitation after stroke. *Topics in Stroke Rehabilitation*, **18**, 35–39.

Nochi, M. 1998. Struggling with the labeled self: people with traumatic brain injuries in social settings. *Qualitative Health Research*, **8**, 665–681.

Pollock, A., Baer, G., Campbell,. P, Choo, P. L., Forster, A., Morrie, J., Pomeroy, V. M., and Langhorne, P., 2014. Challenges in integrating international evidence relating to stroke rehabilitation: experiences from a Cochrane systematic review. *International Journal of Stroke*, **9**, 965–967.

Prigatano, G. P., 1999. *Principles of neuropsychological rehabilitation*. Oxford: Oxford University Press.

Prigatano, G. P. and Summers, J. D., 1997. Depression in traumatic brain injury patients. In M. M. Robertson, C. L. Katano, eds. *Depression and physical illness*. New York: Wiley. pp. 341–358.

Randall, W. L., 2009. The anthropology of dementia: a narrative perspective. *International Journal of Geriatric Psychiatry*, **24**, 322–324.

Shadden, B., 2005. Aphasia as identity theft: theory and practice. *Aphasiology*, **19**, 211–223.

Simmons-Mackie, N. and Elman, R. J., 2011. Negotiation of identity in group therapy for aphasia: the Aphasia Café. *International Journal of Language and Communication Disorders*, **46**, 312–321.

Stewart, J. E., 2013. *Living with brain injury: narrative, community, and women's renegotiation of identity*. New York: New York University Press.

Struhkamp, R., 2004. Goals in their setting: a normative analysis of goal setting in physical rehabilitation. *Health Care Analysis*, **12**,131–135.

Wade, D. T., 2009. Goal setting in rehabilitation: an overview of what, why and how. *Clinical Rehabilitation*, **23**, 291–296.

Weatherhead, S. and Todd, D., eds., 2013. *Narrative approaches to brain injury*. London: Karnac Books.

Weston, S. and Liebmann, M., 2015. *Art therapy with neurological conditions*. London: Jessica Kingsley Publishers.

Ylsivaker, M., 2003. Context-sensitive cognitive rehabilitation after brain injury: theory and practice. *Brain Impairment*, **4**, 1–16.

Chapter 10

Illness narratives in the workplace

Ernst von Kardorff

Introduction

In 1981, medical sociologist Irving Kenneth Zola, who later became the founder of disability studies, published his biography *Missing Pieces—A Chronicle of Living with a
Disability*. In this personal account of his experience of chronic pain, Zola criticizes the
deficits of a medical system that disables ill persons by ignoring their perspectives and feelings. At the same time, the book was a self-critical reflection on the exclusion of personal
experiences, feelings, and the body from the realm of 'objectivity' of science. Zola argued
for the dignity of personal experience as an object of sociological analysis in its own right.
His book could thus be seen as a programmatic 'illness narrative' *avant la lettre*. Since
psychiatrist Arthur M. Kleinman's (1988) famous book *The illness narratives: suffering,
healing, and the human condition*, the idea of telling and reconstructing 'illness narratives'
gained the status of a new paradigm in qualitative medical sociology (Charmaz, 1991,
2008; Bury, 2001), cultural studies (Hydén and Brockmeier, 2008; Reiffenrath, 2016),
and—to a lesser extent—clinical psychology (Lucius-Hoene, 2000, 2008). In their classical study *Unending Work and Care* (1988), Corbin and Strauss analysed the challenges of
Managing Chronic Illness at Home (the subtitle of their book) by using the theoretical concepts of *work* (illness, biographical, and everyday centred lines of work) and *trajectories*
from normalcy to the new status of living with chronic illness. In this context, the need for
constant conscious endeavors throughout life was highlighted. Since then, innumerous
studies on narrations of coping with illness and other critical life events have been published (cf. Pierret, 2003; Schaeffer, 2009). They have proven the importance of changes
in identity, body-image, social relations, everyday conduct of life, etc., that go along with
chronic illness and disability. But rather little has been published on illness narratives in
the workplace. This is astonishing enough as a lot of narratives can be found on worksite conditions in the tradition of industrial sociology (cf. Hien et al., 2001, 2007) and in
the analysis of workers' movements (Kern and Schumann, 1970). In these contexts, the
experience of illness—if narrated at all—is embedded in narrations on the conditions of
safety, strain, and conflict at work and is seldom analysed by researchers in its own right.
In the bulk of literature on somatic and psychosomatic strain and stress in the workplace
(cf. Cox, Griffiths, and Rial-Gonzáles, 2000; Lohmann-Haislah, 2012; Siegrist, 2015), the
subjective experience of the workers is not presented in illness narratives. Albeit their

increase and their presence in companies, illness and disability are seemingly 'closed' topics in the workplace on some reasonable grounds. On the part of the affected persons there is the wish to avoid stigma, not to be taken as a slacker, the fear of being fired or bullied by colleagues, and the desire to avoid negative self-perception. On the part of the employers there is a motivation to avoid conflict about the conditions of work and costs for improving the health-related quality of the workplace, to look for 'smooth' solutions like paying a dismissal wage, lack of information, and insecurity in dealing with chronically ill employees. Some of these aspects will be addressed by the results of narrative case-studies on return to work after vocational retraining (Meschnig, von Kardorff, and Klaus, 2018).

The relevance of illness narratives at the workplace

The number of employees with a poor health status, often carrying the burden of chronic illnesses, tenacious aches, or discomfort, is increasing in modern Western societies (Knieps and Pfaff, 2015; Yach et al., 2004). This is partly due to the effects of demographic ageing of the workforce in conjunction with a later retirement age, partly to unhealthy lifestyles, and to a growing sensitivity of the population towards both physical and (increasingly) psychic work-strain and stress. Further precipitating factors are the rapid changes and challenges of working conditions, including workload compression, tightened schedules, night turns, permanent disposability, multitasking, digitalization of work processes, and expectations regarding simultaneous self-reliant decision-making/fear of making the wrong decision in the situation. Besides the economic burden and the challenges for social policy, the issue of increased rates of chronic illnesses at the workplace, high rates of both work absence and presenteeism, increasing rates of early retirement, burn-out due to lack of esteem, effort–reward imbalance, stigmatization, and bullying (Siegrist 2015; Badura et al., 2015) calls for a deeper analysis of workplace situations and an embedded understanding from within, i.e., from the subjective perspective of the employees. In the considerable research on work-related illnesses and stress (Loisel and Anema, 2013), the experiences of the employees to date have mainly been subject to studies with standardized scales (Weber, Peschkes, and de Boer, 2015). Very little qualitative research on illness narratives in the workplace has been conducted until now. Some rare exceptions include German studies by Uta Gerhardt (1986, 1999) on workers in need of dialysis and workers who had undergone bypass operations; in Sweden, see, for example the Study on Public Service Workers by Thunman and Persson (2015). These studies show how changing patterns of work and their perceived relation to health are reflected and how workers react to health discomfort, aches, and disabilities in everyday situations in the workplace (Haubl, Hausinger, and Voß, 2013). The analysis of illness narratives in the workplace could help to create a more targeted and individualized prevention. This could be at the level of the organization of work, work-settings, working tools, or the culture within working organizations. Prevention could also target the level of individual coping with strain and stress as well as collective strategies to create conditions of 'Good Work'[1] for employees with chronic illnesses, disabilities, aches, discomfort and/or in poor health conditions.

Illness narrations and workplace narrations

The world of labour and the world of illnesses and their semantic referents belong to different universes of perception, sentiment, and approved and prevailing discourses. Work is associated with performance, strength, aspiration, fitness, flexibility, hardship, and hardiness, but also with satisfaction, success, social approval, status, and income; illness is associated with absence from work, reduced working ability, weakness, vulnerability, the suspicion of self-inflicted or malingering illness, and the need for compensation by colleagues. Illnesses are (unconsciously) perceived as threatening and damaging to the idealization of the 'I can do it again' assumption (Schütz, 1973) prevailing in the everyday world of the healthy. Talking about illness at the workplace seems to be taboo, although disclosure might open ways of accommodating workplace conditions (Charmaz, 2010). Nevertheless, disclosing (chronic/chronified) illnesses may lead to uncertain consequences, including stigmatization or dismissal, and only seldom in a search for continuation of the employment (cf., Prince, 2015)—especially for employees with behavioural adjustment or mental disorders.

The predicament of hiding illness at work and of disclosure should be embedded theoretically in the organizational context of work, for example, by using the concept of *closed awareness* and *awareness*; this dimensional concept emerged from the data of Glaser and Strauss' 1965 study on dying. The degree of awareness depends on the concrete manifestations and the visibility of illness and injuries at the workplace on the one hand, and on the corporate culture in the firms on the other. *Closed awareness contexts* that hinder the disclosure of illness at the workplace may also be influenced by the rapid change of the organization of the work to be performed, by work intensification, by job anxiety, and by new normative standards of functioning within the new economy that have reinforced the individualization of malfunctioning in the workplace. Thus, the employees become increasingly more anxious about being victimized as 'low performers' and a perceived threat of the loss of their job.

Different understandings and uses of narratives in the workplace context

Bury's (2001) classification of *contingent, moral*, and *core narratives* is useful for understanding workplace narratives. It is especially helpful for unveiling the deeper connections between the changing challenges of modern types of work and the inherent cultural norms of work—i.e., in Western societies still underpinned by the Protestant ethic (Weber, 1930). This classification may also help to uncover the still-remaining traces of self-consciousness of the working class (Schumann, 2003) and its transformation into 'subjective solidarity' (Hoose and Schütte, 2013)—including a temporary, situational, and thematic solidarity in working groups, as, for example, in the case of the illness of a colleague. In the history of labour, innumerable narrations about the hardships of work have been documented, thus strengthening worker solidarity as well as creating a means of scandalizing health damage and degrading working conditions (van der Linden, 2008). For example, since the 1960s many systematic case studies in different and changing working cultures in industry, service work, and administration have been conducted in Germany by the Göttingen Institute of Social Research. These included numerous qualitative interviews with workers (cf. http://www.sofi-goettingen.de). Although work-related illnesses were not at the heart of these interviews, a lot of comments on unhealthy working conditions and work-related strain are present, as well as personal accounts for workplace-determined causes of diseases. In these studies, illnesses usually do not appear in separate biographical narrations, but often as fragmented pieces of suffering associated with repeated situations of strain, be it harmful substances, extreme noise, constrained postures, multi-tasking, or bullying. In some of these narrations, hardships, dangers, illnesses, and aches sometimes show up as embedded in mindsets of virile narrations of working heroes—proud of being able to accomplish the simultaneously loved/hated work though connected with detrimental effects on health (Hien et al., 2007).

In quite a different organization research approach, narratives are developed as instruments for creating a corporate culture (Fasula and Zucchermaglio, 2008). Staff may use narratives to inform new members about the culture of the firm, proven routines, and no-goes. Furthermore, narratives are used as therapeutic devices to reframe experiences of stress in the workplace by international health insurance companies (MAXIS, 2014). Davies (2016) shows from a critical perspective how these therapeutic uses of workplace narratives produce effects of depoliticization of workplace distress by blaming the subjects for their stress experiences. Last, but not least, illness narratives can veil or unveil collective narratives of expropriation and suppression (Brown, 2006).

Illness narratives in the workplace—accountings and functions

When looking at illness narratives to account for the aetiology of diseases, three main factors appear: hereditary endowment, environmental pollution, and the workplace; to a lesser extent factors relating to personal lifestyle, like cigarette smoking, drug abuse, or personal stress caused by workmates or family members, are mentioned (cf. Williams, 1984). The logic of the subjectively felt aetiological relation between chronic illness and the workplace is evidenced in a 1984 narrative study by Williams: the model of the workers' 'lay' explanations roughly seems to equal the causal logic of the medical model. However, from a wider perspective, workers connect their own bodily experiences and suffering through the observation of their workmates' discomforts. If the illness can be seen as an accountable result of identifiable causes, shortfalls, or conditions of the workplace, it can be integrated in a meaningful context. It thereby strengthens a 'sense of coherence'(Antonovsky, 1987) and self-consciousness, both of which can lead to a perspective for agency and action in the future.

Two examples from a mixed-method study on return to work

Getting to illness-narratives in the workplace: barriers in the field

Interviewing at the workplace comes with practical barriers: researchers are confronted with the argument that interviewing may provoke concerns about already-known problems or about deficiencies that should better remain undiscussed. Interviewing is time consuming and may not be allowed during working hours; motivation to participate past working hours may be limited. Backstage, research on work-related health problems touches on structural conflicts between employers' and employees' interests as far as questions of better working conditions, protection of labour, and health prevention are addressed. Talking with employees about current chronic health problems and their methods of coping with them at work is still taboo and calls for the acknowledgement of 'weakness' and failing in the world of labour (Dew et al., 2002). The readiness to narrate about illnesses at the workplace often occurs only after an acute breakdown, so that most knowledge stems from interviews in clinics and in rehabilitation settings after people have lost their job or on websites designated to self-reported experiences (cf. http://www.healthtalk. org). Job-related experiences and strategies of coping with discomfort and disability have to be recalled using narration-generating questions that focus on the worksite; if they are not focused, the narrations will concentrate on the 'private' side of the illness and its consequences. As in any narration, the retrospective view is always intertwined with situational psychological needs for stabilizing the self and with explanations, excuses, and apologies for malfunctioning at work or for reduced working ability. Furthermore, the narrations depend on the concrete situation at the workplace, on the phase in the worker's (family) lifecycle, the conditions of the regional labour market, and on the worker's subjective expectations on health, work, and plans for the future. Thus, narrations (of illness in the workplace) are representations of conditions of risk and success at a certain moment. They present the trajectories—from work to clinical treatment to medical rehabilitation and/ or to vocational retraining, and then back to the workplace—as a sequence of decisions within the framework of subjective experiences, wishes, assessments, symptoms of disease (aches, relapses, etc.), prospects of the workplace, and demands of the family. The following section draws on selected results from a mixed-method study on trajectories of rehab patients after vocational rehabilitation on their way back to work.

Trajectories after return to work: biographical resources, conditions of risk, and barriers

The study 'Trajectories from vocational retraining back into the labour-market' (von Kardorff, Meschnig, and Klaus, 2016) funded by the German Statutory Pension Insurance Scheme—focused on the trajectories of participants from a two-year vocational retraining into new workplaces, thereby identifying facilitators and barriers for successful return to work in distinctive case constellations. The mixed-method follow-up design included 214 rehab patients who participated three times over a period of 3.5 years by filling out a questionnaire (t_0 = during vocational retraining, t_1 = six month, and t_2 = 18 months after finishing the training). Thirty persons consented to participate in two narrative-episodic interviews (t_1 and t_2) on their vocational biography, their illness experiences at work, and their return to employment. High identification with the new vocation, coming to terms with the remaining health problems, effective and disclosing arrangements with the disabilities at the workplace and in everyday-life, a positive anticipation towards a stable health condition in the future, plans for the future, and existing and satisfying social relations were positive predictors for return to work. Specific risk conditions included lack of partnership, unfinished mental coping with the illness, negative subjective health prognosis, and a more passive attitude to life with the tacit expectations of being looked after by professionals in the sheltered environment of a rehab facility, and relapses (Meschnig, von Kardorff, and Klaus, 2018).

Illness in the workplace after vocational retraining: two stories

The aliases Mrs. Bender and Mr. Vogel stand for contrasting cases with respect to their ways of coping with their illness and their views on the workplace. Both participants completed the two-year vocational retraining, successfully completed the final exams for an administrative service occupation, and both had succeeded in finding a new job. Mrs. Bender has been diagnosed with bipolar disorder; although she had been treated pharmacologically and with psychotherapy, a high psychosocial vulnerability, self-stigmatization, and social anxieties remained—especially the fear of not 'passing as normal' (Goffman, 1963) in the workplace. Mr. Vogel suffers from a chronic heart disease with recurring acute respiratory distress that needs immediate aid from colleagues.

Self-positioning: working with a chronic health condition

Coping and creative transformation of a critical life event like a chronic illness (Corbin Hildenbrand, and Schaeffer, 2009) calls for doing biographical work to find a new way to come to terms with the thereby 'spoiled identity' (Goffman, 1963). People have to manage the respective emotions and rearrange their self-images in relation to their work and their working ability. Mrs Bender expresses her disappointment on the normalizing expectations of the vocational retraining centre:

> … and finally you should be recovered and return to the normal working process … eh, if it was that simple, then we could have done a normal education and apprenticeship before (Bender, line number [LN] 327ff.).

Mrs Bender feels that the remaining cutbacks of her illness put her in a marginalized position, and her statement reflects a characteristic experience of many people with mental disorders (Bezborodovs and Thornicroft, 2013). As Mrs Bender (in her own words) did not experience a substantial change of her health condition, she has not adopted new coping strategies.

Quite in contrast stands Mr Vogel's narration of his experience of the training:

> … and this has also been a really great learning success for me during all this time of the retraining […] before I struggled with the problems […] eh, and now I see it that way. You have the task […] and if you don't get on or so you start asking someone for help (LN 426–430).

His adaptation of new strategies and his retrospective view that the vocational retraining was not intended as time for convalescence but for intensive work of readjustment and adaptation stands for a realistic reframing of his situation. Illness enforces learning processes that are supported by the retraining (Seltrecht, 2006). One reason for Mr. Vogel's success may be attributed to the fact that his illness is physical in nature while Mrs. Bender's is mental, the latter being perceived as more precarious for herself and more ambiguous and erratic for her workmates and her superiors.

Between 'normality' and 'deviance'

Chronic illness is not only a critical life event, but it is also characterized by its duration and its unpredictable developments (Schütze, 1999). Thus, the classical model of the sick role (cf. Parsons, 1951) fits neither chronically ill nor disabled persons; nonetheless, Parsons' (1975) idea of the *moral economy* of coping with illness in society as part of the sick role model remains important (see also Varul, 2010). Importantly, how can remaining impairments be integrated with the normative expectancies that go along with employment? The lived experience of the impact of the moral discourse on illnesses on the worksite is clearly addressed by Mrs. Bender:

> ... you simply try to be a normal person, although you aren't ... and it is sad, that one does not belong to the normal people, isn't it? (LN 537).

The fear and the expectations of patients with mental disorders of being stigmatized show up as almost universal, with a special impact on labour-market inclusion (Brohan and Thornicroft, 2010; von Kardorff, 2017). Mrs. Bender sees herself as a victim not least due to her self-attribution as not being normal; the self-devaluation has become a part of her negative self-image. In contrast, Mr. Vogel declares:

> ... at the moment I would see myself as healthy regardless of my impairment (LN 323f.).

In the same breath he admits that his health status is unstable, but that he has learned to ask for help in critical situations. Nonetheless, Mr. Vogel experiences discrimination as well; he reports low payment for his work in comparison to his colleagues and attributes this fact to the supposed prejudice that connects his illness and his performance in a negative circle. He opposes discrimination by proving to be a very good performer and thus he argues for equitable payment:

> ... now salary negotiations are coming up again [...] presumably nobody would have hired me for the average earnings at the beginning [...] but now after one and a half years [...] people are very chuffed about my work ... (LN 700–717).

Strategies of arrangement and calibration between closed awareness and disclosing

Talking about illness in the workplace remains risky and presupposes a trustful relationship with superiors and workmates, as well as an openness of the organization towards elderly and disabled persons. As Mrs. Bender is well aware of these risks, she chooses the way of passivity: she is anxiously waiting for the inevitable crisis:

> ... the day will come when I have to explain it to [my boss] [...] presumably not before the negotiation about a permanent contract, I won't explain it earlier ... (LN 689–692).

Her strategy could be understood as a hazardous, but nevertheless reasonable, attempt to maintain *information control* (Goffman, 1963). However, her permanent anxiety of being blamed prevents Mrs. Bender from focusing on creative solutions for her illness and vulnerability. On the contrary, Mr. Vogel confirms:

> I won't let myself get stressed, but simply follow my plan in the way how I can manage my tasks and duties albeit my disease … without putting myself under high time pressure or getting stuck too much in a problem and then getting roped into stress (LN 351–355).

This exemplifies a self-caring way of arrangement with his illness in the workplace. He has learned from the vocational retraining to perceive symptoms of distress at an early stage and to act respectively.

Social support and the feeling of social embeddedness

Questionnaire data as well as evidence from interviews confirms the crucial role of social support, especially by spouses and family members. Many studies from industrial sociology confirm the important role of esteem by workmates and superiors (Siegrist, 2015). In Mrs Bender's case, she feels her boss's appreciation is ambiguous:

> My boss tells me again and again that, that I am doing my work well … and that she really appreciates me […] but on the other hand I quite often receive a setback … eh, without anyone asking me (LN 229–232).

She complains that nobody is asking her about the motives and reasons of her behaviour and her expressed emotions. This may be a result of her hiding policy, which creates a spiral of closed awareness contexts for all actors in the workplace. Again, Mr. Vogel explains his positive experience with his disclosing strategy:

> … and this is what my employer knows, and he still asks me every time when I come into his office occasionally […] 'did you need assistance or are you able to manage it by yourself?' (LN 414ff.).

The openness on both sides creates the opportunity to negotiate the conditions of working with impaired health. This does not mean that Mr. Vogel's status is 'normal'; he still finds himself in the position of a 'marginal man' (Park, 1928), even though he is accepted by his superior as well as by his workmates, who give him a feeling of security and being integrated.

Conclusion: workplace illness—balance when walking the line

The inevitable challenge to perform at work despite a chronic illness produces a lasting ambivalence that stabilizes the workplace role of Park's (1928) and Stonequist's (1937; cf. Gehrmann, 2015) 'marginal man'; it could be used here as a *sensitizing concept* (Blumer, 1954) to describe how employees with chronic health problems are constantly balancing at the margins of health and illness, of efficient and reduced working ability, and of acceptance and rejection in the workplace. Beneficial conditions for a creative rearrangement at work can be identified not only in the person itself, nor exclusively in external circumstances, but in the interplay of both at a certain moment of the life cycle. By reconstructing pieces of illness narrations in the workplace within the overall biographical narratives, characteristic patterns of constellations (not to be confused with Weber's 'ideal-types') emerge. These patterns provide clues to be derived for specific support by health professionals as well as by chief executives or shop stewards. The extracts from this chapter's case studies should be understood as a plea for intensified research on illness narratives in the workplace, and at a theoretical level for reaching a better understanding of the ways workers experience working with an illness in the context of changing working conditions. In the field of health policies, illness narratives could inform companies, rehabilitation services, and occupational health and safety agents how to create accepted conditions for 'Good Work'. At the level of methodology, analyses of illness narratives in the workplace unveil aspects of otherwise hidden structures of conditions and relations in the workplace.

Note

1. The term det goda arbetet (good work) developed in the 1980s by the Swedish Trade Unions stands for developing better working conditions on a national and global scale within the Agenda of Trade Unions and International Labour Organization (Sengenberger 2013; for the German Trade Unions, see Hoffmann and Bogedan, 2015).

References

Antonovsky, A., 1987. *Unraveling the mystery of health—how people manage stress and stay well.* San Francisco: Jossey-Bass Publishers.

Badura, B., Ducki, A., Schröder, H., Klose, J., and Meyer, M., eds., 2015. *Fehlzeitenreport 2015. Neue Wege für mehr Gesundheit—Qualitätsstandards für ein zielgruppenspezifisches Gesundheitsmanagement.* Heidelberg: Springer.

Bezborodovs, N. and Thornicroft, G., 2013. Stigmatisation of mental illness in the workplace: evidence and consequences. *Die Psychiatrie,* **10,** 102–107.

Blumer, H., 1954. What is wrong with social theory? *American Sociological Review,* **18**(1), 3–10.

Brohan, E. and Thornicroft, G., 2010. Stigma and discrimination of mental health problems: workplace implications. *Occupational Medicine,* **60**(6), 414–415.

Brown, A. D., 2006. A narrative approach to collective identities. *Journal of Management Studies,* **43**(4), 731–753.

Bury, M., 2001. Illness narratives: facts or fiction? *Sociology of Health and Illness,* **23**(3), 263–285.

Charmaz, K., 1991. *Good days, bad days. The self in chronic illness and time.* New Brunswick, NJ: Rutgers University Press.

Charmaz, K., 2008. Views from the margins: voices, silences, and suffering. *Qualitative Research in Psychology,* **5**(1), 7–18.

Charmaz, K.,2010. Disclosing illness and disability in the workplace. *Journal of International Education in Business,* **3**(1/2), 6–19.

Corbin, J. and Strauss, A. L., 1988. *Unending work—unending care: managing chronic illness at home.* San Francisco: Jossey-Bass.

Corbin, J., Hildenbrand, B., and Schaeffer, D., 2009. Das Trajektkonzept. In: D. Schaeffer, ed. *Bewältigung chronischer Krankheit im Lebenslauf.* Bern: Huber. pp. 55–74.

Cox, T., Griffiths, A., and Rial-Gonzáles, E., 2000. *Research on work-related Stress. European Agency for Safety and Health at Work.* Luxembourg: Office for Official Publications of the European Communities.

Davies, J., 2016. Back to balance: labor therapeutics and the depoliticisation of workplace distress. *Palgrave Communications,* **2,** 16027. doi: 10.1057/palcomms.2016.27.

Dew, K., Keefe-Ormsby, V., and Small, K., 2002. Narratives of Illness and Injury in the Workplace. *Labour, Employment and Work in New Zealand*, **6**, 30–35.

Fasula, A. and Zucchermaglio, C., 2008. Narratives in the workplace: facts, fictions, and canonicity. *Text & Talk*, **28**(3), 351–376.

Gehrmann, M., 2015. *Betriebe auf der Grenze. Integrationsfirmen und Behindertenwerkstätten zwischen Markt- und Sozialorientierung.* Frankfurt a.M: Suhrkamp.

Gerhardt, U., 1986. *Patientenkarrieren. Eine medizinsoziologische Studie.* Frankfurt a.M: Suhrkamp.

Gerhardt, U., 1999. *Herz und Handlungsrationalität. Biographische Verläufe nach koronarer Bypass-Operation zwischen Beruf und Berentung. Eine idealtypenanalytische Studie.* Frankfurt a.M: Suhrkamp.

Glaser, B. G. and Strauss, A. R., 1965. *Awareness of dying.* Chicago: Aldine.

Goffman, E,. 1963. *Stigma. Notes on the management of spoiled identity.* Englewood Cliffs: Prentice Hall.

Haubl, R., Hausinger, B., and Voß, G. G., eds., 2013. *Riskante Arbeitswelten. Zu den Auswirkungen moderner Beschäftigungsverhältnissse auf die psychische Gesundheit und Arbeitsqualität.* Frankfurt a.M: Campus.

Hien, W., König, C., Milles D., and Spalek, R., 2001. *Am Ende ein neuer Anfang? Arbeit, Gesundheit und Leben der Werftarbeiter des Bremer Vulkan.* Hamburg: VSA-Verlag.

Hien, W., Palek, R., Joussen, R., Funk, G., von Schilling, R., and Helmert, U., 2007. *Ein neuer Anfang wars am Ende nicht. Zehn Jahre Vulkan-Pleite: Was ist aus den Menschen geworden?* Hamburg: VSA-Verlag.

Hoffmann, R. and Bogedan, C., eds., 2015. *Arbeit der Zukunft. Möglichkeiten nutzen—Grenzen setzen.* Frankfurt a.M: Campus.

Hoose, F. and Schütte, P., 2013. Fragmentierte Solidarität. Das Ende des organischen Zusammenhaltes durch subjektivierte Erwerbsarbeit. *Arbeits- und Industriesoziologische Studien*, **6**(1), 49–63

Hydén L. C. and Brockmeier, J., eds., 2008. *Health, illness, and culture. broken narratives.* New York: Routledge.

Kern, H. and Schumann, M., 1970. *Industriearbeit und Arbeiterbewusstsein—eine empirische Untersuchung über den Einfluss der aktuellen technischen Entwicklung auf die industrielle Arbeit und das Arbeiterbewusstsein.* Frankfurt a.M: Suhrkamp.

Knieps, F. and Pfaff, K., 2015. *Langzeiterkrankungen. BKK-Gesundheitsreport 2015.* Berlin: Medizinisch Wissenschaftliche Verlagsgesellschaft.

Lohmann-Haislah, A., 2012. *Stress-Report Deutschland. Psychische Anforderungen, Ressourcen und Befinden.* Berlin: BAuA.

Loisel, P. and Anema, J. R., eds., 2013. *Handbook of work disability. prevention and management.* New York: Springer.

Lucius-Hoene, G. and Deppermann, A., 2000. Narrative identity empiricized. A dialogical and positioning approach to autobiographical research interviews. *Narrative Inquiry*, **10**(1), 199–222.

Lucius-Hoene, G., 2008. Krankheitserzählungen und die narrative Medizin. *Rehabilitation*, **47**, 90–97.

MAXIS—Global Benefits Network, 2014. *Stress—reframing the narrative.* Available at: <http://www.maxis-gbn.com/maxis-global-benefits-network-thought-leadership-details?id=a00w000000UZPK4AAP> (Accessed 10 January 2017).

Meschnig, A., von Kardorff, E., and Klaus, S., 2018. Von der beruflichen Vollqualifizierungsmaßnahme zurück in Arbeit. Eine Langzeitanalyse individueller Verlaufskarrieren und ihrer biografischen und strukturellen Bedingungen. *Rehabilitation*, [online first March 2018]. DOI: 10.1055/s-0044-101814.

Park, R. E., 1928. Human migration and the marginal man. *American Journal of Sociology*, **33**(6), 881–893.

Parsons, T., 1951. *The Social System.* London: Routledge.

Parsons, T., 1975. The sick role and the role of the physician reconsidered. *The Milbank Memorial Fund Quarterly: Health and Society*, **53**(3), 257–278.

Pierret, J., 2003. The illness experience: State of knowledge and perspectives for research. *Sociology of Health and Illness*, **25**(3), 4–22.

Prince, M. J., 2015. *Workplace accommodation of persons with invisible disabilities: a literature review* [online]. Available at: <https://www.crwdp.ca/sites/default/files/documentuploader/draft_manuscript_-_lit_review_on_persons_with_invisible_disabilties_in_workplaces_prince_2015.pdf>.

Reiffenrath, T., 2016. *Memories of well-being. rewriting discourses of illness and disability.* Bielefeld: Transcript-Verlag.

Schaeffer, D., ed., 2009. *Bewältigung chronischer Krankheit im Lebenslauf.* Bern: Huber.

Schütz, A., 1973. *Collected papers I. The problem of social reality.* The Hague: Nijhoff.

Schütze, F., 1999. Verlaufskurven des Erleidens als Forschungsgegenstand der interpretativen Soziologie. In: **H.-H. Krüger** and **W. Marotzki**, eds. *Handbuch erziehungswissenschaftliche Biografieforschung.* Bielefeld: VS-Verlag. pp. 205–237.

Schumann, M., 2003. *Metamorphosen von Industriearbeit und Arbeiterbewusstsein.* Hamburg: VA-Verlag.

Seltrecht, A., 2006. *Lehrmeister Krankheit. Eine biographieanalytische Studie über Lernprozesse von Frauen mit Brustkrebs.* Opladen: Barbara Budrich-Verlag.

Sengenberger, W., 2013. *The International Labour Organization: goals, functions, and political impact.* Berlin: Friedrich-Ebert-Stiftung.

Siegrist, J., 2015. *Arbeitswelt und stressbedingte Erkrankungen. Forschungsevidenz und präventive Maßnahmen.* Munich: Urban and Fischer.

Stonequist, E. V., 1937. *The marginal man. A study in personality and culture conflict.* New York: Charles Scribner's Sons.

Thunman, E. and Persson, M., 2015. Justifying the authentic self. Swedish public service workers talking about work stress. *Forum Qualitative Research (FQS)*, **16**(1), Art. 13.

Varul, M. C., 2010. Talcott Parsons, the sick role and chronic illness. *Body and Society*, **16**(2), 72–94.

van der Linden, M., 2008. *Workers of the world. Essays toward a global labor history.* Leiden: Brill-Acad.-Publ.

von Kardorff, E., 2017. Diskriminierung seelisch beeinträchtigter Menschen. Zur Paradoxie der fortlaufenden Diskriminierung 'Ver-rückter'. In: **A. Scherr, A. El-Maafalani**, and **Y. E. Gökcen**, eds. *Handbuch Diskriminierung.* Heidelberg: Springer.

von Kardorff, E., Meschnig, A., and Klaus, S., 2016. Wege von der beruflichen Qualifizierungsmaßnahme in das Beschäftigungssystem. Berlin: Institut für Rehabilitationswissenschaften. Available at: <https://www.reha.hu-berlin.de/de/lehrgebiete/rhs/forschung/copy_of_abs>.

Weber, M., 1930. *Protestant ethic and the spirit of capitalism.* New York: Allen & Unwin.

Weber, A., Peschkes, L., and de Boer, W. E. L., eds., 2015. *Return to work—Arbeit für alle. Grundlagen der beruflichen Reintegration.* Stuttgart: Genter Verlag.

Williams, G., 1984. The genesis of chronic illness: narrative re-construction. *Sociology of Health and Illness*, **6**(2), 175–200.

Yach, D., Hawks, C., Gould, L., and Hofman, K. J., 2004. The global burden of chronic diseases. overcoming impediments of prevention and control. *JAMA*, **291**(21), 2616–2622.

Zola, I. K., 1981. Missing pieces: a chronicle of living with a disability. Philadelphia: Temple University Press.

Narratives in training of communication and empathy

Chapter 11

Using narratives for medical humanities in medical training

Alexander Kiss and Claudia Steiner

Introduction

In recent decades our understanding of the mechanisms of disease and the technology for diagnosing and treating disease has become increasingly complex. These advances have led to a proliferation of scientific thinking in medicine and to medicine being represented more scientifically (Louis-Courvoisier, 2003). Medical education has also become increasingly scientific and technical while the narrative skills (Charon, 2001) necessary to grasp the uniqueness of patients' individual illnesses have been neglected. Because the arts and humanities can illuminate human experience in a way that so-called hard science cannot, medical humanities were introduced into medical education curriculums in the late 1960s and early 1970s in the United States and Canada. In the following decades, medical humanities have become established parts of the medical education curriculum at schools around the world (Dittrich, 2003).

During the 1997 academic reform, the form and content of medical studies at the University of Basel underwent fundamental change. Whether medical humanities were at all necessary and whether to integrate them into medical history or ethics was a subject of controversy. In the end, medical humanities were introduced into the medical curriculum as an independent teaching programme in 1998. The rationale for introducing medical humanities was that a space for 'thinking outside the box' was missing in the Basel medical curriculum, and that the humanities and arts could offer tools to think about and reflect on medicine. The programme did not start with predefined learning goals, but instead developed medical humanities through a process of 'learning by doing' and taking the local circumstances into account.

One major goal was for some elements of the medical humanities curriculum to be mandatory for all students in order to not only 'preach to the converted', i.e., only address the students drawn to the humanities. It is challenging to navigate between the inherent complexity of medical humanities and the limited interest some students show. Evaluations of each medical humanity course have proved useful in this context and determined that courses where movies are shown are better accepted than those with literature readings or reflective writing. Regularly including clinicians in medical humanity courses also substantially enhanced students' acceptance of medical humanities. Currently, the medical humanities curriculum comprises a mix of mandatory and elective courses from the first through to the final year of the medical university curriculum in Basel (Table 11.1).

From the start, the collaboration and involvement of artists, experts from the humanities, and medical doctors was of great importance for the planning and implementation of the courses. Presently, the medical humanities are organized by a small group of interested persons who receive support from an advisory committee that meets twice yearly and comprises medical and humanities faculty members, members of the dean's office, and senior clinicians. One of the guiding principles is (and was) that a clinician always be involved in the teaching of the courses in order to show how medical humanities are relevant for and can be transferred into clinical practice.

The ultimate learning goal of the medical humanities curriculum as taught in Basel is to foster narrative competence (Charon, 2001). In order to co-create an illness narrative together with the patient over time, a good doctor needs to be a good listener and a good storyteller. Over the course of the years, the learning objectives have been reformulated to simplify the message in order to get it across. Currently, students are told that most of their regular curriculum views disease as being unambiguous, evidence-based, and impersonal. This *concept of disease* is basic and necessary. What is missing in the regular curriculum is the *concept of illness*, i.e., the individual suffering and search for meaning, which is a personalized, individualized, and narrative-based concept. While the diagnosis and treatment of a disease has to be as clear as possible, being ill with the same disease may differ substantially from one person to another. Watching a movie, listening to an author reading, and writing about a patient encounter are opportunities to listen to and to reflect on people's illness stories. The programme hopes to foster an interest in ambiguity by exposing the students to the diverse views of fellow students, experts in the humanities, artists, and clinicians on the same subject.

Table 11.1 Medical Humanities in Basel

Academic Year	Course	Mandatory/Optional	Hours
Bachelor Year 1	Film and Medicine	2 of 3 mandatory	2 x 4 hours
Bachelor Year 2	Literature and Medicine	2 of 3 mandatory	2 x 4 hours
Bachelor Year 3	Medical Mindfulness	optional	20 hours
	Transcultural Competence	optional	20 hours
Master Year 1	Reflective Writing	mandatory	
Master Year 2 and 3	Internet Forum: Reflective Writing	optional	? hours

Reproduced courtesy of Claudia Steiner.

First and second year of study

Medical humanities in the first bachelor year consist of three four-hour 'Film and Medicine' courses. In each course students watch a movie that deals with stories of illness, medical institutions, treatments, or procedures. In addition, a media expert and a medical expert provide short (15 to 20 minute) lectures on the film. The students are required to attend two out of three of these courses.

After a brief introduction on the learning goals, the students and experts watch the entire movie together. One such movie is *The Fault in our Stars*, which tells the (love) story of two adolescents with cancer. After viewing the film, students are asked to voice their spontaneous thoughts on it; different views are welcomed and discussed. Afterwards, a film critic shares her viewpoint in a short lecture, asking questions about from whose perspective is the story told, if it follows classical Hollywood conventions, or how the movie's narrative is constructed. This lecture is followed by a discussion and a question and answer session. Thereafter, the medical expert provides a short lecture. For *The Fault in our Stars* this was the head of the Paediatric Haematology/Oncology unit at the Children's Hospital Basel. In the ensuing discussion and question session, the students were keen to know how the paediatric oncologist copes with existential situations like those depicted in the film. The oncologist answered by telling his personal story:

◆ In contrast to adult oncology, many young patients can be cured—something most students did not know.

◆ Working in oncology always means working in a team and interacting with other professionals. When a patient dies, grief is not only a private issue, but is part of a coping process of the whole team, which may in turn be helpful for individual team members.

◆ Working part-time in a research lab is a useful personal coping strategy to find some distance from all the losses due to treatment failures by searching for better treatment options in the lab.

Our aim is that the students confront their own personal perspectives with those of their peers and with the perspectives of experts in the fields of media and medicine. In doing so, they may better understand that perspectives are multifaceted, that they can be ambiguous, and that they matter.

The selection of films is discussed in the advisory committee. Most often, fictional films are shown. However, occasionally documentary films are shown that provide insight into illness narratives. In 2015, for example, the documentary film *At the Doctor's Side* was shown in the presence of the filmmaker and general practitioner, Sylviane Gindrat.

Literature and Medicine, which students attend in their second bachelor year, is structured similarly. Recognized literary authors of novels which deal with stories of illness, medical institutions, treatments, or procedures are invited to give a 45-minute reading. The novels are usually based on their own illness experience as patient or doctor, or on the experience of someone close to them, for example, that of a family member. Most of the authors invited accept the invitation despite the modesty of the fee offered, and despite the fact that medical students attending a mandatory reading may be more challenging than their usual audience. In the best of cases, this format leads to passionate discussions about illness narratives, for example, with the author David Wagner, whose prize-winning novel *Life* is based on his experience with a serious autoimmune disease that led to a liver transplantation. The reading is followed by a discussion between the author and the students and short lectures by a scholar of literature and a medical doctor with discussions after each lecture.

Both Film and Medicine and Literature and Medicine have the same learning objectives. Both strive to teach the students to be good listeners, to know what the film or text is telling them, and to understand how the story is told. In terms of competence, both courses promote storytelling by asking the students to articulate their thoughts of the film or text, to listen to peer opinions and attitudes, and then to discuss these different perspectives in a constructive manner. In terms of attitudes, the courses strive to promote inquisitiveness for the unknown and foreign, self-reflection, and to foster an interest in illness narratives. They provide multiple perspectives that lead to ambiguity, which the students are encouraged to deal with. All this supports the development of their professional role.

At the end of each class, students fill out evaluation questionnaires to assess their satisfaction with the courses and whether they believe that the learning objectives are met. Furthermore, the evaluation questionnaires show whether the course assessments change over time. According to Kirkpatrick and Kirkpatrick (2006), training and educational programs can be evaluated on four levels: 1) the reaction to the course or training (for example, satisfaction); 2) learning; 3) behaviour; and 4) results or outcomes. The first two levels for Film and Medicine and Literature and Medicine were evaluated with respect to satisfaction with form and content of the courses, and learning was evaluated with respect to the learning objectives of the courses. The questions were answered using a Likert scale (from 1 = does not apply at all to 6 = fully applies; Figures 11.1 and 11.2).

The results, which cover a period of seven years, are gratifying. For Film and Medicine, for example, the students were particularly satisfied with the choices of film and the contribution of the medical experts. The aim to provide a novel approach to certain topics (e.g., death and dying, dealing with illness) through the cinematic experience also met the students' pronounced approval. An increase in mandatory attendance from one to two courses explains the increase in the number of students evaluated in 2014. Having to participate in two courses rather than one did not affect the students' satisfaction, and in comparison to the previous years, subjective learning success even increased.

The students also have the opportunity to write personal comments on the evaluation questionnaires. These are examples of the reactions received to Film and Medicine, and to Literature and Medicine:

> The film was most important to me. It was very impressing, really touching, and showed me how diverse geriatric medicine is. (*Amour*, 2015).

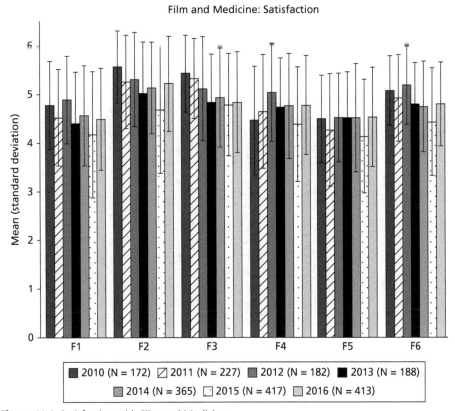

Figure 11.1 Satisfaction with Film and Medicine.
Students answered on a scale from 1 to 6: 1 = not at all satisfied to 6 = totally satisfied. Satisfied with:
F1: the introduction.
F2: the choice of film.
F3: the medical contribution.
F4: the contribution by the film critic.
F5: the discussions.
F6: the afternoon course in its entirety.
Reproduced courtesy of Alexander Kiss and Claudia Steiner.

For me the most important thing was the presence of the professionals (psychosomatic medicine, paediatric oncology, and film critic) who gave us their input. I really enjoyed the course–it was inspiring! (*The Fault in our Stars*, 2015).

That many voices were heard and contributed to the interesting discussion was most important to me. (*Life*, David Wagner, 2015)

I have never looked at a book in this way. I think that becoming a doctor is going to change the way I read. (*Life*, David Wagner, 2015)

This 'Literature and Humanities' was moving! Despite the author's dry and sober style, his and the literary expert's (great choice!) discussion showed us how complex the story really is. (*Life*, David Wagner, 2015)

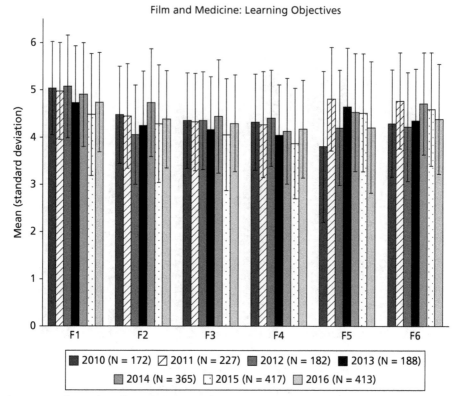

Figure 11.2 Film and Medicine: learning goals.

Items were assessed on a six-point scale ranging from 1 = does not apply at all to 6 = fully applies. N = the number of filled-out questionnaires returned.

The course was useful to:

F1: take another approach to medical subject matter.

F2: reflect on how one's viewpoint influences the relationship to patients.

F3: deal with different perspectives.

F4: analyse the film.

The film:

F5: moved me.

F6: motivated me to deal with the patients' perspectives rather than only disease.

Reproduced courtesy of Alexander Kiss and Claudia Steiner.

Fourth year of study: reflective writing

Reflection is essential to learning from experience (Chretien et al., 2012). At the University of Basel, fourth-year medical students are required to actively participate in one-on-one tutorials in a general practitioner's office one half day per week over two semesters. The aim of the one-on-one tutorials is to improve students' practical and communicative skills, provide a problem-based learning opportunity, and the opportunity to apply medical knowledge day by day in the tutor's practice (Isler et al., 2009). To promote reflection on this learning experience mandatory reflective writing was introduced in 2011. The students are asked to write a short essay about a patient encounter in the one-on-one tutorial. While the precise subject of the essays changes from year to year, the learning objectives of reflective writing are always:

1. to observe patient encounters precisely;

2. to describe the situation accurately;

3. to reflect on the encounter; and

4. to draw conclusions for the future.

To write their essays, the students are provided with a template with the essay theme. Over the years, they have been asked to write about encounters with a memorable patient, a patient from whom they have learned something, a patient for whom they had little or no empathy, or a difficult patient. The students are provided with written instructions to increase observational acuity and descriptive accuracy (e.g., patient description, first impressions, interaction with patient). Prompts are given to encourage reflection on the encounter (e.g., 'What made me feel little or no empathy for this particular patient?' and 'What was so special about the patient or my own behaviour?'). Students are asked to reflect on the impact the encounters could have on their professional behaviour with similar patients in the future.

The students then discuss their essays with their general practitioner tutor. Finally, they fill out two questionnaires, one on their satisfaction with the feedback (adapted from Reis et al., 2010) and the other on the reflective writing learning objectives.

Satisfaction with tutor feedback to the reflective essays has been very high from the very start. Satisfaction was assessed with six items on a six-point scale ranging from 1 'does not apply at all' to 6 'fully applies'. Mean satisfaction scores were never below five. Although the general practitioners cannot give the same feedback to a written text as would a literary expert, they do have a number of advantages over literary experts. They are trained and versed in giving feedback to students' clinical skills, they have a personal relationship with the student who has written the text, and furthermore, they know the patient. This can be important, for example when discussing how to maintain a professional demeanour when dealing with a specific patient for whom the student felt little or no empathy.

Also assessed are the subjective learning objectives via an eight-item questionnaire. Figure 11.3 shows that the students feel that the reflective assignment sharpened their sense of observation, helped them describe with greater accuracy, and motivated them to think about patients more.

Some of the reflective writing essays were analysed within the framework of master and doctorate theses. For example, the 134 essays written by students in 2011, on an encounter with a patient for whom they felt little or no empathy, were analysed using thematic analysis (Braun and Clarke, 2006) for a master thesis (Notter, 2013). Three main themes were found in the encounters in which students felt little or no empathy.

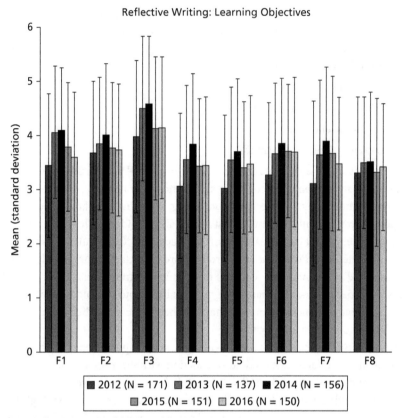

Figure 11.3 Reflective writing learning objectives.

Items were assessed on a six-point scale ranging from 1 = does not apply at all to 6 = fully applies. N = the number of filled-out questionnaires returned.

Reflective writing:

F1: sharpened my sense of observation.

F2: helped me describe the patient with greater accuracy.

F3: motivated me to think about patients more.

F4: helped me better understand my thoughts on, feelings for, and attitude towards certain patients.

F5: provided me with new insight.

F6: helped me draw conclusions for future patient contacts.

F7: is an appropriate method to come to terms with and reflect on patient encounters.

F8: is suitable to train and improve doctors' narrative competence.

Reproduced courtesy of Alexander Kiss and Claudia Steiner.

1. Challenging patient characteristics

Examples of challenging patient characteristics are *the demanding patient* who, for example, literally demands 'just give me a prescription for an antibiotic; I don't want another kidney infection!'; or *the passive and non-compliant patient* who the student feels 'takes it easy and lets the others do all the work (. . .) and then the doctor has to listen to her complain about pain'; or *patients who seem to exaggerate*, who, as one student writes, 'made such a big deal out of her symptoms, you would think she was about to die'.

2. Non-acceptance of the student

Students have a hard time feeling empathy with *patients who do not accept them*. One student wrote that 'although the patient agreed that I could be present during the interview and the medical exam, she was pretty hostile towards me'. Another wrote of an encounter where the patient addressed the tutor asking, 'Does she even know what she's doing?'; another wrote that 'He just sat on his chair looking bored without answering my questions. I was baffled and tried to apply the different techniques we learned in communication skills training, with no success. There was nothing I could do but wait for the doctor. When she entered the room, Mr F. was suddenly very cooperative.'

3. Stressful interactions

Stressful interactions also hamper students' empathy. Often they occur when difficulties with communication arise, for example, when there is a *language barrier*: 'I have to admit that the language barrier may be the reason why he didn't describe his pain precisely but just repeated the same words over and over again'; when patients are reluctant to communicate: 'She rarely answers questions but makes a face and we have to interpret what she may think of the question'; or in the presence of a relative: 'She ... constantly interrupts Mr S. (patient), which makes a conversation impossible'.

The majority (86%) of the students reported what they felt that they had learned from the patient encounter and how they would handle it differently in the future.

To transfer her findings back into medical training, Notter (2013) concludes her thesis with the suggestion that these possible obstacles to medical students' capacity for empathy be addressed in communication skills training. Furthermore, tutors should be informed on how they can help their students develop their empathy skills, e.g., by discussing difficult encounters with them afterwards, or by being a good role model.

Fifth and sixth year of study: Internet forum

In Basel, medical students spend nine months of their tenth and eleventh semesters rotating in three-month clerkships (internal medicine, surgery, and a field of their choice) in different hospitals. In 2015, a closed Internet forum was launched to provide a space for them to reflect on their first work experiences in writing and to share these experiences with their peers. The submissions were commented by Alexander Kiss, head of the Department of Psychosomatic Medicine at the University of Basel, and Dr Edy Riesen, general practitioner and regular author of a reflective column in the Swiss medical journal *Primary and Hospital Care*. In addition to comments and feedback, articles were provided to the authors and other forum participants on the subject matter under discussion.

The themes treated in the students' contributions are many and multi-faceted. The following examples provide some insight:

> At the beginning, a lot of hospital day-to-day life is impressing, touching, or even frightening. So it was, when I started working in a locked psychiatric ward (...). At the beginning of my clerkship, a lot of things preoccupied me; but routine comes quickly; it's normal that I can move about freely while my patients need a special permit for each excursion. (...) Mr. L is convinced that he has to

save the world as a peace knight. (…). For him this situation is a great injustice; in his reality he belongs to the 'good guys' and yet he can only take half hour walks, accompanied by the security staff. (…). So he sits on a sofa day in, day out, waiting. What quickly becomes normal is actually quite sad. (…)"

(…) Epicurus once said 'Death does not concern me, because when death comes, I am no longer here'. This also applies to anaesthesia. If the breathing tube were pulled, the patient could not defend himself. He could not protest. He would not even care. He would never know, never suffer from it. After a few days, I realized just how much this thought traumatized me; how great my own fear was of the moment when the propofol flows into the veins and one knows that within a few seconds one reaches a state that, at least philosophically, corresponds to brain death.

I was astonished that many patients even preferred general to a local anaesthesia. They saw the first as a state of deep sleep, which hardly corresponds to reality. You can be awakened from sleep when the house is burning down. (…)

After a few detours, I landed in a rural family practice this month, after spending the entire summer experiencing the OP life in diverse hospitals. 'Not my world', was my preliminary conclusion. Now, in this double family practice everything is so colourful and lively. No mask, no hood and no rubber boots, and between my hand and the patient, usually no layer of latex. Not even a white coat as a protective cover. Just me, alone, face-to-face with the patient. I also feel somewhat help-less. What do I know? I am often scrutinized—I often scrutinize back. Automatically. Sometimes I need the protection of the keyboard and then hammer almost every statement into the computer. That gives me time to think and just a little protection. Protection from what? Protection from an encounter on eye level with a fellow human being? Why do I sometimes fear it?

Originally, it was planned to publish the three best submissions in *Primary and Hospital Care*. However, given the high quality of most of the reflections, the journal chose to pub-lish excerpts from a larger number (Studierende der Universität Basel, 2017).

Conclusion

The University of Basel has developed a longitudinal medical humanities curriculum that strives to sensitize medical students to illness narratives and to narrative medicine with a combination of mandatory and elective courses. It tries to provide a blend of evidence-based medicine (concept of disease) with narrative-based medicine (concept of illness) and thereby give medical students the opportunity to develop and practice narrative medicine over the course of the six years they spend studying medicine.

References

Braun, V. and Clarke, V., 2006. Using thematic analysis in psychology. *Qualitative Research in Psychology*, **3**, 77–101

Charon, R., 2001. The patient-physician relationship. Narrative medicine: a model for empathy, reflection, profession, and trust. *JAMA*, **286**, 1897–1902

Chretien, K. C., Chheda, S. G., Torre, D., and Papp, K. K., 2012. Reflective writing in the internal medicine clerkship: a national survey of clerkship directors in internal medicine. *Teaching and Learning in Medicine*, **24**, 42–48.

Dittrich, L. R., 2003. Preface. *Academic Medicine*, **78**, 951–952.

Isler, R., Romerio, S., Halter, U., Heiniger, S., Persike, M., Röers, B., Martina, B., Tschudi, P, and Bally, K., 2009. One-on-one long-term tutorials in general practitioners' practices—a successful new teaching concept in primary care medicine. *Swiss Medical Weekly*, 139, 161–165.

Kirkpatrick, D. L. and Kirkpatrick, J. D., 2006. *Evaluating Training Programs. The four levels*. San Francisco: Mcgraw-Hill Professional.

Louis-Courvoisier, M., 2003. Medical humanities: a new undergraduate teaching program at the University of Geneva School of Medicine, Switzerland. *Academic Medicine*, 78, 1043–1047.

Notter, J., 2013. *When medical students lack empathy—a qualitative analysis of reflective writing essays*, Master Thesis, University of Basel, Department of Medicine.

Reis, S. P., Wald, H. S., Monroe A. D., and Borkan, J. M., 2010. Begin the BEGAN (The Brown Educational Guide to the Analysis of Narrative)—a framework for enhancing educational impact of faculty feedback to students' reflective writing. *Patient Education and Counseling*, 80, 253–259.

Studierende der Universität Basel, 2017. Erste Erfahrungen im medizinischen Alltag. Auszüge aus Texten des Lehrgangs «Reflective writing» der Universität Basel. *Primary and Hospital Care/Allgemeine Innere Medizin*, 17, 57–58.

Chapter 12

The 'narrative spirit'

Narratives for training doctors in Korea

Yeonok Jeoung, Gabriele Lucius-Hoene, and Yong Ik Bak

Medical culture and contemporary communication behaviour of Korean doctors

Until recently, doctors enjoyed a prosperous life style and commanded high esteem in Korean society. Lately, however, a strong shift among patients and the whole population towards discontent and antipathy against doctors has taken place. A survey among 1,069 citizens in 2001 showed that only 19.6% of respondents rated their doctors as friendly, and 33.9% of respondents judged them to be unfriendly;[1] 13% rated them as likable, and 45.5% as unlikable.[2] The altogether negative image increased further after doctors participated in a series of strikes against the legal separation between the rights to prescribe drugs for doctors and to prepare them for pharmacists.[3]

Several studies with patients, doctors, and nurses investigating doctors' communication behaviour shed further light on the negative image of doctors. Ahn and colleagues' investigation of the doctor–patient relationship and of doctors' communication skills (2006, 282) asked 90 inpatients and outpatients of a university clinic to rate their content and discontent in their meetings with doctors. Just under 17% of respondents rated doctors as authoritarian and unfriendly. Table 12.1 shows the most difficult aspects of the doctor–patient relationship according to Ahn et al. (2006, 282).

Due to the authoritarian and unfriendly attitudes of doctors, patients not only feel uneasy when meeting their doctors, but also find it difficult to ask for details regarding any diagnosis or treatment; they complain that their explanations are difficult to understand and insufficient, and 8.1% of patients reported that consultation time is too short. Thus, patients' chances to express their concerns are inadequate and the meetings fall short of their expectations to get sufficient information from their doctors.

In a qualitative investigation of communication behaviour of Korean doctors, expert interviews with ten doctors and ten nurses focused on communication experiences with other doctors. Most of the participants described their colleagues' communication styles as authoritarian, aggressive, disrespectful, unfriendly, impersonal, unjust, rude, inconsiderate, and unlikable (Lee, 2014; Lee et al., 2014; Lee et al., 2016).

An exploration of communicative behaviour of head physicians and junior physicians during morning conferences using conversation analysis showed that head physicians

Table 12.1 The most difficult aspects of the doctor-patient relationships.

Patients' responses (N=86)	Number (%)
Doctors are authoritative and unkind	16 (18.6)
Explanations are too difficult to understand	9 (10.5)
Not enough explanation	7 (8.1)
Excessive wait-time	7 (8.1)
Insufficient interview time	4 (4.7)
Hard to trust doctors	1 (1.2)
No such experience	5 (5.8)
No response	37 (43.0)

Source: data from Ahn, S W, Lee Y-M, Ahn DS. A Study on How Young Doctors and Patients Perceive the Doctor-Patient Relationship. Korean Journal of Medical Education,18(3), 279–287. Copyright ©2006 Korean Journal of Medical Education. All rights reserved.

initiated all topics discussed, whereas other physicians only reacted. Pieces of advice and opinions of the chiefs were accepted by their subordinate doctors without questions or discussions (Bak et al., 2014). Communication between head physicians and junior physicians may therefore be characterized as unidirectional and authoritarian.

Bak and colleagues (2013) further analysed conversations of 26 medical students with standard patients. They had already been trained in medical communication, and they all were preparing for their final examinations, which also focus on their communication skills. They achieved only 8 out of 100 points for friendliness and sympathy, and 32 out of 100 points each in active listening and in considering psychosocial aspects of their patients. The data indicate that shortly before becoming practicing physicians students still lack skills in patient orientation, empathy, and listening.

These findings suggest that in Korea the public, patients, nursing staff, and even medical doctors themselves do not rate highly doctors' communicative behaviour. This is also backed by analytical examinations of conversation. Indications are that a considerable majority of South Korean physicians tend to communicate in an unfriendly, inconsiderate, authoritarian, impersonal, and unsympathetic mode. This can lead to interpretations by patients that they are egocentric, impersonal, and play out their feelings of superiority and predominance over both their patients and their hierarchically subordinated staff, which in turn may result in their negative communicative behaviour and their bad image.

These poor communicative behaviour skills, however, seem to be similar across many different cultures. Explorations of medical communication in western countries report the same phenomena, specifically that:

- doctors assume the dominant and active role in communication;
- they prevent patients from talking;
- they do not listen to patients;
- they explain too little and when they do, their explanations are incomprehensible;
- they do not show enough empathy;

and so on (Dwamena, Fortin, and Smith, 2005; ten Have, 1991, 141f.; Lalouschek, 2002, 17; Silverman, Kurtz, and Draper, 2004, 57f.).

Using narratives in training Korean doctors

Recently, Korean doctors' awareness of their poor public reputation, lack of respect, and the growing antipathy of their patients has increased. In taking these phenomena seriously, doctors took measures to improve their social acceptance and to regain respect and patient goodwill, one of which was the introduction of communication training in medical degree programmes (Noh, 2009). Medical communication has become a mandatory subject in medical schools. Since 2009, competency in medical communication is part of the medical state examination (the Clinical Performance Examination, or CPX). Additionally, the Korean Society for Medical Communication was founded in 2006. These concrete measures seem to have improved the awareness of the problematic aspects of communication among Korean doctors and implemented some change; these improvements have tended to be superficial, however. This process of change is undoubtedly a long-term goal, and unfortunately at most Korean universities, medical communication training is restricted to very few hours. The content of the medical communication course is based on training medical students in communication skills. While originally the training addressed aspects of patient orientation and empathy, the main goal is to establish the use of various actions and behavioural tools and to demonstrate how they can be introduced into patient conversations. To date, it appears that students' interest in the class seems to be restricted to achieving the necessary marks for passing the examinations. Problematic attitudes towards patients, underlying role perceptions, and aspects of the doctor–patient relationship are barely addressed. Also, the negative effects of poor communication and behaviour on patients, colleagues, and doctors themselves are rarely discussed. Therefore, the doctors' traditional ethical foundations in learning how to interact with patients presumably remain untouched, although they should be the baseline for both verbal and nonverbal actions in doctor–patient relationships and medical communication skills as a whole. Without changes in ethical attitudes, substantial improvements in building relationships and communication patterns with patients and colleagues cannot be expected.

Thus, alternative and complementary concepts to overcome weaknesses and limitations in learning communication skills are needed. They can be found in the wake of the emergence of narrative medicine (Greenhalgh and Hurwitz, 1998), which in the use of patients' illness narratives plays an invaluable part in broadening understanding and commitment as a basis for developing better communicational skills.

Charon (2001, 2007) has shown that narrative competence enables doctors and students to actively listen to and appreciate patients' narratives. It allows them to understand and acknowledge significant aspects of their patients' messages, enables them to feel and acknowledge the emotional impact of illness, and thereby allows them to act on behalf of their patients. Narrative competence can be considered and defined as listening, understanding, feeling respect and empathy, and acting from the perspective of the other. The goal of introducing narrative competence into medicine is to increase feelings of partnership between doctor and patient and to increase doctors' compassion for their patients' suffering. Charon suggests that 'Narrative medicine focuses on our capacity to join one another as we suffer illness, bear the burdens of our clinical power-lessness, or simply, together, bravely contemplate our mortal limits on earth' (2007, 267). This definition of narrative medicine proposes the existence of basic human attitudes and virtues like altruism, compassion, respect, loyalty, humility, courage, and trustworthi-ness (Charon, 1999, 2001; Hudson Jones, 1999). Fundamental conditions for putting these attitudes and virtues into practice are the ability and the willingness to perceive and judge matters not only from one's own perspective, but also to see, think, and feel from the perspectives of others. This requires the maturity and empathy to assign one's own perspective, values, and interests lesser prominence to that of others. DasGupta (2007, 1385) calls this 'emptying of self', i.e., ignoring or limiting one's egocentric self. 'Emptying the self' gives room for something else to appear; in medicine, this would foremost be the fear, voice, and presence of the patient. This tears down the border be-tween human beings and installs a social and emotional alliance. Referring to Levinas, DasGupta states 'What lies beyond the comprehension of the self, Levinas teaches us, is the other' (2007, 1388). It is only in this 'empty' state that we are able to recognize ex-periences, attitudes, and emotions of others in the way they want their narratives to be understood. Thus, the best tool in medicine is 'the self, which is attuned to the patient through engagement, on the side of the patient through compassion, and available to the patient through reflection' (Charon, 2001, 1899).

This basic idea and goal of using the beneficial effects of telling and listening to stories in medicine could be named a 'narrative spirit'. The 'narrative spirit' entails the capacity to limit one's own ego and to adopt the perspective of the other and the insight into the fundamental fellowship of humans, which is actualized by empathic listening. This 'narrative spirit' is diametrically opposed to the documented negative set of attitudes and communicational habits of many Korean doctors, which makes it an appropriate tool for initiating change and improvement in their communication skills and behav-iour. Table 12.2 shows various changes, including their attitudes, roles, and communi-cation behaviour, that may occur in doctor–patient encounters when doctors learn to use narratives in training.

'Narrative spirit' in Korean tradition of thought

The 'narrative spirit' is not a new philosophy that opposes traditional medicine. Many of its characteristics are deeply rooted in Korean philosophy and culture and mirror central aspects of Buddhism and Confucianism which have shaped and imbued thinking cul-tures and daily life in East Asia. In his first lecture after his enlightenment, Buddha spoke about the interdependent arising of existence, or *Pratītyasamutpāda*: 'all beings arise through the existence of other beings' (Lee, 2002, 104). According to Buddhism, which

Table 12.2 Changes that may occur in doctor–patient encounters when doctors learn to use narratives in training.

Scientific medicine	Narrative medicine
Orientated towards illness symptoms	Orientated towards illness experiences
Paternalistic doctor–patient relationship	Cooperative doctor–patient relationship
Doctor as questioner	Doctor as listener
Patient as listener	Patient as narrator
Patient as lay person	Patient as expert
Based on doctor's perspective	Orientated towards patient's perspective
Objectivity-orientated	Subjectivity-orientated
Fact-orientated	Emotion-orientated
Standard-orientated	Individuum-orientated

Source: data from Emanuel, EJ., et al. Four models of the physician-patient relationship. *JAMA* 267(16), 2221–2226. Copyright © 1992 JAMA; Klemperer, D. (2003). Wie Ärzte und Patienten Entscheidungen treffen. Konzepte der Arzt-Patient-Kommunikation. Berlin, Wissenschaftszentrum Berlin für Sozialforschung. (accessed 22 October 2017); Dwamena FC, Fortin VI AH, Smith RC (2005). Patient-Centered Interviewing. In Tierney Jr LM, Henderson MC (eds.), *The Patient History. Evidence-Based Approach* (pp.9–16). New York, Lange Medical Books. Copyright © 2005 Lange Medical Books; Charon, R. Narrative Medicine: A Model for Empathy, Reflection, Profession, and Trust. *JAMA.* 286(15), 1897–1902. Copyright © 2001 JAMA; DasGupta S (2007). Between stillness and story: lessons of children's illness narratives. *Pediatrics* 119(6), e1384-91. Copyright © 2007 American Academy of Pediatrics; Lucius-Hoene G, Deppermann A (2004). *Rekonstruktion narrativer Identität. Ein Arbeitsbuch zur Analyse narrativer Interviews. 2. Aufl.* Wiesbaden, VS Verlag. Copyright © 2004 VS Verlag.

does not acknowledge an independent and subjective 'I', no being can exist on its own independently from others; all beings are inter-related existentially within a network called 'Indrajala', or Indra's net. According to Indrajala, the whole universe comes from one root and all beings share the same body; thus, the awakened person (Bodhisattva or Buddha) suffers when the non-awakened beings (sattva, or other living beings) still suffer (Jeong and Lim, 2014). Its central tenets are the concepts of the great loving kindness (metta, wishing peace and happiness for everybody) and compassion (karuna, wishing the ending of suffering and losses for all), which are central in Buddhism (Moon, 2012, 17).

The central term and concept in Confucianism is 'jen' (仁 'goodness, kindness'), which Confucius defines as 'love of the other' (愛人) (Lunyu 12.12). Realizing goodness requires conquering the egotistic self: 'when you conquer the egotistic self and return to morality, goodness is realized (克己復禮爲仁)' (Lunyu 15.8); 'goodness is acquired by sacrificing one's self (殺身以成仁)' (Lunyu 12.1). Self-conquest in the Confucian sense means getting rid of one's own will, of obstinacy, rigidity, and self-love within one's self. It is by self-conquest that the noble person as the ideal of Confucianism creates space for other human beings, thus enabling him not only to verify his own self but also the others' selves: 'he wants to let the others achieve and gain, when he himself wants to achieve and gain (己欲立而立人, 己欲達而達人)' (Lunyu 6.28); the 'noble person does not push on others what he himself does not want for himself (己所不欲, 勿施於人)'

(Lunyu 15.23). For Confucians, recognizing the wishes and preferences of others as a prerequisite for acting in their sense is not difficult, because they can be derived from the own self. To realize them adequately, it is necessary to 'reflect on them three times a day (吾日三省吾身)' (Lunyu 1.4). These prerequisites for altruism are closely connected to another central concept in Confucianism, i.e., sympathy.[4] For Confucius, sympathy should be maintained across a person's whole life. Sympathy entails the capacity to look at matters from the perspective of others and to act for their benefit by conquering and emptying oneself. Thus, when encountering others the noble person is polite, generous, trustworthy, eager, and considerate. This creates resonance with the other, who answers with acknowledgement, respect, friendliness, and love.[5] In this context of reciprocity of respect and love, Mencius maintains: 'Who loves others, will be loved by others (愛人者, 人恒愛之)' (Mencius, Li Lou II. 56). These basic concepts of ancient East Asian thinking traditions like Buddhism and Confucianism are echoed in the 'narrative spirit'. By overcoming and emptying one's self, the self can then be connected with the other person. This enables a person to perceive the others from their own perspective and to act on their behalf, which creates appreciation and friendly resonance from without, which is the basis for contentment and happiness.

Korea has been strongly influenced and imbued by these traditions on all levels of everyday life and is regarded as a society steeped in Buddhism and Confucianism. Therefore, Buddhist philosophy and its healing practices left traces on Korean indigenous medicine (In, 1996). Thus, it is expected that ethical attitudes and behaviour of Korean doctors should mirror these basic traditional ideas as regards their patients. As mentioned, however, doctors do not exhibit these behaviours when dealing with patients. This may be due to the fact that the old ethical codes and the 'narrative spirit' as well ask for very high standards of morality, which may also not have been maintained on an everyday basis in the times of Buddha and Confucius. Confucius confirms this by saying that the whole world becomes benignant when the self is overcome on one single day and returns to morality. This implies the huge effects of self-conquest as well as the immense difficulties in realizing it. But although it is understandable that the communication skills of Korean doctors do not mirror the 'narrative spirit' perfectly, their huge distance from this ideal remains a problem. Therefore, it is likely that the 'narrative spirit' will remain as a predominantly unattainable ideal concept of humanity; it is a state reachable only by a very few. However, as an ideal concept the 'narrative spirit' can stimulate and spur our endeavours to attain this mindset as much as possible, and thus the use of narratives in medical education and training is necessary in order to make future physicians realize what might be possible in establishing sympathetic and more equal relationships with their patients.

Methods to develop the 'narrative spirit'

'Narrative spirit' is not part of the narratives themselves, but is expressed when they are used in interactions between doctors and patients, and when doctors try to understand the patient perspective and to act from this vantage point. Doctors display 'narrative spirit' when they encourage patients to tell the stories of their illness experiences, and when they respect and appreciate these stories, listen to them carefully, and consider them thoroughly. The stories offer an insight into the inner worlds of patients, and this glimpse enables doctors to build an alliance departing from their experiences and to act on their patients' behalf (Lucius-Hoene, 2008).

In Korean medical practice, making use of patients' narratives is well known already. However, in training programmes for doctors and students, their use is only recent. To date, the Korean authors of this paper and their co-workers are the only group to implement the use of patients' narratives for training medical staff in workshops for health communication at meetings of the Korean Society for Medical Communication. Often participants included teachers from the faculties of medicine.

Training materials for developing the 'narrative spirit' which are used in the training programme include literary texts, interviews aimed at illness experiences of patients, and transcripts of interactions between patients and doctors during consultations. In the workshops, the written materials are closely read to encourage active listening, to enhance deeper understanding, and to access the inner worlds of patients. To improve doctors' skills in eliciting patients' narratives by active listening and displaying signs of empathy, the narrative interview is used as elaborated by Fritz Schütze (1976), who describes the many benefits of its use when applied to training people in listening and empathy skills. During the narrative interview, storytellers are given free rein and are encouraged to tell what has happened from their own perspective and to assume the role of being the expert for his/her specific and unique experiences. In contrast, the interviewer acts in a supportive, attentive, and non-judgmental way, showing his/her willingness to listen, to appreciate the story, and to take seriously what is told in the story. To assume this role successfully, the listener must set aside his/her own perspective, relevancies, and priorities (Lucius-Hoene and Deppermann, 2004, 77, 301). It is these requirements which make the narrative interview a very apt and beneficial training tool.

The workshop programme, which is based on the aptitude and benefits of narrative interviews as training materials for listening and developing empathy, consists of both a theoretical and a training part. The theoretical part starts with discussing the problematic communication behaviour of Korean doctors, as many of them do not realize these deficits, perceiving the critical styles and faults as adequate and normal. These doctors are so used to the 'normal abnormality' that they first must be made aware of the ensuing problems and negative consequences of this mindset; however, heightened awareness of the problems is necessary for any kind of change. Secondly, terms and concepts of active listening and empathy (Rogers and Farson, 1957) are discussed as the main basis for the ethical stance of the 'narrative spirit'. Afterwards, the characteristics of narratives in general and their therapeutic effects are discussed. Based on the scientific literature on illness narratives in medical communication, concrete methods are then introduced for evaluating narrative interviews by looking at their patterns with the help of evaluation sheets. During the practical parts of the workshops, there is discussion of the methods and procedures of eliciting patients' narratives, e.g., in research narrative interviews, but these are slightly adapted for the communicational requirements of medical encounters. Participants form teams of three people, and each plays a different role—teller, listener and observer—which is rotated. In three training units, every participant occupies one of the roles successively. The 'Interviewer' tries to use active and empathic listening skills and to elicit stories of illness experience. The third participant observes the interview and fills in the evaluation sheet. Afterwards, observations, problems, and experiences of all three participants are exchanged and discussed. Rotating the roles enables each person on the team to experience the perspectives of the interviewer, the narrator, and the observer.

The third part of the workshop focuses on training to understand and interpret patients' narratives, and uses authentic videos and verbatim transcripts of narrative interviews that have been recorded with the consent of patients, doctors, and the responsible ethics committee of the clinic (IRB, Institutional Research Board) for teaching purposes. Thus, nonverbal communication, including breaks, eye contact, gestures, and expressions, supplies further emotional and psychological information to understanding subtle meanings beyond the concrete spoken word. Using the corresponding transcripts in addition to watching the videos has many advantages: phrases can be read slowly and thoroughly many times, enabling in-depth understanding; different parts of the texts can be compared and participants can name precisely on which expressions they base their interpretations and inferences. Participants are asked to work on the transcripts with the following tasks and discuss their results:

◆ Give an oral or written summary of the interview's content in their own words.

◆ Which episodes are narrated?

◆ What is the communicative purpose of each of the episodes?

◆ What is the connection between the different episodes?

◆ What is the patient's main problem?

◆ How does the patient position him/herself in the narrative?

◆ How does (s)he evaluate his/her experiences?

◆ How would you respond after the interview if you were this patient's doctor?

The authentic narratives can also be used to analyse doctors' acts of and competency in active listening and of showing empathy. Single interactions can be closely watched, reread, and discussed in terms of appropriateness, consequences, and communicative alternatives. This fine-grained analytical work is a very useful training for developing problem awareness and sensitivity for the impact of language and communicative acts.

During the last few years, several workshops have taken place in cooperation with different medical societies. Participants provided positive feedback in discussions afterwards; however, a systematic evaluation is still required.

Many participants conveyed that the workshops not only made them understand the concepts of the 'narrative spirit' and the preconditions and the method of listeners' activities and empathy, but also helped to incorporate them through the practical tasks. Feedback showed that they intended to practise these attitudes not only with patients, but also with colleagues and their families. The medical professors would have liked to introduce the concept to their faculties, but as novices to narratology they did not feel capable of implementing it after two three-hour workshops; this may be the reason for lack of comments or questions after the workshops. Only one university professor implemented the method for improving listening skills and evoking empathy. During his course, guest speakers give an introductory lecture about narrative medicine and the method of the narrative interview. After some practical tasks, his students perform an interview with a patient; his students' feedback for this task is positive.

Despite these positive records, limitations of the programme must be discussed (Bak and Park, 2009). Firstly, the duration of the workshops is limited to three hours, as the participating medical societies do not allow longer training times. Thus, time is very short to introduce and discuss the foundations of the 'narrative spirit' and the methods of the narrative interview thoroughly. Secondly, the participants are not practicing physicians, but mostly professors from university teaching staff who teach medical communication or humanities in medicine. Most professors had no training or experience with the subject matter of the course and showed more interest in didactics, contents of courses, and training materials for medical communication and medical humanities than in understanding and realizing the 'narrative spirit'. Thirdly, the number of medical staff who can make use of this training is very small, as this is the only group to offer this kind of communicational training or lectures, which limits impact on the usual communication styles. Chances to change the awareness of problematic behaviour on a bigger scale are still few and far between. However, hopefully others will follow and narrative methods, including approaches such as the 'narrative spirit', can eventually be implemented in training curricula at medical faculties, so that systematic evaluation with standardized material is possible.

Conclusion: 'narrative spirit' as a fusion of traditional philosophy and narrative medicine in Korea?

As in other countries, the ideals and ideas of narrative medicine still await integration into Korean standard medical practice. But regarding it simply as a trend in holistic and communicative medicine from western medical culture may fall short. The narrative spirit as a joint venture and an overarching philosophical and communicative tie may not only imbue the relationship between professionals and patients with empathy, but also overcome the differences among practitioners from various traditions and backgrounds (Hong, 2001). In returning to Korean cultural and social philosophical roots, backing patients' own cultural backgrounds in their personal stories and taking up their participation in a collective memory of suffering and healing on one side (Hwang and Kim, 2013), and the patient-orientated approach inherent in western narrative medicine on the other, may find a common denominator in the appreciation of illness stories. However, finding ways to integrate the use of illness stories into medical education and advanced training for professionals in the tight teaching and working schedules of modern medicine remains a challenge.

Notes

1. http://www.kossda.or.kr/kpoll/view2.asp?tp=0&no=00003904.
2. http://www.kossda.or.kr/kpoll/view2.asp?tp=0&no=00003906.
3. 52.9% of interviewees stated that their image of doctors had deteriorated after the strikes (http://www.kossda.or.kr/kpoll/view2.asp?tp=0&no=00003808).
4. The Chinese symbol for sympathy 恕 is made up of 如 'same', and 心 'heart'. The concept of sympathy in the Chinese language is based on the idea that sympathy is a state of the same heart in two or more persons.
5. 'When you are polite, you are not despised. When you are generous, you win many people over. When you are trustworthy, other people believe in you. When you are eager, you can achieve many things. When you are considerate, you can assign tasks (恭則不侮, 寬則得衆, 則人任焉, 敏則有功, 惠則足以使人)' (Lunyu 17.6).

References

Ahn, S. W., Lee, Y-M., and Ahn, D. S., 2006. A study on how young doctors and patients perceive the doctor-patient relationship. *Korean Journal of Medical Education*, 18/3, 279–287.

Bak, Y. I., Jin, J. K., Lim, I. S., Jeoung, Y. O., and Kim, C. W., 2013. Analysis of criteria to evaluate patient doctor relationships in a clinical performance examination—linguistic dialog analysis approach. *Health Communication*, 8/1, 13–25.

Bak, Y. I. and Park, E. W., 2009. Problems of the Curriculum for the Improvement of the Medical Communication in Korean Medical Schools. *Health Communication*, 4/1, 34–42.

Bak, Y. I., Sin, S. E., Kim, T. G., and Lee, J. W., 2014. A study on the structure of dialog sequences in the physicians' morning conferences. *Discourse and Cognition*, 1/2, 55–80.

Charon, R., 2001. Narrative medicine: a model for empathy, reflection, profession, and trust. *JAMA*, 286, 1897–1902.

Charon, R., 2007. What to do with stories. The sciences of narrative medicine. *Canadian Family Physician*, 53, 1265–1267.

Charon, R., 2008. *Narrative medicine: honoring the stories of illness*. Oxford: Oxford University Press.

DasGupta, S., 2007. Between stillness and story: lessons of children's illness narratives. *Pediatrics*, 119(6), e1384–e1391.

Dwamena, F. C., Fortin VI, A. H., and Smith, R. C., 2005. Patient-centered interviewing. In: L. M. Tierney Jr. and M. C. Henderson, eds. *The patient history. Evidence-based approach*. New York: Lange Medical Books. pp .9–16.

Emanuel, E. J. and Emanuel, L. L., 1992. Four models of the physician-patient relationship. *JAMA*, 267, 2221–2226.

Greenhalgh, T. and Hurwitz, B., 1998. *Narrative based medicine: dialogue and discourse in clinical practice*. London: BMJ Books.

Hong, C. D. C. D., 2001. Complementary and alternative medicine in Korea: current status and future prospects. *The Journal of Alternative and Complementary Medicine*, 7, 33–40.

Hwang, I. I. K. and Kim, H. H. Y., 2013. The encounter between oral history and narrative medicine: a preliminary study. *Korean Journal of Medical History*, 22, 357–388.

Hudson Jones, A., 1999. Narrative based medicine. Narrative in medical ethics. *British Medical Journal*, 318, 253–256.

In, S. Y., 1996. Buddhism and Medicine in Three Kingdom Period. *Korean Journal of Medical History* 5(2): 197–214

Jeong, R. and Lim, G. J., 2014. On the interdependent relationship of sharing life in Buddhism. *Bumhan Philosophy*, **75**, 1–24.

Klemperer, D., 2003. *Wie Ärzte und Patienten Entscheidungen treffen. Konzepte der Arzt-Patient-Kommunikation*. Berlin: Wissenschaftszentrum Berlin für Sozialforschung.

Lalouschek, J., 2002. 'Hypertonie?' oder das Gespräch mit PatientInnen als Störung ärztlichen Tuns. In: R. Fiehler, ed. *Verständigungsprobleme und gestörte Kommunikation*. Wiesbaden: Verlag für Gesprächsforschung. Available at: <http://www.verlag-gespraechsforschung.de /2002/probleme/ probleme.pdf, 97–115> (Accessed 22 October 2017).

Hwang, I. and Kim, H., 2013. The encounter between oral history and narrative medicine: a preliminary study. *Korean Journal of Medical History*, **22**(2), 357–388.

Lee, H. K., 2002. On the relations between the idea of Brahma-ātma-aikya and Pratītyasamutpāda. *Korean Indian Philosophy*, **12**(1), 99–118.

Lee, J. W., Bak, Y. I., Baek, S. J., Lee, J. U., Lee, H. Y., and Jeoung, Y. O., 2014. How hospital nurses communicate with physicians? *Journal of Humanities*, **71**(1), 345–385.

Lee, H. Y., 2014. Suggestion to address a communication problem between doctors in hospitals: Focus on experiences of hierarchical communication. *Language and Linguistics*, **65**, 133–162.

Lee, H. Y., Sok, S. H., Park, S. C., Bak, Y. I., Lee, J. W., Jin, J. K., and Jeoung, Y. O., 2016. How members of a medical center communicate with each other. *The Sociolinguistic Journal of Korea*, **24**(1), 213–239.

Lucius-Hoene, G., 2008. Levels of narrativity in doctor-patient-interaction. *Health Communication*, **3**/ 2, 81–90.

Lucius-Hoene, G. and Deppermann, A., 2004. *Rekonstruktion narrativer Identität. Ein Arbeitsbuch zur Analyse narrativer Interviews. 2. Aufl.* Wiesbaden: VS Verlag.

Lunyu (論語). Available at: <http://www.confucius.org/lunyu/lange.htm> (Accessed 22 October 2017).

Mencius (孟子). Available at: <http://ctext.org/mengzi> (Accessed 22 October 2017).

Moon, E. S., 2012. Developing aspects on conception of Maitrī-karuṇā in Buddhism Scriptures. Focused on conception to be expressed in early Buddhist scriptures and Abhidhamma Buddhist scriptures. *Buddhist Studies*, **37**, 9–42.

Noh, Y. K., 2009. The current state of medical communication education in the Korean medical school. *Proceedings of the 6th Korean Academy on Communication in Healthcare Conference*, (pp. 20–21), March, 2009, 3–7. Seoul

Rogers, C. R. and Farson, R. E., 1957. *Active listening*. Chicago: Industrial Relations Center of The University of Chicago.

Schütze, F., 1976. Zur Hervorlockung und Analyse von Erzählungen thematisch relevanter Geschichten im Rahmen soziologischer Feldforschung—dargestellt an einem Projekt zur Erforschung von kommunalen Machtstrukturen. In: Arbeitsgruppe Bielefelder Soziologen, eds. *Kommunikative Sozialforschung: Alltagswissen und Alltagshandeln, Gemeindemachtforschung, Polizei, politische Erwachsenenbildung*. Munich: Fink. pp. 159–260.

Silverman, J., Kurtz, S., and Draper, J., 2004. *Skills for communicating with patients*. 2nd ed. Oxford: Radcliff Medical Press.

ten Have, P., 1991. Talk and institution: a reconsideration of the 'asymmetry' of doctor-patient interaction. In: D. Boden and D. H. Zimmerman, eds. *Talk and social structure. Studies in ethnomethodology and conversation analysis*. Cambridge: Polity Press. pp. 138–163.

Chapter 13

How to use illness narratives in medical education

First teaching experiences with the German DIPEx website project

Alexander Palant and Wolfgang Himmel

Background

To be effective, (future) clinicians should gain an understanding of patients' perspective on his or her illness, including patients' key concerns, values, experiences, cultures, and preferences (Teutsch, 2003). If healthcare providers were trained to use more patient-centred approaches and to focus on the patient as a person with individual preferences situated within social contexts instead of focusing on diseases and their management alone, positive effects would be observed on a range of measures. These include clarifying patients' concerns and beliefs, talking about treatment options, and display of empathy (Dwamena et al., 2012). Similar effects could be observed as live presentations of patients during lectures or hospital rounds during provision of clinical care are a sort of 'tacit curriculum' to learn more about people's perceptions of illness (Teutsch, 2003; Bell et al., 2009).

Case presentations are the most frequently used teaching and learning techniques. Ideally, these should balance biomedical and psychosocial approaches to health during medical education. Knowing how patients experience their illness significantly improves medical students' clinical performance and skills (Snow et al., 2016). For example:

♦ There are different ways to teach students about patients' perspectives and how to understand the patient from a holistic viewpoint (Onishi, 2008).

♦ Working with simulated patients is another strategy to make students aware of a patient's perspective, especially when simulated patients are trained to give feedback and evaluate student performance (Cleland, Abe, and Rethans, 2009). This approach facilitates perspective-taking and reflection and is of particular importance when learning, for example, about the experiences and needs of patients with disabilities (Long-Bellil et al., 2011).

◆ Finally, real patient contact is a central point of learning and deepens the students' perceptions of patients' illness experiences (Graungaard and Andersen, 2014). As undergraduate students put it in their free text responses in a study in a study conducted by researchers from the University of Manchester, real patients provide a 'different perspective', and 'a view from the other side' (Bell et al. 2009).

However, there are several limitations in these exercises. Firstly, medical rounds and live presentations focus mostly on the clinical manifestation of the disease, without a specific focus on communication skills or learning more about the patient's perspective (Teutsch, 2003). Additionally, the descriptions of patients in case presentations mostly follow commonly accepted standards with a focus on the 'clinical database', whereas the social history and the impact of the medical illness on the patient play only a minor role (Green et al., 2009). Furthermore, the work with simulated patients has the advantage to provide professional feedback to students from a simulated patient perspective. Yet simulated patients sometimes lack authenticity, even if they incorporate their experiences as real patients into their roles (Bokken et al., 2010). Some studies failed to show effectiveness of simulated patients in facilitating communication skills development in general (Williams and Song, 2016). Lastly, real patients are difficult to recruit (Bokken et al., 2010).

The most important limitation, however, is that exercises with simulated patients—and even exercises with real patients—do not systematically reflect the broad spectrum of physical, social, and emotional experiences of *different* patients. As Dwamena et al. (2012) and Snow et al. (2016) show, knowing, or at least being aware of, this broad spectrum helps to develop a better patient-centred approach in clinical practice. For example, type 2 diabetes may mean different things to different people when it comes to the impact or the consequences of the condition on a patient's life.

Although it is neither necessary nor possible for medical teachers to show the complete spectrum of illness experiences, medical students need to have seen/heard a sample of illness experiences from the patient perspective. It might be sufficient to convey to the students the necessity of listening carefully to the patient and to make sure—in an exemplary way—that they understand how different patients experience their illness, what it means for a particular individual to have this condition, and how the students, as future doctors, can help this person and treat him/her and not just the disease.

How patients experience their illness is best represented in illness narratives. Illness narratives are stories about people's experiences with a medical condition (Leal et al., 2016). They are typically collected through open interviews and illustrate physical, social, and emotional experiences of different patients. Such illness narratives can be found on www.krankheitserfahrungen.de (Lucius-Hoene et al., 2013; see also Figure 13.1), the German version of the international DIPEx website www.dipexinternational.com. These websites contain a variety of interview fragments of people suffering from various health conditions in video, audio, or text format (Ziebland and Herxheimer, 2008).

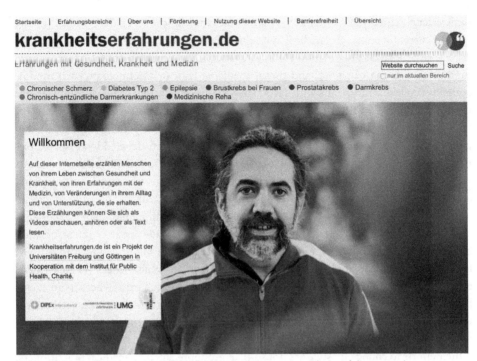

Figure 13.1 Front page of the website project http://www.krankheitserfahrungen.de.
Reproduced from www.krankheitserfahrungen.de with kind permission from Britt Schilling. © 2017 Britt Schilling.

Originally intended to help fellow sufferers and their families, the DIPEx projects have also been used for professional training and seem well suited for use in medical education, for example, to teach students about the patient's perspective. By watching a sample of videos, medical students may gain a better understanding of each unique patient's situation and the spectrum of different experiences of the illness within a social and psychological context. Watching and talking about these types of videos in the medical curriculum may be an alternative to real patient contacts, may teach students things that cannot be learned from books, such as empathy, responsibility, and professional identity, and may help them build integrated skills for clinical reasoning, communication, and medical history taking (Bokken et al., 2009).

Concept development

The authors developed a teaching unit using video material from a website project. The idea of the teaching unit was to expose students to patient experiences using one of the diseases of the module; we chose diabetes in the endocrinology module of the second clinical semester. The teaching unit was aimed to be implemented during the clinical science section of the medical curriculum. The curriculum in Germany is structured in semesters or trimesters and it takes a student usually about six years to finish (two years of basic science, three years of clinical science, and one clinical year). The clinical science section currently covers 21 medical specialties. Previously each subject was taught separately. Now subjects are often taught in interdisciplinary teaching modules, e.g., a 'head module' combining ear, nose, and throat medicine with ophthalmology. Each module contains single teaching units with several lessons about different topics. A unit's lessons usually address the same essential questions about different diseases (Chenot, 2009). For the pilot, we chose illness narratives about weight loss from five patients with type 2 diabetes. This topic was selected because it demonstrates an often-debated issue during primary care visits (Buchmann et al., 2016). The unit's aim was to provide medical students with authentic experiences from patients' perspectives. They were supposed to identify and work out different subjective views of, and reactions towards, the pressure to give up a previous lifestyle in diabetic management and learn how different patients experience and talk about their struggles. Many of the patients are already aware of the association between lifestyle and their condition, but still experience an intensive pressure to show abstinence and feel misjudged when their efforts have no visible effect (Lucius-Hoene et al., 2013). Our intention was for students to understand such experiences in an exemplary way. They were supposed to realize that informing and motivating diabetic people repeatedly to change their life, to exercise more, to eat less, and to lose weight, might do more harm than good. This can happen because patients often feel hurt and disappointed if their efforts to change lifestyle are not sufficiently appreciated by medical practitioners. Our teaching unit was not meant to be a replacement for what was already being taught in medical courses, but rather an addition to it from the perspective of the patients.

The teaching unit consisted of four stages, lasting approximately 35 to 40 minutes in total; eight minutes for watching the videos, the rest for the tasks and discussions.

First stage

The teacher explains the course of action and gives the students a handout with the transcripts of the clips and a small task (Box 13.1).

Box 13.1 Task for the first stage

Please write down or mark in the text during the presentation at what point you felt:

◆ *amused*

◆ *annoyed with the patients*

◆ *surprised/astonished*

◆ *sympathy for the patients*

Second stage

After reading the handout, the students watch the videos (Figure 13.2).

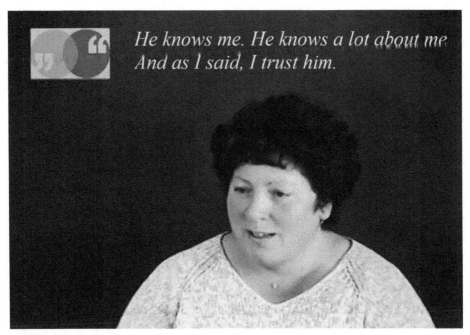

Figure 13.2 Screenshot from one of the videos from the teaching unit.
Reproduced from www.krankheitserfahrungen.de with kind permission from Britt Schilling. ©2017 Britt Schilling.

Third stage

The teacher initiates a discussion within small groups, during which the students talk about their observations following the questions and guidelines as outlined in Box 13.2.

Box 13.2 Task for the third stage

Form small groups (3–4 people) and discuss the following questions (8–10 min):

- *Did you notice any differences between the statements of the interviewees and your knowledge from textbooks (regarding medical facts, but also psychosocial aspects)? If yes, what specifically? What could be the reasons?*
- *What characteristics about the patients' experiences surprised you?*
- *What makes these people 'tick'? What do they wish from their doctors?*

Fourth stage

At the end of the exercise, the teacher encourages discussion among the whole group. The session should end with a take-home message for the students (Box 13.3).

> **Box 13.3 Task for the fourth stage**
>
> Group discussion and take-home message (8-10 min):
>
> ◆ *How can you—as future doctors—respond better to the specific situation of each patient from the film or other patients in similar situations?*

Pilot

The student group for the pilot was chosen by the coordinator of the endocrinology module. It consisted of approximately 40 people; one quarter of all students of the semester. To test our concept, this sample seemed appropriate.

The teaching unit was designed in such a way that the developers of the concept did not necessarily need to be present or conduct the lesson. There was detailed documentation of the concept, including a script for teachers which explains step by step how to execute the exercises, which important issues should be kept in mind during the discussions, and how to formulate a take-home message.

Educational objectives of our concept were:

◆ To give the students a better understanding of the patients' situations and experiences with a disease; and

◆ To improve communicative skills for a better doctor–patient relationship.

These objectives are in line with the educational objectives of the current National Competency-based Learning Objectives Catalogue in Medicine (Fischer et al., 2015). This catalogue contains an entire chapter about doctors as communicators. The authors state that it is crucial for medical students to understand the importance of the doctor–patient communication. Overall, they appeal for an improvement of patient-orientated communication skills so that students become aware of emotionally demanding situations for the patients and consider socio-cultural and socio-economic influences.

Preparing the videos

Five short videos were arranged to tell a 'story' about communication with doctors in regard to losing weight. They were designed to be a narrative of their own.

The video selection follows theories of health behaviour such as the 'Health Belief Model' and related models that try to predict health behaviour. They cover, for example, why people take part in preventive activities, exercise, go on a diet, or take their medicine (O'Dea and Saltman, 2004). The chosen videos show different levels of perceived severity of a disease, in this case type 2 diabetes, and perceived benefits, barriers, or cues of action, with a special focus on the doctors' role. The viewers witness a vast spectrum of experiences with doctors when it comes to discussions about lifestyle changes (Box 13.4). The patient in the first video tells the audience about not being understood and feeling frustrated because he does not get any support from his doctors. The second and third patients speak about wanting and trying to change things, but not getting the help they need. The next patient speaks about the behaviour he would appreciate from his doctor: being supportive,

Box 13.4 Excerpts from the five videos

Video 1: Günther Brockmann experienced quite a few doctors who spoke to him very harshly. However, this did not surprise him.

[...] Weight reduction is certainly the issue number one in all these discussions with various doctors. [...] I know all the verbal abuse; because there are doctors who do it quite dramatically. [...] I cannot be shocked by that.

Video 2: Antonia Winkler is frustrated because she does not lose weight. Her doctors see no evidence of her attempts and she does not feel supported by them in this process.

Every time I look at my scale, I say: 'Shit! Put on some weight again!' This is really frustrating because you are trying so hard and doing a lot. And then there is no result, it gets even worse. [...] And every time I hear from the doctors, especially from different doctors: 'You have to lose weight' and stuff like that. [...] Because then I say: 'What more can I do? I'm already exercising and eating less. [...] That is pure stress!' But this stress is made by the doctors, because they say: 'You have to lose weight somehow.'

Video 3: Bettina Neumann also felt unsupported by her doctor.

Well, it is always about weight. She (the doctor) wanted me to lose about five kilos every four weeks. [...] So I became more depressed. [...] Then I ate a piece of chocolate or cake again. [...] I was so motivated and I wanted to, but if you get absolutely no support ...

Video 4: Sedat Gencay has been directly advised by his doctor about the risks of his being overweight. At the beginning, he still refused to believe it.

[...] The doctor did—he always told me [...] 'You need to exercise, because you have to do something.' [...] I did not want to believe. I understood everything he said. [...] So he could not cage me up and say 'Now you do it.' Actually, it would have been great, if he had done that. [...] Why should I blame others? It was me who screwed up.

Video 5: Regina Mosbach trusts her doctor and gets the support that she needs.

He knows me. [...] He often talked to me about losing weight. He was right and he is still right. [...] But I cannot stand it anymore to hear him say it. I say, 'Doctor, you're right.' I say, 'But you also have to see my point of view.' [...] I like to eat. [...] But I cannot stop it completely. [...] Sometimes it needs harsh words. Of course. But he understands. He knows how I am and how I act. And I think he accepts that. And then he says: 'We'll figure it out.' He helps me. [...] And then he leaves me on my own. [...] This is a matter of trust. And if you do not trust the doctor then even the best treatment does not help anyway. [...] Because that depends on cooperation.

but at the same time applying some pressure. The last patient speaks about a good relationship with, and a lot support from, her doctor, who accepts her as she is but nonetheless addresses her problems in an open and frank manner. These narratives should make the listeners understand how very difficult and stressful it can be for patients to lose weight and that they need help rather than lectures or condescending words and attitudes.

Working with the videos

All four stages of the pilot were successfully performed during the exercise. During stage three there was a lively discussion among the students. We did not intervene, answered only a few questions, and listened to the discussions. The students seemed to have understood the different patient experiences as entangled in the 'narrative' and were talking about how patients in the videos were affected by the disease. They were especially concerned about the doctors who were mentioned in the videos. While discussing whether the doctors behaved appropriately, the students seemed to be on the patients' 'side' and clearly demonstrated empathy for their struggles. Some of the students shared their experiences with patients in similar situations during work experiences in hospitals.

Assessment of the teaching units

After the end of the unit, the author asked the students as well as the module coordinator for oral and written feedback. Most comments were positive. The participants reported that the teaching unit successfully shows the patients' perspective and helps to better understand their problems. Furthermore, the module coordinator agreed that this type of exercise would be a welcome addition to the portrayal of the disease and the patients' problems. A major point of criticism was the length of the unit.

Discussion

A new teaching unit was developed for the medical curriculum at the University of Göttingen using carefully edited sequences of video interviews from the website project www.krankheitserfahrungen.de. Although this was a pilot project without elaborate evaluation, it seems that two of the main aims can be realized:

◆ To raise awareness for the patient perspective; in this case, for their struggles to live a healthier life.

◆ To start a discussion about how students, as future doctors, could better meet patients' expectations about their treatment and to give students a deeper understanding of the patients' situation and their experiences with a chronic illness.

However, we did not manage to implement this teaching unit in the regular curriculum of the clinical sciences part of medical education—for several reasons.

The main reason was a very tight schedule that seemed too dense to allow for additional courses and teaching units to be integrated. Although behavioural and social sciences are considered important, it is well known that medical faculties have problems integrating these in the general medical curriculum due to limited time availability (Tabatabaei, Yazdani, and Sadeghi, 2016). Similarly, Henry, Holmboe, and Frankel (2013) concluded from their review about improving communication skills in medical education that faculty members have little time to evaluate students' skills in these areas in light of working hour restrictions and productivity demands.

Historically, because of the dominance of the biomedical model, communication skills were considered less important than technical aspects (medication, surgery, etc.) in medical education. However, the focus seems to have shifted in the last decade, especially because of studies investigating the effectiveness of good patient–doctor communication on the patients' well-being (Loureiro et al., 2011).

Engbers et al. (2016) analysed the difficulties in implementing medical teaching policies in university hospitals and developed three levels of obstructions: individual, departmental, and institutional. The results overlap with our observations. First, difficulties were noted in the implementation of the teaching unit on the individual level mainly because those responsible for reforming the curriculum may not be passionate about teaching communication skills. They might understand the value of these skills, but still consider such teaching units as complementary, i.e., not absolutely necessary, and perhaps even as a burden. Second, the departmental level and especially the social context of the departments play an important role. The department structure, strategy, and culture need to be changed towards a focus on improvement of communication skills. This can be achieved in various ways: 'creating dedicated medical teaching profiles; offering supportive preconditions that help to balance workload; appointing a dedicated teaching contact or committee; communicating (successes in) medical teaching policy; and structural follow-up on performance agreements in medical teaching' (Engbers et al., 2016). Finally, the institutional level needs to be considered. Similarly to the departmental level, the authors believe it is a question of general attitudes or even philosophy about how important the dean of the faculty or other people in positions of authority consider communication to be in medical education.

The authors still believe that this concept—and illness narratives in general—are well-suited to convey the patient perspective to medical students. To better meet this challenge, we see three options:

1. Shortening the exercise: In this case, shortening the narrative—the most important part of the teaching unit—would probably result in a failure to achieve educational objectives.

2. Offering the exercise as a voluntary course: This option is unlikely to be realized, especially because students would probably not wish to sign up for an additional course due to their already tight schedule.

3. Expanding the teaching unit to a more general communication exercise for role play and case story presentation. Instead of implementing the teaching unit in the clinical core subjects such as internal medicine, surgery, or gynaecology, it may be worth incorporating the unit in the clinical skills training, especially in those parts of the

training where students foster their narrative competence. For example, the Mayo Medicine School programme 'Telling the Patient's Story' (Hammer et al. 2011) works together with theatre techniques to offer students a chance to reflect upon patients' experiences. They teach, among other topics, the ability to actively and generously observe and listen to each other, as well as a performance sensibility that ensures the delivery of a good story. We think that our teaching unit could deliver exactly the 'material' needed to learn about the vast variety of patient experiences. This material could be tied to a sample of case presentations with the focus on the patient perspective.

In conclusion, the results of the pilot teaching unit were mixed. While students and teacher appreciated the exercise, external and internal conditions circumvented the implementation of the concept into the medical curriculum. Despite a patient-orientated turn in clinical medicine, there still seems to be a clash between, as Mishler put it, the 'voice of medicine' and the 'voice of the lifeworld' (see Barry et al., 2001). The voice of the lifeworld means concerns with health and illness as they relate to everyday experiences and can be heard in the narrative organization of the needs of patients. The voice of medicine reflects a technical approach with the aim to decontextualize a patient's personal and social contexts. While the patients express their condition as a lifeworld problem, especially in the case of chronic conditions, Barry and colleagues (2001) observed that many doctors treat the condition as a physical issue with the need to block or ignore the voice of the lifeworld.

As long as doctors—and medical teachers—are reluctant to include patients' feelings, experiences, and biographical situations in the consultation and in the medical core curriculum, teaching initiatives that use patient narratives are welcome in theory, but blocked by the realities of a tight schedule. The authors are therefore forced to look for alternatives to incorporating our teaching unit in the medical curriculum. At the moment, it could be integrated into a larger context of learning case presentations skills together with already implemented communication exercises. In the end, since the decision to change teaching policy is ultimately made at the individual level, we hope to motivate and persuade medical teachers of the importance of teaching communication and of the important role of narratives within the medical core curriculum.

References

Barry, C. A., Stevenson, F. A., Britten, N., Barber, N., and Bradley, C. P., 2001. Giving voice to the lifeworld. More humane, more effective medical care? A qualitative study of doctor-patient communication in general practice. *Social Science & Medicine*, 53(4), 487–505.

Bell, K., Boshuizen, H. P., Scherpbier, A., and Dornan, T., 2009. When only the real thing will do: junior medical students' learning from real patients. *Medical Education*, 43(11), 1036–1043.

Bokken, L., Rethans, J. J., van Heurn, L., Duvivier, R., Scherpbier, A., and van der Vleuten, C., 2009. Students' views on the use of real patients and simulated patients in undergraduate medical education. *Acad Med*, 84(7), 958–963.

Bokken, L., Rethans, J. J., Jöbsis, Q., Duvivier, R., Scherpbier, A., and van der Vleuten, C., 2010. Instructiveness of real patients and simulated patients in undergraduate medical education: a randomized experiment. *Academic Medicine*, 85(1), 148–154.

Buchmann, M., Wermeling, M., Lucius-Hoene, G., and Himmel, W., 2016. Experiences of food abstinence in patients with type 2 diabetes: a qualitative study. *BMJ Open*, **6**(1), e008907.

Chenot, J. F., 2009. Undergraduate medical education in Germany. *GMS German Medical Science*, 7, Doc02.

Cleland, J. A., Abe, K., and Rethans, J. J., 2009. The use of simulated patients in medical education: AMEE Guide No 42. *Medical Teacher*, **31**(6), 477–486.

Dwamena, F., Holmes-Rovner, M., Gaulden, C. M., Jorgenson, S., Sadigh, G, Sikorskii, A., Lewin, S., Smith, R. C., Coffey, J., Olomu, A., and Beasley, M., 2012. Interventions for providers to promote a patient-centred approach in clinical consultations. *Cochrane Database of Systematic Reviews*, **12**(12), CD003267. DOI: 10.1002/14651858.CD003267.pub2

Engbers, R., Fluit, C. R., Bolhuis, S., de Visser, M., and Laan, R. F., 2016. Implementing medical teaching policy in university hospitals. *Advances in Health Science Education*, **22**(4), 985–1009.

Fischer, M. R., Bauer, D., Mohn, K., and NKLM-Projektgruppe, 2015. Finally finished! National Competence Based Catalogues of Learning Objectives for Undergraduate Medical Education (NKLM) and Dental Education (NKLZ) ready for trial [in German]. *GMS Zeitschrift für Medizinische Ausbildung*, **32**(3), Doc35.

Graungaard, A. H. and Andersen, J. S., 2014. Meeting real patients: a qualitative study of medical students' experiences of early patient contact. *Education for Primary Care*, **25**(3), 132–139.

Green, E. H., Durning, S. J., DeCherrie, L., Fagan M. J., Sharpe, B., and Hershman, W., 2009. Expectations for oral case presentations for clinical clerks: opinions of internal medicine clerkship directors. *Journal of General Internal Medicine*, **24**(3), 370–373.

Hammer, R. R., Rian J. D., Gregory, J. K., Bostwick, J. M., Barrett Birk, C., Chalfont, L., Scanlon, P. D., and Hall-Flavin, D. K., 2011. Telling the patient's story: using theatre training to improve case presentation skills. *Medical Humanities*, **37**(1), 18–22.

Henry, S. G., Holmboe, E. S., and Frankel, R. M., 2013. Evidence-based competencies for improving communication skills in graduate medical education: a review with suggestions for implementation. *Medical Teacher*, **35**(5), 395–403.

Leal, E. M., Souza, A. N., Serpa Júnior, O. D., Oliveira, I. C. D., Dahl, C. M., Figueiredo, A. C., Salem, S., and Groleau, D., 2016. The McGill Illness Narrative Interview—MINI: translation and cross-cultural adaptation into Portuguese. *Ciencia & Saude Coletiva*, **21**(8), 2393–2402.

Long-Bellil, L. M., Robey, K. L., Graham, C. L., Minihan, P. M., Smeltzer, S. C., and Kahn, P., 2011. Teaching medical students about disability: the use of standardized patients. *Academic Medicine*, **86**(9), 1163–1170.

Loureiro, E., Severo, M., Bettencourt P., and Ferreira, M. A., 2011. Third year medical students perceptions towards learning communication skills: implications for medical education. *Patient Education and Counseling*, **85**(3), 265–271.

Lucius-Hoene, G., Groth, S., Becker, A. K., Dvorak, F., Breuning, M., and Himmel, W., 2013. What it means for patients to have their illness experiences published in the Internet [in German]. *Rehabilitation*, **52**(3), 196–201.

O'Dea, N. and Saltman, D. C., 2004. Health beliefs. In: R. Jones, ed. *Oxford textbook of primary care. Vol 1*. Oxford: Oxford University Press. pp. 103–106.

Onishi, H., 2008. Role of case presentation for teaching and learning activities. *Kaohsiung Journal of Medical Sciences*, **24**(7), 356–360.

Snow, R., Crocker, J., Talbot, K., Moore, J., and Salisbury, H., 2016. Does hearing the patient perspective improve consultation skills in examinations? An exploratory randomized controlled trial in medical undergraduate education. *Medical Teacher*, **38**(12), 1229–1235.

Tabatabaei, Z., Yazdani, S., and Sadeghi, R., 2016. Barriers to integration of behavioral and social sciences in the general medicine curriculum and recommended strategies to overcome them: A systematic review. *Journal of Advances in Medical Education & Professionalism*, **4**(3), 111–121.

Teutsch, C., 2003. Patient-doctor communication. *Medical Clinics of North America*, **87**(5), 1115–1145.

Williams, B. and Song, J. J. Y., 2016. Are simulated patients effective in facilitating development of clinical competence for healthcare students? A scoping review. *Advances i Simulation*, **1**(6). https://doi.org/10.1186/s41077-016-0006-1

Ziebland, S. and Herxheimer, A., 2008. How patients' experiences contribute to decision making: illustrations from DIPEx (personal experiences of health and illness). *Journal of Nursing Management*, **16**(4), 433–439.

Chapter 14

Using patient narratives as source material for creative writing

Paula McDonald

Why create fictional narratives?

Why should we create fictional narratives? After all, access to authentic narratives in the form of autobiographies, blogs, and websites such as http://www.healthtalk.org has never been more readily available. The challenge, however, lies in getting doctors and other healthcare workers to read these narratives.

The schism between doctors and patients

The websites http://www.teambloodglucose.com/TeamBG/About.html and https://www.facebook.com/gbdoc.co.uk are online communities for people with diabetes in Great Britain, and illustrate the schism between health professionals and their patients (Figure 14.1).

Paul Buchanan, BMJ patient columnist and founder of http://www.gbdoc.co.uk, comments:

> People who live with chronic conditions are lifelong users of the services provided by health care, and whilst clearly not experts in a medical sense, are the most qualified to talk about their experience and lessons learnt in living well with their condition. It is frankly astonishing that such a depth of lived experience, of knowledge and of applied healthcare is disregarded quite so vociferously by medical professionals for being 'anecdotal'. Just because there is no RCT demonstrating the rise of the sun in the east doesn't mean it isn't true.

Healthcare workers may not realize how little they know about the experience of living with a health problem until a personal experience of illness brings the point home. A BMJ feature called 'Personal Paper' allowed authors to share their insights about an aspect of medicine. A recurrent theme of these articles was the illuminating (and often chastening) experience of healthcare workers who had developed health problems. An article written by Trevor Howell, a consultant geriatrician, 'How my management of stroke would change after my own', described solutions to problems he had never thought about, such as how to tear off a piece of toilet paper with only one functional hand:

> At first, it may be necessary to place the head firmly on top of the toilet roll before trying to detach a section with the stronger hand ... (Howell, 1984).

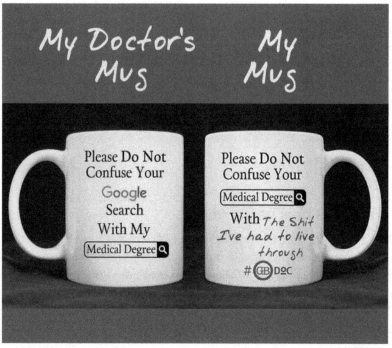

Figure 14.1 The schism between doctors and patients.
Reproduced courtesy of Paul Buchanan.

Consultant physician C. D. Shee (1983) developed an ulnar nerve palsy after an accident, and then remembered the patient he had taught on shortly before his accident:

> I realised that although I had demonstrated the deformity and listed the muscles affected, I had not discussed the resulting disability, which to the patient is the most important aspect. On that wet summer day, the patient must have thought it strange that we did not ask him how his injury interfered with ordinary activities.

More recently, in *Here Comes The* Sun, a blog by 'Lindsay', an oncology nurse turned cancer patient, its author commented:

> Dear every cancer patient I ever took care of, I'm sorry. I didn't get it …

She lists the many things she didn't get, including how hard it is to wait for test results, how awkward it is to tell other people the news that you have cancer, how much patients hang on to every word that professionals say to them, and how crippling the tiredness is:

> I didn't get that when you said you were tired, you really meant so much more. Sure there are words like exhaustion and extreme fatigue—but there should really be a separate word just for cancer patients, because it's crippling. Really. Some days you really wondered how you'd trudge forward. I'm sorry. I didn't get it' (Lindsay, 2017).

Doctors have distanced themselves from listening to patients

William Osler famously said 'Just listen to your patient, he is telling you the diagnosis'. However, over the last century, as technological advances offered new diagnostic and treatment options, doctors began to lose interest in listening to patients. Liao (2016) points out that medieval physicians had a humanistic approach to medicine, but in modern times, 'the technical mind-set and the promulgation of naive optimism that it (modern technology) can solve all our problems' has distanced doctors from patients. As Frank (1995) suggests, 'The chart became the official story of the illness'.

Partnership and empathy: what patients want from their doctors

More recently, there has been a growing recognition that technology does not have all the answers. Frank (1995) points out that in recent times patients 'have reclaimed the capacity for telling their own story, a personal voice telling them (the professionals) what illness has imposed on them'. Having had their experiences colonized by medicine, post-colonialism has emerged: 'The demand to speak rather than being spoken to and to represent oneself rather than being represented, or in the worst cases, rather than being effaced entirely'.

Listening to patients is not just good for patients: it is good for doctors as well, especially for doctors in training. Research has shown that involving patients and carers in medical education can lead to better outcomes such as improvements in students' knowledge, attitudes, and confidence (Morgan and Jones, 2009, Jha et al., 2009, Jha et al., 2010, Spencer et al., 2011, Snow et al., 2016).

Perhaps unsurprisingly, research suggests that authentic interactions with real patients are more valuable in teaching than interactions with simulated patients. (Clever et al., 2011). It has been suggested that including authentic patient experience makes teaching more relevant and helps students prepare for the complexities of real life patient encounters (Morgan and Jones, 2009).

In acknowledgement of this, patient and public involvement in medical education has been advocated in the UK by the General Medical Council since 2009.

How have medical schools responded to this?

Medical schools have been slow to react to this shift in expectations. A 2017 BMJ editorial entitled 'Medical student training: five year backward view' commented:

> We know of (no medical schools) teaching co-management with patients as a core principle despite a high profile Supreme Court ruling in 2015 emphasising the importance of involving patients in decisions about their care (Oldham and Everington, 2017).

Whilst some medical schools might argue that they are doing their best to involve patients in different areas of their courses (Lancaster, 2017), the reality is that patients able and willing to become involved in teaching are in short supply in some areas—as Snow (2016) comments, 'It is not always feasible or ethical to ask patients to describe what may be unpleasant or upsetting experiences to successive cohorts of clinicians in training'.

There is a vast amount of online material documenting the lived experience of patients with health disorders in the form of written accounts, blogs, videos, and patient forums. This resource is currently under-used in medical education. This chapter describes a creative writing module for medical students which forces students to consult these materials and discusses the potential benefits.

Use of creative writing in medical schools

Creative writing has been used in a number of different contexts, including acting as a vehicle to encourage reflection, as a curricular device, to encourage personal growth, to enhance professionalism and to help develop 'soft skills' such as compassion and empathy. (Cowen, Kaufman, and Schoenherr, 2016)

Use of clinical realism with creative writing at two medical schools

This chapter discusses a creative writing module which has run at Manchester and at Brighton and Sussex Medical Schools (between 2010–2013 and 2014–2017 respectively). Like many creative writing modules, it is an opt-in module for a group of six to eight students. At Manchester, it ran as part of a four-week full-time narrative medicine option. In Brighton and Sussex, it was a stand-alone module which ran for either an hour a week or a session a week for six to eight weeks, depending on the year of the students involved. At the start of the module, the students 'create' a character with a health disorder. All of their writing exercises on the module are written 'in character', writing in the first person.

What is clinical realism?

During this course, students write in a genre that I have entitled 'clinical realism'. This is defined as 'fictional writing where health problems are systematically represented, not as a metaphor, not as a plot point, and not as the central topic of the writing, but as a part of a character's personal identity and day-to-day experience' (McDonald et al., 2015).

Intended outcomes of the module

The intended outcomes of the module are:

1. Improved writing skills;
2. Learn more about a specific health condition by researching it for your character;
3. Stress reduction; and
4. Increase in empathy.

The first three may seem self-evident, but it may be helpful to discuss the theoretical basis for the fourth intended outcome.

Theoretical basis for a possible increase in empathy

Empathy is generally thought to have two basic components; affective empathy and cognitive empathy. *Affective empathy* is the ability to experience the emotions the other person is feeling, while *cognitive empathy* or perspective taking, is the ability to put oneself in another's shoes. (Hojat et al., 2002, Halpern, 2003). Neurobiology is starting to support these distinctions: research suggests that there is a core neural network involved in empathy and that different parts of the brain are activated by the different forms of empathy (Fan et al., 2011, Bernhardt and Singer, 2012).

Gottschall, pointing to the plasticity of the brain, comments that the realistic rehearsal of any skill leads to enhanced performance (Gottschall, 2013). During the module, the students create a fictional character with a given health condition. They research the condition by looking at patient narratives online and then write about the character in different situations, writing in the first person and weaving in some aspects of living with their health condition. The research and writing done by the students during the module forces them to take the patient's perspective, i.e. put themselves in the patient's shoes. In other words, they are rehearsing cognitive empathy

They also have the opportunity to experience affective empathy when writing about and discussing their character. Repeatedly writing about the same character and discussing them in the writing workshops may reinforce this cognitive process (Gottschall, 2013).

Is there any evidence that this happens?

At first sight, it might seem counter-intuitive to suggest that writing about fictional patients might help students to understand real life patients. However, the exercise forces students to get much more involved in living with an illness than just listening to a patient. Box 14.1 shows examples of the creative writing outputs from students on the module and demonstrates perspective-taking, with students including authentic details of living with their disorders, and examples of 'their' characters reflecting on their situation, and on how it had affected their personal and social identity.

There were also examples of affective empathy in essays that students wrote about the experience of creating their character:

> What I did not foresee was how much I would care about Kain. In each situation he was written into, no matter the genre, I found myself rooting for him (Louise Francis).

Students often commented themselves that they felt that the course had made them more empathic:

> Co-incidentally, after writing this section of the story, I had a placement in cancer outpatients. I felt far more involved in the patients in the clinic and understanding of their experience after reading about opinions of going through similar situations (Tom Wild).

> Interpreting the clinical realisms the other students incorporated into their pieces helped me to understand the conditions in a way that felt closer to the perspective that a patient might have. The messages seemed clearer and stuck in a way that they otherwise might not (Sanjay Noonan).

Box 14.1 Examples of clinical realism written by medical students.

Day-to-day experience of living with a health problem

I'm still gasping for breath and I get random looks from the other passengers not of concern but annoyance. I'm breaking the law of train travel in which silence has to be observed. (Aderinsola Alatishe)

I had my usual recurring dream. The one in which it's Nazmin in the wheelchair and I'm telling him to get out and play rounders with us. He keeps saying he can't get out and we keep encouraging him to just try once more. Try once more. Go on. You can do it. (Zara Rochfort)

I stare at the door handle. When I have my own home, the door handle will be long, flat, easy. The cylindrical gold globe that greets me is one of my daily punishments. (Stephanie Mulhern)

After that, I got to be more careful, bars on the windows, child safety covers on every edge, nothing decorative that isn't made of less than 95% cushion. It's like I'm making a prison from the inside out, she can't get out, but who would want to come in? (Susanna Elsesser)

This must have been the seven thousandth occasion when I've needed to end a conversation abruptly to deal with my stomach, so I'm used to the tuts and disapproving looks, and honestly? I just don't care any more. (Louise Francis)

And tonight my planned small but helpful dose of pill popping (painkillers and sleeping tablets) is not an awful lot different from some other twenty something's Friday night party pill popping. (Susie Wincell)

I could smell the salbutamol in the nebuliser—it reminded me of Sharon's perfume. I would not go so far as to say that this contributed to my dislike of Sharon. I disliked Sharon long before I knew she had the aroma of Ventolin. However, it did contribute to my seeing her as the living embodiment of an asthma attack. (Georgia Blackwell-Green)

I stay awake for most of the night. This is a bad sign. I'm desperate to get up and do something; cook maybe, or paint. Instead I stare at the dark lump in the corner of the room that is Simon and feel restricted. I'm not the only one who knows the warning signs, and to get up now would be to lose my independence for at least a week, probably more. (Jamie Tye)

And then I remembered the story of a local farmer's son who had suddenly caught a disease of the stomach and died soon after. I hadn't paid much attention at the time, and was now trying to frantically fish through my memory to draw or rule out any similarities. (Zeeshan Saeed)

Wait, carefully, I told myself. I thought of the green fluorescent leaflet. 'Be extra cautious round sharp objects, e.g., scissors and keys'. The keys were now lying in my palm like a dagger. (Megan Sambrook-Smith)

Cheer up. Weekend ahead! You are worrying over nothing. Well, maybe nothing. But what if it's more than nothing? ... and we're back to square one, and I'm thinking about cancer and dying and operations and going bald. (Edward Rice)

Some students initially found it difficult to relate to the character they had been allocated—because they found them boring, because they had a stigmatizing disorder such as Hepatitis C or a head injury, or because they had a psychiatric condition that was difficult to imagine.

> Initially I struggled to create an authentic character that I believed in—I had little knowledge of Hepatitis C from the patient's perspective … (Dorrie Imeson).

> In terms of writing about stigma I had initially planned to have strangers treat my character differently on account of her disorder but upon reading the blogs it was clear that the most common and most hurtful examples of stigma came from the blogger's loved ones. As a result in my story all the peripheral characters, such as the woman at the supermarket checkout and Jack's school mates and her co-workers are all very friendly or at least indifferent to her. The examples of stigma that I included were from her brother and parents, people who love her very much but are struggling to understand her disease. It was easy to see how this would be the case to me as I struggled with the same things trying to write this story (Jamie Tye).

However, students generally reported feeling closer to 'their' character as the course progressed:

> I have realised through getting to know my imaginary character that he faces many problems with stigma and as a result of this he has withdrawn into his shell and does not interact with anybody (Amos Meir).

Garden (2007) and Lamm and Majdandzic (2015) have written about affinity, the tendency that we have to empathise with other people like us, while Lamm and Majdandzic contend that empathy is sensitive to deeply-rooted parochialism and in-group bias, with research showing that humans have reduced neural responses to pain being inflicted on ethnic outgroup members and higher altruistic helping for ingroup members, such as fellow football team fans. Researching and repeatedly writing about characters they had little in common with helped the students to understand them better and feel more empathic towards them. The exercise breaks down the traditional doctor/patient roles and forces the students to see the patient as a person in their own right. This goes beyond the communication skills training usually done in medical schools (McDonald et al., 2015).

One student summed up her experience as follows:

> Although creative writing may initially seem like something far removed from medicine as a subject and also as a way of thinking, I have found it to be a valuable experience in trying to gain an understanding of another person. After all, doctors predominantly deal with people, not conditions (Georgia Blackwell-Green).

Other researchers have demonstrated similar effects. Elizur and Rosenhelm (1982) looked at the effect of group experience on the empathy and attitudes of students studying psychiatry and found that group experience consolidates and deepens genuine empathy, a change that persisted at the six-month follow-up. DasGupta and Charon (2004) found that a group of medical students who discussed their own personal illness narratives subsequently reported an increased sense of empathy for patients while Shapiro and colleagues (2006) showed that a group of students trained in point-of-view writing showed significantly more awareness of the emotional and spiritual aspects of a case in an end-of-year writing assignment than did a control group who had had training in clinical reasoning.(Shapiro, Rucker, Boker, and Lie, 2006).

Planning a clinical realism creative writing course: practical aspects

In which year of the course should it run?

Cowen, Kaufman, and Schoenherr reviewed the use of creative writing in US medical schools, and reported that the writing activities they identified 'did not seem to be intimately connected to the formal curriculum and competencies required of medical students'(2016). This is a missed opportunity, because 'learners connect new knowledge with lived experience and weave it into existing narratives of meaning' (Easton, 2016). Easton also suggests that stories could be an effective way to promote understanding and embed new ideas in the narrative component of the long-term memory. It makes sense to run the creative writing alongside courses where students are learning about chronic disorders—respiratory, cardiac, neurological, and so on. This is often in early years at the medical school.

Venue

The ideal venue is a quiet, pleasant room with comfortable chairs so students can sit in a circle to workshop their writing and have other discussions, plus a table they can sit at for writing exercises. Unfortunately, few such rooms exist in medical school premises!

Some groups like to play music in the background when they are doing writing exercises, so equipment for this is helpful.

'Forming' the group

As with all groups, icebreaking exercises are needed—discussing favourite novels, films, and characters works well. The discussion can move on to how many of the students' choices include characters with health problems.

Character creation

Working on the principle that students will get the most benefit from getting to 'know' a character they have little in common with, students do not choose their own character's diagnosis, but are instead allocated one of a range of diagnoses, for example:

- A chronic condition, such as asthma, diabetes, or arthritis;
- A deteriorating or possibly progressive one such as cancer or multiple sclerosis;
- A 'visible' condition e.g., severe psoriasis, hemiplegia;
- An 'invisible' condition, e.g., Hepatitis C;
- A genetic disorder;

◆ A condition that is a result of an injury, e.g., head injury;

◆ A stigmatizing condition, e.g., incontinence, colostomy, facial scarring;

◆ A condition that the character has to keep explaining to others because it is rare or ill-understood, such as myalgic encephalitis or antiphospholipid syndrome;

◆ A carer of any of the above.

Students create their character by choosing from a series of envelopes containing slips of paper. These contain their diagnosis, age, sex, what sort of property they live in, and who they live with. They choose a name for their character and then spend some time researching the condition and completing a 'character creation sheet' with their character's history, physical characteristics, and medical history. After doing all of this, they start their writing exercises.

Writing exercises

The exercises should be interesting, but fairly generic, so that students can use their own creativity. Basing them around day-to-day events such as meals, birthdays, journeys, etc., gives scope to build in the clinical realism. The first exercise is the most daunting for students, so it helps if it is started during the first workshop.

Workshopping the creative writing

The writing workshop is a central element of the course. Students carry out a variety of homework assignments and each piece of writing is discussed in the workshop, looking at both the technical aspects of the writing and at the clinical realism—how well they have represented the day-to-day experience of living with 'their' condition.

People invest a lot of themselves in what they write. It is important to have ground rules for the workshop, especially that criticism must be constructive. Students are usually very respectful of this.

There may not be time to read out each piece in full, so it helps if they can be circulated beforehand, with a deadline to allow time for everyone to read it and reflect on it.

On the day of the workshop, the author can introduce the piece by reading out the first few lines, followed by a discussion of the story and of the clinical realism contained in it. This may lead on to discussion of other aspects of dealing with a chronic disorder. Different students will raise different issues, but the workshop format means that they will be considered by all students.

Is the module teacher qualified to teach creative writing?

Does it matter if the teacher is qualified to teach both medicine and creative writing?

There is little research in this area. A review of 54 outcome studies examining the use of creative writing in medical schools in the United States found that the instructors or facilitators of the writing activities were often not specified or were vaguely referenced across the literature.

From a practical point of view, it certainly helps if the teacher can pick up on healthcare issues, for example, discussing if prostate symptoms are storage or voiding symptoms, and pointing out that if someone has a disease with autosomal dominant inheritance, then it is not very likely that all five siblings would be unaffected.

It also helps if the teacher can cover basic principles of creative writing, such as use of dialogue, plot, genre, characterization, arc of the plot, etc., and can pick up on issues that come up in the workshop. A doctor with an English degree or a creative writing qualification would be well-placed to run this sort of workshop, and a combination of a doctor and a creative writing teacher would also work well. However, the main benefit is in the student researching and developing 'their' character, and in the group discussion at the workshop, where students learn from each other. It would still be possible for someone from a different background to facilitate this.

Should creative writing be offered to all medical students?

The feedback from the (self-selected) groups of students who took the module was generally very positive indeed, with some suggesting that this should be part of the mainstream curriculum. However, it should be acknowledged that not all students are comfortable with creative writing. In response to an evaluation question asking if the student would recommend this course to another student, one medical student wrote 'Yes—if they like that sort of thing'. Some students struggle with writing exercises and find the reflective portfolios used in many medical schools difficult to complete. They might be more comfortable with a different task which encourages them to research patient experiences.

Conclusion

Creative writing can be integrated into the medical curriculum to help students learn about chronic disorders. Using clinical realism to construct fictional narratives encourages students to research not only the medical aspects of a disorder, but also the lived experience of patients suffering from the disorder. Writing repeatedly about the same character may encourage students to feel more empathic towards patients who are unlike them.

Acknowledgements

I sincerely thank Kaye Tew, my creative writing tutor on the Manchester Metropolitan University MA course in Creative Writing, for her help in creating this course, Paul Buchanan for permission to use the photograph in Figure 14.1, and the various students who have attended the course, especially those who have allowed me to quote from their work.

References

Clever, S., Dudas, R. A., Solomon, B. S., Yeh, H. C., Levine, D., Bertram, A., Goldstein, M., Shilkofski, N., and Cofrancesco Jr., J., 2011. Medical student and faculty perceptions of volunteer outpatients versus simulated patients in communication skills training. *Academic* Medicine, **86**, 1437–1442.

Cowen, V., Kaufman, D., and Schoenherr, L., 2016. A review of creative and expressive writing as a pedagogical tool in medical education. *Medical Education*, **50**(3), 311–331.

DasGupta, S. and Charon, R., 2004. Personal illness narratives: using reflective writing to teach empathy. *Academic Medicine*, **79**, 351–356.

Easton, G., 2016. How medical teachers use narratives in lectures: a qualitative study. *BMC Medical Education*, **16**(1), 3.

Elizur, A. and Rosenheim, E., 1982. Empathy and attitude among medical students: the effects of group experience. *Journal of Medical Education*, **57**(9), 675–683.

Fan, Y., Duncan, N., de Greck M., and Northoff, D., 2011. Is there a core neural network in empathy? An fMRI based quantitative meta-analysis. *Euroscience & Biobehavioral Reviews*, **201**(35), 903–911.

Frank, A., 1995. *The wounded storyteller. body, illness and ethics*. 2nd Edn. Chicago: The University of Chicago Press Ltd.

Garden, R., 2007.The problem of empathy: Medicine and the humanities. *New literary history*, **38**(3), 551–567

Gottschall, J., 2013. *The storytelling animal-how stories make us human*. New York: First Mariner Books

Halpern, J., 2003. What is clinical empathy? *Journal of General Internal Medicine*, **18**(8), 670–674.

Health Talk. Available at: http://www.healthtalk.org. (Accessed 22 April 2018).

Hojat, M., Gonnella, J., Nasca, T., Masngione, S., Vergara, M., and Magee, M., 2002. Physician empathy: definition, components, measurement, and relationship to gender and specialty. *American Journal of Psychiatry*, **159**(9), 1563–1569.

Howell, T., 1984. How my teaching about the management of stroke would change after my own. *British Medical Journal*, **289**(6436), 35.

Jha, V., Quinton, N., Bekker H., and Roberts, T., 2009. Strategies and interventions for the involvement of real patients in medical education: a systematic review. *Medical Education*, **43**, 10–20.

Jha, V., Sentra, Z., Al-Hity, A., Quinton, N., and Roberts, T., 2010. Patient involvement in teaching and assessing intimate examination skills: a systematic review. *Medical Education*, **44**, 347–357.

Lamm, C. and Majdandžić, J., 2015. The role of shared neural activations, mirror neurons, and morality in empathy—a critical comment. *Neuroscience Research*, **90**, 15–24.

Lancaster, T., 2017. Re: medical student training: five year backward view. *BMJ*, **356**, j294.

Liao, L., 2016. Opening our eyes to a critical approach to medicine: the humanities in medical education. *Medical Teacher*, **39**(2), 220–221.

Lindsay. (2016) Dear every cancer patient I ever took care of, I'm sorry. I didn't get it. *Here comes the sun*. Available at: <https://herecomesthesun927.com/2016/11/14/dear-every-cancer-patient-i-ever-took-care-of-im-sorry-i-didnt-get-it/>. (Accessed 22 November 2016).

McDonald, P., Ashton, K., Barratt R., Doyle, S., Imeson, D., Meir, A., and Risser, G., 2015. Clinical realism: a new literary genre and a potential tool for encouraging empathy in medical students. *BMC Medical Education*, **15**(1), 112.

Morgan, A. and Jones, D., 2009. Perceptions of service user and carer involvement in healthcare education and impact on students' knowledge and practice: a literature review. *Medical Teacher*, **31**, 82–95.

Oldham, J. and Everington, S., 2017. Medical student training: five year backward view. *BMJ* 2017 j294. https://doi.org/10.1136/bmj.j294.

Shapiro, J., Rucker, L., Boker, J., and Lie, D., 2006. Point-of-view writing: a method for increasing medical students' empathy, identification and expression of emotion, and insight. *Education for Health*, 1, 96–105.

Shee, C. D., 1983. Personal View. *BMJ*, **286**, 1742.

Snow, R., Crocker J., Talbot K., Moore, J., and Salisbury, H., 2016. Does hearing the patient perspective improve consultation skills in examinations? An exploratory randomized controlled trial in medical undergraduate education. *Medical Teacher*, 12, 1229–1235.

Spencer, J., Godolphin, W., Karpenko, N.,and Towle, A., 2011. *Report: Can patients be teachers?* London: The Health Foundation. Available at: <https://www.health.org.uk/sites/health/files/CanPatientsBeTeachers.pdf>. (Accessed 22 April 2018).

Chapter 15

Engaging the vulnerable encounter

Engendering narratives for change in healthcare practice by using participatory theatre methods

Chris Heape, Henry Larsen, and Merja Ryöppy

Identifying issues of practice

By exploring and working with a range of healthcare projects, such as chronic pain, patient falls in hospital, cancer doctor-patient communication, general practitioner(GP)-patient existential conversations, and nursing education, the discovery is that healthcare practitioners are often caught in fixed notions of what their practice entails, and most are reluctant to change that practice. In particular, issues of professional identity seem to influence what practitioners feel they can or cannot allow themselves to do. This appears to be particularly prevalent in situations where a sense of vulnerability arises between doctors and patients, or 'the vulnerable encounter'. This chapter investigates how the use of participatory improvised theatre (henceforth: improvised theatre) can encourage change in healthcare practices and explore how those involved could otherwise interact in vulnerable encounters.

Informing the improvising

The use of improvised theatre is mainly engendered by four perspectives:

1. Theatre: Based on our professional theatre practice developed over two decades and based on forum theatre (Boal, 1979) and theatre improvisation (Johnstone, 1981, 1999), we developed a practice (Friis, 2006; Larsen, 2006, 2008, 2011; Larsen and Friis, 2006, 2017) that serves as an invitation to share experiences and stimulate reflexivity between those involved (Cunliffe and Easterby-Smith, 2004).

2. The Relational: Our practice and research is highly influenced by a focus on complex responsive processes of relating as initiated by Stacey, Griffin, and Shaw (2000), who understand social interaction as transformative. First described in 2000, their theories build on those of George Herbert Mead (1934) and Norbert Elias (1956).

3. Narrative: Jack Coulehan (2005) appeals for a 'narrative based professionalism' whereby medical practitioners can foster 'the ability to acknowledge, absorb, interpret, and act on the stories and plights of others' (Charon, 2001, p. 1897). Shapiro (2008) advocates an understanding of professional healthcare practice as an 'ethics

of imperfection' that allows for the expression of vulnerability, sharing mistakes, and incorporating not-knowing as a part of professional medical practice where practitioners 'are aware of and transparent about their emotional reactions to patients and about working on the edge between intimacy and detachment; and most importantly, who acknowledge common bonds of humanity with their patients' (Shapiro, 2008, p. 7). Arthur Kleinman suggests that medical practitioners should be better able to engage the 'interpretation of narratives of illness experience ... ' and develop the ability to 'understand how illness has meaning' by 'witnessing and helping to order that experience'(1988, pp. xiii–ix).

We also wished to explore the possibility of engendering narratives that work with past, present, and future life expectations and the relationships involved. We were inspired by the work of Ochs and Capps, who consider the use of narrative as a means of sense-making in which 'narrative ... is a fundamental means of making experience.... Narrative activity provides tellers with an opportunity to impose order on otherwise disconnected events and so create continuity between past, present and imagined worlds' (Ochs and Capps, 1996, p. 19) where 'we use narrative as a tool for probing and forging connections between our unstable, situated selves' (Ochs and Capps, 1996, p. 29). With this in mind, the final perspective entails:

4. Temporality: As our interest lies more in the processes of how people bring narratives to life as opposed to thinking of narrative as an after-the-fact account, we were interested in exploring how we could better account for the dynamic, relational, and temporal nature of how narratives emerge as a sense-making process. To this end we were inspired by John Gatewood (1985) who, having identified a 'disregard of action in cognitive anthropology' and a 'more fundamental lack of concern with the temporal dimension of knowledge,' suggested that 'we change our analytical language habits. Rather than speaking of ideas, concepts, categories, and links, we should speak of flows, contours, intensities, and resonances' (Gatewood, 1985, p. 216).

Exploring the relational through theory and practice

Informing the practice: complex processes of relating

Our investigations are informed by a focus on complex processes of relating (Stacey et al., 2000; Stacey, 2001; Stacey, 2003; Shaw and Stacey, 2006). This perspective understands the sociality of people's collective actions and participatory practice by noticing the complex and processual nature of human knowing, doing, making, relating, and organizing. In this context, new meaning and learning (Buur and Larsen, 2010) arises from the on-going gesture and response interactions between those involved (Mead, 1934) and are as such situated in that practice (Lave and Wenger, 1991). Lave and Wenger consider 'learning and knowing as social participation, in which person, activity, and world are mutually constitutive, rather than on cognitive processes or conceptual structures. We do not learn about a practice, they say. Our learning, as the experience of engaging day-to-day as bodily persons in sustaining and developing meaningful activity with others, is practice. Practice and personal identity emerge together as our experience of co-created patterns of meaning' (Shaw, 2002, p. 166).

The view that social interaction is transformative had a major influence on our work. Of particular importance to us is the pragmatist George Herbert Mead's notion of the simultaneous shaping of mind, self, and society. Mead (1934) understood this creation of mind, self, and society as emerging in local, social interaction. This understanding shifts the focus from the individual and their relation to the overall situation to a focus on the processes of relating, which Mead called iterations of gesturing and responding. Instead of understanding communication as sending and receiving messages to convey what is already thought, Mead saw communicative interactions as transformative; as creating and changing mind, self, and society in one and the same action. In this gesturing and responding, we re-interpret our own gesture according to the response we get. This idea is similar to Johnstone's (2012) understanding, according to which the role of the actor in theatre improvisation emerges in the re-acting towards the other actors (Larsen and Friis, 2006).

Following Mead and Johnstone, conversation and bodily communication is an act of gesturing and responding in ongoing improvisation. Similarly, in improvisation one spontaneously responds to another's gestures. As such we do not know the full meaning of what we are doing until we have done it. Meaning emerges through the process of having intentions, acting, and getting a response. This is a social process where we create meaning together by what we are doing, in the act of doing it.

Doing the practice: improvised participatory theatre workshops

Improvised theatre enables professionals', patients', and lay people's narratives to be co-constructed. Participant reflections are brought into play with actors as real-time improvisations to explore the relational issues that emerge. We call this process 'working live' (Larsen and Friis, 2006, pp. 21–39), which is mainly carried out in theatre workshops.

Working live confronts participants with challenges and issues in their social life and creates space for the emergence of alternative forms of being. It provides a means through which participants and actors can experiment with and capture the emergence of understanding through live, improvised exploration (Larsen and Friis, 2006, pp. 21–39). This theatre-orientated workshop method allows important issues to surface, which participants might not otherwise identify or be willing or able to express (Larsen, 2006; Larsen and Bogers, 2014). Theatre workshops also provide a forum that supports the reflexivity required for a change in attitudes and practice (Pässilä, Oikarinen, and Harmaakorpi, 2015). Participatory theatre methods have unique capacities for 1) sharing perspectives, 2) using fiction as a way of dealing with difficult and conflictual topics, 3) making sense by coming to recognize the perspective of the other, and 4) providing opportunities for working with many people (Larsen, 2011).

Improvised theatre is used to play out small vignettes based on real-life situations, after which people are invited to comment on what they have seen, how it relates to their own situation, and how they think the piece should proceed. Actors then improvise around the original situation by incorporating the suggestions of those present. The audience may improvise by taking over from one of the actors or playing another character to show their perspective or explore alternatives. This allows actors, audience, and researchers to run and re-run narratives to explore nuances of relating, of gesture, and response, and, in particular, to demonstrate how sense-making and meaning emerge from moment-to-moment interactions.

People can see how they actively or passively influence the going-on, 'rehearse the future' (Binder, Brandt, and Halse, 2009) by imagining future scenarios and explore alternatives by using 'narrative as a tool for probing and forging connections' (Ochs and Capps, 1996) in the unknown. Over time this collaborative layering of situated experience and informed experiment generates narratives that reflect a diverse range of participant perspectives on present and future healthcare practice, situations, and experience.

Although improvisations may be fictional, they are based on empirically gleaned accounts and informed by rich experience from previous workshop encounters. Our aim is to bring as diverse a range of perspectives as possible into play by encouraging disparate voices to be raised, of professionals as well as patients, and lay people. We wish to demonstrate how various attitudes influence, constrain or enable a sense of identity and practice and, in particular, we wish to challenge attitudes that are fostered by current approaches to healthcare situations. As indicated above, 'practice and personal identity emerge together as... co-created patterns of meaning' (Shaw, 2002, p. 166). Healthcare professionals often find themselves in situations where they create meaning with patients and, for example, with a patient's family members. As such, we are not only interested in involving healthcare professionals in our workshops, but also patients, their families and or friends, and work colleagues. Participant numbers range from ten to fifty.

The theatre workshops allow the sharing of experiences that promote finding alternative ways of acting in a particular situation. Issues of fixed attitudes and sense of self inevitably surface. Through iterations of improvisation, discussion, reflection, and suggestion, participants experience first-hand the frustration, hesitation, and doubt of engaging in an unexpected interaction. They sense the dilemma of how to otherwise act in a vulnerable situation and gain new insights as they actively play out alternatives.

From moment to moment

This section briefly describes two instances from two improvised theatre workshops. The first deals with chronic pain, where those involved explore the knock-on, relational issues that can arise when a family member suffers from chronic pain. The second deals with GP–patient existential conversations and describes a situation where a patient is wondering if he will meet his now-deceased wife in the next life.

Chronic pain—but how to talk about it?

The following incident occurred at a theatre workshop held at the International Conference on Narratives of Health and Illness 2016 on Tenerife. Keynote speakers were, among others, Professor Brian Hurwitz, Director of the Centre for Humanities and Health, King's College London, UK, and Arthur Frank, Emeritus Professor at theUniversity of Calgary, Alberta, Canada, and author of *The Wounded Storyteller* (1995). Conference delegates were, for the most, healthcare professionals and illness narrative researchers.

The workshop began with a three-minute scene that was part of a fuller narrative developed over the past three years (an abbreviated version of which is in Larsen et al., 2017). The main characters in the scene are Peter and Hannah; Peter is a 63-year-old man with chronic back pain who lost his job as a result and now helps his daughter, Hannah, by picking up her children from daycare. As Peter is usually medicated, Hannah expects her father to take the bus to pick up the children. When Hannah gets home from work she discovers that her father has picked the children up in his car. A strained conversation takes place, where little is said, but it is clear this is an unresolved issue that has arisen before.

After the scene, the facilitator asked the audience to discuss what they saw. For the next ten minutes there was a lively discussion that focused on the implicit nature of the nonverbal interaction, driving the car, safety, lack of trust between father and daughter, the children being looked after by a medicated grandfather, and lack of communication. The people in the audience, all medical professionals and researchers, tended to suggest solutions rather than pursue the relational implications of what they had witnessed. After the discussion, the facilitator suggested playing a scene where the daughter, Hannah, talks to a friend about her father. A young woman in the front row of the audience offered to act as Hannah's friend. The actress who played Hannah and the woman who played the friend did not otherwise know each other.

What followed was a four-minute scene between the two. Hannah, played by a trained actor, was clearly distressed, yet reluctant to share her situation with her friend. She initiated the conversation by indicating how overwhelmed she is feeling with work. The friend encouraged her to 'tell me more.' Instead of answering, Hannah turned to the audience and asked, 'What do I say?' The following suggestions were given:

Audience: It's my dad.

Hannah turns to her friend : It's my dad. (She shakes her head slightly.)

Friend: Oh …

Hannah: Yeah.

Friend: Is everything ok?

Hannah: Well… (Turns to the audience with opens arms) Can you help me?

Audience: He won't use the seat belts in the back seat.

Hannah: He won't use the seat belts in the back seat.

Audience: The children.

Hannah: (To her friend) Yeah, because he won't use the seat belts in the back seat with the children. He's risking the twins. I mean … I feel so upset about it. (Hannah slumps in her chair, clearly in despair.) But how to talk about it? I mean, he's my father who has brought me up. He's always been there for me. And now I think like it's changing. Something is changing and I don't know how to talk with him. To be honest, I don't know.

At this point the friend turned to the audience to ask for help. The audience laughed as she had clearly adopted the same technique as Hannah.

At this point the facilitator intervened to ask the 'friend' how she would act in real life. 'Brutally honest', was her reply to the facilitator. 'Say it, say it', he suggested. As the conversation continued, Hannah became more upset. The person playing the friend turned to the audience, lifted the back of her hand to the side of her mouth as if she was trying to hide a secret from Hannah, laughed a little and whispered: 'I want to give her a hug.' The friend then turned to Hannah and they both embraced in a long hug. The response to this genuine expression of compassion was quite palpable. The audience laughed and clapped. Those on stage smiled and clapped.

Existential conversations—will I see my wife again?

At the start of the workshop the participants, 25 GPs, were introduced to a short vignette that described how a doctor ignored a patient's request for sleeping tablets and prescribed tranquillisers instead without asking the patient why he is troubled, which he clearly is. After a discussion between the participants as to what the issues might be, the patient-actor, Jorgen, interacted in three separate situations with three of the GPs present. Each tried to find a way of engaging Jorgen, with various results. In the vignette, the patient Jorgen is 65. His wife died two years ago after suffering from multiple sclerosis for many years. A couple of years before she died he stopped working to take care of her. During this period he lost contact with his friends and workmates, and is now feeling rather lonely.

Although we invented this story as a baseline for the actor, the development of the conversation was genuinely improvised as he needed to react to the response from the GP. The actor was very experienced in this kind of improvisation, so he was able to stick to the role as well as relating to the GP's response.

1. The first doctor ('Alice') offered to interact with Jorgen. Jorgen became very emotional, and said: 'My wife was very strong, and what made her strong was her trust in God.… Her last words to me were: we'll meet again!' He tried to hold back his tears then looked directly at the GP. 'But will we?' he asked.

Alice attempted to engage Jorgen, but was rather hesitant and non-plussed by the conversation. After a few minutes she turned to the facilitator and asked for a time out. Although the conversation was short, it still raised a number of issues.

The facilitator asked the participants to discuss what happened. The question as to why Alice stopped the conversation at that particular moment came up. It was clear to many in the audience that she twice avoided the question of whether she believed Jorgen would meet his wife again. The facilitator gestured to Alice to comment: 'I understood what was going on,' she said. 'I felt it intensely ,,, but what can one do?' Her question resonated with similar struggles the other participants had experienced.

This disclosure initiated a conversation about the difference between a GP's professional role and their presence as a fellow human being. As one participant pointed out, 'Sitting here in the audience I was very touched by what was going on. If I'd been the GP in that conversation, I couldn't have just sat in front of the patient with tears in my eyes. I would have had to put on my professional mask.'

2. The facilitator suggested 'So let's continue the conversation with Jorgen,' but he is interrupted by one of the course leaders who suggested a coffee break. This was immediately vetoed, as the participants wanted to contine. Another GP ('Beatrice') accepted the invitation to continue the conversation with Jorgen. She decided to improvise a consultation that happened a week after the first, and she has put 20 minutes aside.

   At first their exchange was a little hesitant, but it created a sense of trust. Beatrice, picking up on the thread from the week before, began to discuss with Jorgen whether he will meet his wife again. 'Will I?' he asked. She returned the question: 'Will you?' He shook his head slowly: 'No, I don't suppose I will.' Once again she returned the question: 'You don't think you will?' 'I don't know,' he said after a while. From here the conversation drifted towards more general topics.

Beatrice made several attempts to return to Jorgen's question of faith, but as her questioning continued with the circular or mirroring technique, the intensity of the exchange once again receded.

The facilitator stopped the improvisation and asked the audience to comment, and in the ensuing discussion, the point was again made that Beatrice tried to avoid questions about faith. 'You were asked about your belief, but answered by talking about your sense of community,' the actor said. Beatrice thought for a while and responded, 'Yes, you're right. Community I understand better than faith. I'm more comfortable talking about that. But then of course I could feel how we avoided the main question.'

3. Yet another GP ('Cecilie') wanted to try a conversation with Jorgen. She started by going straight to the point about his wife and her faith that Jorgen now misses.

Jorgen: That's what made her so strong, her faith … do you recognize that?

Cecilie: What do you mean?

J: Well … that faith is something that helps you?

Cecilie hesitated, and then:

C: Are you … are you asking me personally whether to believe helps me … is that what you're asking? If believing helps me?

J: Yes.

Jorgen looked at her intensely waiting for an answer.

C: Yes ... in a way I suppose ... in an unconscious way ... quite often.

J: OK?

Jorgen waited for more to come, and then:

C: It's not something I'm consciously aware of ... but I can sense that it does mean something.

J: (Insistant) But how can you sense it? ...That's just it ... I can't feel it any longer ...

C: No ... Your wife ... That must be difficult.

J: (looks away as if it is not his wife he wants to talk about) Yes ... no, it wasn't that easy with my wife ... but you say you can sense it?

C: Yes!

J: But how?

C: (Once again searching for the right words) I think ... it feels like ... making sense ... in a different way ...

She emphasises the words 'making sense.' Jorgen sits back, nodding slowly.

The facilitator moved onto centre stage and asked the others to comment. The intensity we sensed in the room confirmed for us that this was an important move and needed careful reflection. In other work (Larsen, 2008; Larsen and Friis, 2006; Shaw and Stacey, 2006) we have noticed that conversations that lead to a new understanding usually have the character of half-articulated sentences, to which others then respond.

In the ensuing discussion, the first GP suddenly realised that circular questioning (the so-called 'mirroring' technique), albeit helpful in some circumstances, promoted a 'safe' distance towards the patient. Thus, when working with existential conversations in a doctor–patient relationship, the topics that are interacted with, the roles of patient and physician, the understanding of what ill and healthy means, and what caring is, must be challenged.

Shifting from individual to relational

Challenging attitudes to chronic pain

Current attitudes and practices to chronic pain focus on individual experience, self-motivation, and efficacy (Mann, Le Fort, and Van Den Kerkhof, 2013). Lisa Käll (2013, p. 1) describes pain as the source of sorrow, suffering, hopelessness, and frustration. She contends that there is perhaps no experience that better brings to light the singularity and solitude of our lives than the experience of pain (Käll, 2013, p. 27). However, Kruks (2001) describes a notion of pain as an intercorporeal weave that is established between sufferer and witness to that suffering. In other words, pain can also be considered as relational.

Nanna Johannesen identified a discursive figure, 'the good chronic pain patient' with its attitudes and expectations of control, self-management, mastery, coping, administration, organization, and lonely struggle (Johannesen, 2011, p. 169). These expectations demand that a person to be willing to accept their new situation, take on a new identity, fight, battle on, and altogether manage alone. Johannesen is careful to explain that this approach is not necessarily negative, but its singular focus diverts attention from what else is going on for both the individual and those they relate to, which in turn affects their well-being, such as: 'lifelong and continual identity construction and reconstruction; a lack of a linear sense of time, thereby limiting a person's ability to structure their self-narrative as a chronological account; a lonely position as a self-reliant and self-organising individual; a lack of witnesses to a person's struggle and subjective relationship to pain' (Johannesen, 2011, p. 168). Nuances of suffering are often hidden or silenced by the widespread notion of acceptance and control. Johannesen makes the point that those involved in a chronic pain situation are interdependent on each other and that the individual, even when alone, is in relation to others. Relation and sociality are closely intertwined with identity and sense of self, as on a very basic level identity can be considered something that is established in relation to others.

As became clear in the workshop snippet above, a person's chronic pain can have an almost predatory influence on the relationships it ensnares. Chronic pain weaves its way into the very fabric of people's daily lives, both at work and at home, thus influencing the relational. Chronic pain can be seen as an interdependent, communicative, and relational phenomenon that influences, and is influenced by, patients' quality of life, condition, and interaction with others, both private and professional.

Changing attitudes to practice

As a relational understanding of chronic pain challenges known attitudes, this begs the question as to how it could influence professional healthcare practice. One of the contributions of our theatre workshops is that we are able to identify a degree of nuance that further expands, for example, Kruks' notion of the intercorporeal weave and Johannesen's notion of the sociality of chronic pain. By asking healthcare practitioners to engage in our improvisations, they are able to experience alternative practices.

Common to our theatre workshops were discussions among the professional participants that often led to a greater understanding of the role of the medical practitioner and of what constitutes his/her professionalism. It became legitimate to consider good doctoring as a process that also involves investing oneself in a conversation, in particular in a vulnerable encounter, by surrendering to its emergent quality and relational resonance. Entering this improvised mode of relating with the patient creates a quality in the conversation (Buur and Larsen, 2010) that can lead to a sense of meaning that cannot be otherwise achieved. This demands having an eye for the overall situation while sensing the nature of the moment as it emerges. In other words, at the same time as engaging in a conversation on a personal level, the clinician is able to keep a professional distance. The sociologist Norbert Elias called this the paradox of involvement and detachment (Elias,

1956)—a paradox that could almost be described as being in two temporal attentions at the same time.

In conclusion, this chapter now look more closely at the micro-narrative of practice that such an encounter entails.

Being present by staying present

Both the short exchange between the two friends in the chronic pain workshop and the patient asking the GPs if he will see his wife again touch on the same issue of engaging or surrendering to a shared vulnerability as a natural part of professional practice. Hannah's friend, who turned to the audience and admitted she wanted to give her a hug, was possibly in a similar dilemma. She was suddenly overwhelmed by an urge to express her compassion for Hannah, but was briefly caught by a need to have her professional colleagues in the audience sanction what she wanted to do. One can almost hear her asking if it is 'alright if I give her a hug.' Her secretive hand gesture and whisper strongly suggest this. In the existential conversation situations, it was clear the GPs floundered somewhat as to how to engage a situation where professional distance could not resolve their dilemma. They lacked the means to extend a genuinely compassionate gesture. To do so meant that they, too, had to embrace the vulnerability and risk involved by lowering their professional shield.

Improvised theatre clearly has a role to play in both engaging people and helping them better understand the relational nature of what it means to participate in a vulnerable situation, regardless as to whether it concerns chronic pain, an existential dilemma, or otherwise. But, the theatre is not just describing health and illness narratives that have taken place. It engenders and co-constructs them through its active involvement of all participants as new interpretations and new narratives, while at the same time challenging those involved to fully consider how they both do and can engage a healthcare situation. The interactions described here wavered between a professionally shielded response and an expression of compassion as a surrendering to the situation that emerged. In both the situations sketched above, and in other theatre workshops, it has become clear that in order to improvise, to compassionately surrender to the shared vulnerability of a situation, one has to be present and stay present.

But what is the difference between being present in an improvisation and not being present? Keith Johnstone (1999), who has spent a lifetime training actors in improvisation, defined presence as a degree of listening, but realized it is not enough to be a good listener. Having observed many actors improvising, he comprehended that, apart from listening and being interested in what your partner is telling you, 'you must be altered by what's said' (Johnstone, 1999, p. 59). Being altered in this case means you cannot stay unaffected, but will have to change a little, lose some control, and become someone slightly different from who you are, which may feel scary. The fear here is that you might make a fool of yourself or lose control (Larsen, Friis, and Heape, 2017).

What is needed in an improvisation is to move from something known to something that is unknown that emerges in the collaboration between the actors. Good improvisers are willing to pick up on new ideas, which means they lose some control. They become vulnerable in the unknown situation, as they don't know what they are in the midst of, where they are heading, or how they will handle what they encounter. 'Who am I if I can't handle the situation?' also brings questions of identity into play (Larsen, Friis, and Heape, 2017).

Therefore, in order for an actor to improvise with the GP, he has to be present, be willing to follow the GP, and allow himself to get into situations he may not know how to handle. But if we shift the perspective from the actor to the GP in the improvisation, the demands are the same. To be present in a conversation with an existential topic, the GP cannot stick to the well-known role of GP, but has to be willing to be changed through the interaction with the patient and 'be altered by what's said' by following the invitation from the patient to engage in mutual improvisation.

When the patient asks the GP: 'Will I meet my wife again?', this acts as an invitation to a mutual improvisation with the GP. By following the invitation the GP allows herself to acknowledge, surrender to, and work with her uncertainty in relation to the patient's. He is as uncertain as she is! By acknowledging their mutual uncertainty, albeit unspoken, both GP and patient now find themselves in a common ground of vulnerability—not necessarily equal, but common, as it has emerged from their uncertainty. By staying present in this shared vulnerability, it initiates and legitimizes a positioning and repositioning to each other. A re-patterning of the conversation emerges on which each can act and respond from moment to moment. By surrendering to that vulnerability and improvising with it, they can both recognize, respond to, and meet each other in a spontaneous, empathic, and mutual gesture of understanding.

In their moment-to-moment interaction and improvisation a new co-constructed narrative emerges from the re-patterning of the conversation. By exploring the fictitious situation, which is still linked to known practice, those involved are present in the known and the unknown. Together they weave a new, believable, narrative of practice to life and in the process, through a number of iterations, they change their practice as an improvised response to the resonance of the situation as it unfolds. This change of practice may be barely noticeable, but it is change, nevertheless.

References

Binder, T., Brandt, E., and Halse, J., 2009. Design Laboratories. In: A-L. Sommer, M. Mackinney-Valentin, M. Brobeck, N. Lynge, and T. Binder, eds. *FLUX: Research at the Danish Design School*. Copenhagen: The Danish Design School Press. pp. 150–157.

Boal, A., 1979. *Theater of the Oppressed*. London: Pluto Press.

Buur, J. and Larsen, H., 2010. The quality of conversations in participatory innovation. *CoDesign*, 6(3), 121–138.

Charon, R., 2001. Narrative medicine. A model for empathy, reflection, profession, and trust. *JAMA*, **286**, 1897–1902.

Coulehan, J., 2005. Viewpoint: today's professionalism: engaging the mind but not the heart. *Academic Medicine*, **80**(10), 892–898.

Cunliffe, A. and Easterby-Smith, M. P. V., 2004. From reflection to practical reflexivity: experiential learning as lived experience. In: M. Reynolds and R. Vince, eds. *Organizing Reflection*. Aldershot: Ashgate Publishing. pp. 30–46.

Elias, N., 1956. Problems of involvement and detachment. *The British Journal of Sociology*, **7**(3), 226–252.

Frank, A. W., 1995. *The wounded storyteller: body, illness, and ethics*. Chicago: University of Chicago Press.

Friis, P., 2006. Presence and spontaneity in improvisational work. In: P. Shaw and R. Stacey, eds. *Experiencing risk, spontaneity and improvisation in organizational change: working live*. New York: Routledge. pp. 75–123.

Gatewood, J., 1985. Actions speak louder than words. In: J. W. D. Dougherty, ed. *Directions in Cognitive Anthropology*. Urbana: University of Illinois Press. pp. 199–219.

Johannesen, N., 2011. *Smertens Socialitet—Bidrag til nye forståelser af det lidelsesfulde i liv med kroniske smerter*. Copenhagen: Copenhagen University Press.

Johnstone, K., 1981. *Impro: improvisation and the theatre*. New York: Routledge.

Johnstone, K., 1999. *Impro for storytellers*. New York: Routledge.

Käll, L. F., 2013. Intercorporeality and the shareability of pain. In: L. F. Käll, ed. *Dimensions of pain*. New York: Routledge. pp. 27–40.

Kleinman, A., 1988. *The illness narratives: suffering, healing and the human condition*. New York: Basic Books.

Kruks S (2001). *Retrieving experience: subjectivity and recognition in feminist politics*. Ithaca, NY: Cornell University Press.

Larsen, H., 2006. Risk and 'acting' into the unknown. In: P. Shaw and R. Stacey, eds. *Experiencing risk, spontaneity and improvisation in organizational change*. London: Routledge. pp. 46–72.

Larsen, H., 2008. *Spontaneity and power theatre improvisation as processes of change in organizations*. Saarbrücken: VDM Verlag Dr. Müller Aktiengesellschaft & Co.

Larsen, H., 2011. Improvisational theatre. In: L. B. Rasmussen, ed. *Facilitating change*. Copenhagen: Polyteknisk Forlag. pp. 327–354.

Larsen, H. and Bogers, M., 2014. Innovation as improvisation in the shadow. *CAIM*, **23**(4), 386–399.

Larsen, H. and Friis, P., 2006. Theatre, improvisation and social change. In: P. Shaw and R. Stacey, eds. *Experiencing risk, spontaneity and improvisation in organizational change: working live.*, London: Routledge. pp. 19–43.

Larsen, H. and Friis, P., 2017. Improvising in research, in P. Freytag and L. Young, eds. *Collaborative research design: working with business for meaningful findings*. Singapore: Springer Nature. pp. 341–376.

Larsen, H., Friis, P., and Heape, C., 2017. Improvising in the vulnerable encounter: using improvised participatory theatre in change for healthcare practice. *Arts and Humanities in Higher Education*. Published online ahead of print 2018. DOI: 10.1177/1474022217732872.

Lave, J. and Wenger, E., 1991. *Situated learning—legitimate peripheral participation*. Cambridge: Cambridge University Press.

Mann, E. G., Le Fort, S., and Van Den Kerkhof, E. G., 2013. Self-management interventions for chronic pain. *Pain Management*, **3**(3), 211–222.

Mead, G. H., 1934. *The philosophy of the present*. Chicago: Chicago University Press.

Ochs, E.and Capps, L. B., 1996. Narrating the self. *Annual Review of Anthropology*, **25**(1), 19–43.

Pässilä, A., Oikarinen, T., and Harmaakorpi, V., 2015. Collective voicing as a reflexive practice. *Management Learning*, **46**(1), 67–86.

Shapiro, J., 2008. Walking a mile in their patients' shoes: empathy and othering in medical students' education. *Philosophy, Ethics, and Humanities in Medicine*, **3**, 10. https://doi.org/10.1186/1747-5341-3-10

Shaw, P., 2002. *Changing conversations in organizations: a complexity approach to change*.

Shaw, P. and Stacey, R., 2006. *Experiencing risk, spontaneity and improvisation in organizational change.* London: Routledge.

Stacey, R., 2001. *Complex responsive processes in organisations.* London: Routledge

Stacey, R., 2003. Learning as an activity of interdependent people. *The Learning Organization,* 10(6), 325–331.

Stacey, R., Griffin, D., and Shaw, P., 2000. *Complexity and management: fad or radical challenge to systems thinking.* London: Routledge.

Chapter 16

Drawing on narrative accounts of dementia in education and care

Joyce Lamerichs and Manna Alma

Introduction

In 2012, a review study of care curricula in Dutch secondary Vocational Education and Training (VET) colleges identified a general problem: the courses offered in the VET care curriculum focusing on elderly care and dementia needed structural improvements to better prepare students for a career as professional carers (Hamers et al., 2012). Students who were interviewed mentioned they missed the perspective of experiential knowledge, which would allow them to better understand what it means to live with a particular illness and help to understand how professional care is experienced by elderly patients (Hamers et al, 2012, pp. 11–14). Teachers pointed out that there was little opportunity for a more in-depth focus on particular aspects of elderly care such as dementia. Professional carers working with VET students during their apprenticeships pointed out that students lacked sufficient knowledge about dementia, the appropriate skills to communicate with people suffering from dementia, and an empathetic attitude towards their clients that included aiming for a general sense of well-being and not only perceiving them as ill people (Hamers et al, 2012, p. 16).

Many educational programmes have been developed since then in the Netherlands to repair the above gaps; many focused on dementia care in particular, as one of the most prevalent illnesses in the elderly (VET Board, 2016). However, an analysis of those newly developed programmes in dementia care conducted for the current project showed that what still remained absent in many of them was the perspective of the person with dementia (Lamerichs et al., 2015). The educational materials that were developed did little to include the actual experience of the person with dementia or that of their informal carers. And if they did, it was provided in an indirect way (e.g., by including a poem about dementia written by someone who suffered from dementia) or by asking students to engage in role-play or simulations. Authentic film or video materials to stimulate students' interest in topics to do with dementia were rarely used and were not integrated in the lessons. Thus, the newly developed programmes offered students little insight in what it means to experience dementia from the perspective of the person with dementia, with whom students would get in touch in their work as professional carers in a nursing home or home care. The ability to understand the subjective perspective a person with dementia holds with respect to their illness (or, being able to see the person 'from the inside from the outside') is considered an essential part of carers' professional competence (Hannay, 1997, quoted in Nordhy, 2016; also Coulter, Locock, Ziebland, and Calabrese, 2014).

This chapter aims to report on how videotaped narrative interviews that were collected in a previous project for the Dutch DIPEx website http://www.pratenovergezondheid.nl, which documents how people with dementia and their carers experience and live with this illness, can be used in VET curricula on dementia care. In particular, it aims to show how working with a selection of narrative interview clips in these lessons can offer a contribution to closing the gap between what pupils learn about dementia in theory and an improved understanding of the people they care for in practice.

The affordances of illness narratives

Although working with illness narratives in an educational setting is not new, little is known about the positive changes learners reportedly experience (c.f., Arntfield, Slesar, Dickson, and Charon, 2013, who report on a narrative medicine training project with medical students) or how the underlying processes work that are found to foster recognition, absorption, interpretation, and being moved by illness stories (Charon, 2006). It may thus come as no surprise that scant knowledge is available on what happens when VET students are presented with narrative interviews and how this might contribute to solve some of the problem areas that were identified in the Dutch care curricula in particular.

There is a wealth of research available that has explored the affordances of narratives as instruments for health communication. Our current project can be linked with findings in this research tradition, which has theorized the effects of narrative messages in terms of transportation theory (see Green, 2006 for an overview).

For the purpose of this chapter, two mechanisms are highlighted that explain immersion in a story as the basis for its narrative impact. It is proposed that there may be parallels with the way narratives work in an educational setting that aims to foster learning, and that these parallels need further exploration. First, transportation into narratives is believed to induce emotional responses and may foster empathy with the character in the story. Moreover, the structure of narratives (with a beginning, middle, and end, as well as the fact that actions and implications are combined to form a causal chain) ensures that memorable or touching parts are easily stored in memory and can easily be recalled (Green, 2006). Second, narratives are rich sites for discussion on the topics that are brought up. Interestingly, while the narrative structure allows to infer a sense of causality from the story, its potential for discussion lies more in the fact that the precise nature of the causal connection might be left open, which renders them 'especially viable instruments for social negotiation' (Bruner, 1990, cited in Czarniawska, 2009, p. 9).

These two mechanisms have some explanatory power in a context of learning. This chapter therefore aims to highlight in more detail how narrative clips can be used as part of a course on dementia care offered to VET students. This chapter emphasizes 1) how students engage with a selection of narrative episodes in a classroom setting; 2) how they evaluate this experience; and 3) how working with narrative materials can address some of the still existing gaps in dementia care education.

The next section describes how interview clips from the original set of narrative interviews that were conducted were selected, how these clips were used in two pilot lessons on dementia care, and the results.

Using narratives in teaching: developing a course

The project began with an inventory phase, which formed the basis for further developing a course for dementia care. After mapping the contents of existing and newly developed educational programmes for dementia care (Lamerichs et al. 2015), stakeholders' views were collected to see how they evaluated the current educational programmes in VET and how they saw students' competencies as professional carers during their apprenticeships. The stakeholders interviewed were representatives of patient organizations, healthcare professionals, students and teaching staff in VET, and researchers in educational practice and educational science. Several stakeholders pointed out that students experienced difficulties communicating with people with dementia and with their informal carers. This was sometimes even described as a more general 'fear to act'. Another point that was repeatedly raised was the need to increase students' general awareness of what it means to live with dementia.

The stakeholder interviews, the review of educational programmes on dementia care, and the initial interview collection with people with dementia and their informal carers formed the basis for developing thematic content in eight areas that constitute the basis for the course: 1) knowledge of dementia; 2) pathology of dementia; 3) different approaches to dementia care; 4) the caregiver's role; 5) vulnerability of the caregiving relationship; 6) representations of dementia; 7) managing loss and bereavement; and 8) diversity and dementia. The thematic content was further developed into lessons. The video clips from the narrative interview collection were integrated in these lessons in order to foster learning about dementia care. The next section discusses how these interview clips were selected to develop pilot lessons for Themes 1 and 3.

Selection of interview clips

The interview materials that were used in this project were collected for the pratenovergezondheid website. For this project, narrative interviews were held with 37 people with mild-to-moderate dementia and with 53 informal carers. The interviews aimed to elicit the interviewees' story on experiencing dementia. For this purpose, they were conducted with interviewing techniques that are 'non-restrictive, highly supportive and non-judgemental and aim at eliciting narratives' (Ziebland, 2013, p. 40).

The selection of the interview clips was first informed by the content of the interviews. In line with what Lucius-Hoene, Adami, and Koschack observed in their study, narrative interviews with people with dementia show patients 'treated like objects, stripped of biographical and personal resources, interpersonal competencies and power to stand up for themselves' (2015, p. 107). The contents of all initial narrative interviews were explored to search for content that reflected how people with dementia described their experience living with the illness and on the ways in they were perceived, approached, or talked to by other people. This first selection was guided by three criteria: 1) people with dementia described how they experienced the onset of the disease in their own words; 2) people with dementia described the ways in which they are approached by other people, e.g., friends, family, care staff; 3) informal carers of people with dementia talked about how they and their loved ones are being approached by other people.

Based on this first selection in terms of content, a further selection of video clips to be included in the course was made. For every theme, interview segments were selected in which the interviewees used detailed language (illustrative examples, detailed anecdotes) to describe their day-to-day experience with the illness. In order to ensure that the selected clips offered a rich opportunity to stimulate discussion, 'complete', rounded off anecdotes were also selected that could be presented as standalone examples (i.e., with a beginning, middle, and end).

To explore whether these selected videotaped clips could be used as a vehicle to facilitate learning about dementia care, two pilot lessons were organized with VET students.

Pilot lessons

The pilot lessons were held at two VET colleges in the south and the north of the Netherlands. Although the colleges differed in terms of student population and students' ethnic background, they both offered an educational programme on dementia care in combination with apprenticeships and facilities for learning on the job in nursing homes and home care. The first pilot lesson focused on the theme 'Knowledge of dementia' and was designed as a first introduction into the topic of dementia. The second pilot lesson addressed the third theme of the educational module 'Different approaches to dementia care'. Students participating in the pilot lessons (n = 10) were doing an apprenticeship as nursing assistants in a nursing home and in home care. All students were female, aged 16 to 19 years old.

The next section reports how the pilot lessons were received by the students and illustrates the main findings with relevant quotes from the pilot lessons, which were taped and transcribed. The quotes are translated to English from the Dutch originals and the names of the students (S1, S2, etc.) and the teacher (T) are anonymized. An overview of the video clips that were used, and to which students refer to in the extracts, are also included in Boxes 16.1–16.5.

Effects of a first encounter with 'real' narratives

The pilot lessons showed that VET students had not often been in contact with 'actual' narratives from people with dementia or their caregivers in their study programme. They reported that during their apprenticeship, there were few instances in which they had an opportunity to talk with their clients about what it means to suffer from dementia. One important reason for this is that they worked with clients who were no longer able to engage in such conversations due to the stage of their illness. They also pointed out that in school, they were offered a mainly a 'theoretical perspective' about the condition.

In the light of the above, students pointed out that the narrative interview clips fulfilled an unmet need that offered access and an authoritative voice to the illness experience. It showed how they described their reactions to the story in one of the clips, in which Mrs van Driessel describes how she experiences her childrens' visits (Box 16.1). All pupils expressed how they were touched by this story, in a way similar to what S3 expresses in Extract 1.

Box 16.1 Mrs van Driessel

Mrs van Driessel: Yes, those, those, um, tests that were taken, they had all of them, too. I sent them to them. Because I was thinking, it would be silly not to tell my children. So they all know. And they enter very cautiously because of that. But I don't think that is necessary.

IR: What does that mean, entering cautiously? How do they do that?

Mrs van Driessel: Uhm well just like they are strangers […] Yes well it is like they are not my children. But you know, if they have been here for five or ten minutes, then that disappears. So they find it terrible.

Extract 1

```
S3:    it hits closer to home
       you know to have people - not theory
       because these people tell it themselves
       and also you know
       the lady who told how she felt
       when her children entered the room
       they can describe it best
       you know, what it is like
```

Narratives as vehicles for reflection and deeper understanding

After watching a set of different narrative interview clips the students were asked to formulate some additional thoughts on what they saw and heard. Students then linked the contents of the clips to their working practice as professional carers, for example, when it comes to how they approach their clients and why they do so in particular ways. This can be shown in Extract 2, where S4 presents how in her way of approaching clients, she always tries to stress their self-reliance. This is then linked to what Rien says, who talks about his difficulties accepting the help of his wife (Box 16.2). He explains that he experiences this as restrictive, because it takes away his 'freedom' to make his own mistakes and behave accordingly (i.e., learn from his mistakes).

Box 16.2 Rien

Rien: You see at some point we all become dependent on others, isn't it, and I am not any different. I could just say 'mind your own business', but it comes from a caring heart and I have to—I realize that. Only well, it strikes me as oppressive sometimes and then I think sometimes, just let me be, give me some, even if I would stumble, but then I know, next time, I am not able to do that anymore. See I am not given the opportunity to fall. That is what I mean.

Extract 2

```
S4:   yes because what I just said, you don't address it
      in practice or like now, let's say
      but yes I always try to
      just keep it human, on their own level
S3:   yes
S4:   so that it is not
      like what this other man said like uh
      that people want to take over everything
      let me just stumble first
      before you start helping me
T:    yes
S4:   and that I often keep in mind
      to just keep the self-reliance of people in place
      like well if I really see that it just doesn't work
      then I go on to of- offer help, let's say
T:    yes
```

In a similar vein, the narrative clips also proved very suitable for discussing students' behaviour or attitudes as professional carers towards their clients, and their insecurities and struggles. Extract 3 offers an illustration of such a discussion in which the students (together with the teacher) collaboratively engage in 'sharpening' their ideas of how they perceive their clients, after watching Mien (see Box 16.3), who strongly resists the idea of being pitied. Discussion about how students view their clients can be a valuable means for inviting reflections on their working practices as care staff.

Box 16.3 Mien

Mien: I don't want them to pity me, because I don't feel like I am to be pitied.

Extract 3

```
S5:    and the other woman who said that she wasn't to be pitied
       did not want to be pitied because she wasn't
       yes well I don't know
       I do find it kind of difficult not to see them like that
       because I just think that it is just a pity
       that it happens to them
S2:    well you are not pitiful
S4:    they are not to be pitied but the situation is just harrowing
S3:    yes not as a person but it is just sad
T:     that is a nice difference you point out there now
```

The power of metaphoric language

It turned out that clips that included anecdotes or metaphoric language worked as particularly strong cues for students to recall in class. One example of such metaphoric language was provided by Mien. She describes what her illness feels like when she wakes up and the inside of her head feels like a tangled knot of wool (see Box: 16.4). In Extract 4 below, S4 uses the metaphor introduced by Mien to describe the difficulties children might experience in dealing with the unpredictability of their parent's illness, for which she is now able to express a greater understanding.

Box 16.4 Mien

Interviewer: If Alzheimer's disease was to be seen or felt, how would that be?

Mien: Messy, I think.

Interviewer: Can you explain that?

Mien: Yes a knot that is all tangled and sometimes you have a bit that runs well and a little later it's all knotted again. Because there are days that—and I think that I never have a whole day that I am unwell. But most of the times I feel it in the morning when I wake up, and I think, the woolly knot is there again. But then I get up and get going and then it starts running and I manage.

Extract 4

```
S4:    so yes then I also understand
       for example for the children
       like you see in practice
```

```
           their mother for example is on one day
           like the lady with the ball of knotted wool
T:    yes
S4:   that it is a tangle and that she herself
           you know, doesn't know anything anymore
T:    yes
S4:   and next time they might have found a string
           that runs and then they are able
           to talk about all kinds of things
           so then for the family
           you know for example then they are very well able
           to talk with their mother about all kinds of things
           and if it turns into a knot all of a sudden then it
           is completely different
           so then when the children enter the room
           then it is like ah well how is my mother doing today
```

The metaphor provided by Mien was frequently alluded to in subsequent class discussions and also formed the basis for 'adding on' second stories to address particular concerns. Extract 5 illustrates how S2 uses this image provided by Mien to address a difficult situation she finds herself in when her client repeatedly experiences the pain of losing a loved one. In this sense, the narratives also offer room to discuss potential difficulties the students experience in their work as professional carers, specifically when dealing with people with dementia.

Box 16.5 Wim

Wim: Because there was a woman who called the Alzheimer helpline once. I think that is a very clear example and she said, 'well I don't know what to do. My father is so very aggressive all the time. He had Alzheimer's disease and was in a nursing home'. And then I said, 'well what happens then?' And then she said, 'well he starts xxx and he stands in front of the window looking out into the garden and says "what do these stupid animals do outside. These deer don't belong here". And I say—and what do you say then?—"Ah come on dad, those are not deer"'. And then I said 'you could also try to stand beside him and say, "dad, how many deer do you actually see?"'

Interviewer: Exactly, yes.

Wim: At that time you enter his world of thinking and maybe you will be able to move one little step in the right direction. It is not to say that it will, but it could be a way of getting there.

Extract 5

```
S2:    just like the lady mentioned when she said it was
       like a knotted ball of wool
       that sometimes there is a string that runs
       and the other time it is just all tangled
       that is like it is
T:     is it? do you recognize that from-
S2:    yes I do, from the beginning
       from the first stages of the illness
       because uh there are times that you have clear moments
       and then you can for example say to someone
       I am sorry, your husband passed away
       oh yes I do know that
T:     yes
S2:    while the next day
       she would experiences the same emotion again
       just like she experienced when her husband
       had just passed away
T:     yes
       (5 lines omitted, in which other students confirm
       this experience)
S2:    and then that ball is all tangled again
```

Students also listened to Wim, an informal carer who talks about the advice he gave to a woman who found it extremely difficult to deal with her father's hallucinations as a result of his dementia (he would report seeing deer in the garden of the nursing home). The advice Wim gave was not going against what the woman's father saw, but trying a different approach, by asking: 'dad, how many deer do you actually see?' (see Box 16.5).

Students then reflected how they themselves deal with clients who hallucinate, and how 'stepping into the world of the person with dementia' (using the words Wim used to describe his advice in more general terms) may be a way to offer comfort rather than upsetting a client even more. This is illustrated in Extract 6, where S8 provides a second story. Note how S8 also points out that she is touched by the perspective of Wim (see also Extract 1 for other illustrations of students' emphatic reactions to the fragments shown).

Extract 6

```
S8:    yes I thought it was interesting
       how this man was saying
       that you should help other people
       and think like they do
       I thought that was a beautiful thought
```

```
T:     and how do you do that in the nursing home
S8:    the other day there was this woman
       who said that her car had been stolen
       and then I just said to her no
       it is in the shop
       we took your car to the repair shop
       and then everything was all right again
T:     and don't you feel like you are fooling her
S8:    no because it is- otherwise she would start
       panicking even more and now I am able
       to comfort her
```

Discussion and conclusion

The pilot lessons featured a set of videotaped and highly detailed narrative accounts of how people with dementia and their informal carers both experience dementia. The analysis shows that the narrative form in which these experiences were presented to students in secondary vocational education and training, may contribute to learning about dementia care in a number of ways.

First, the narratives offered recognizable content, which students could not only relate to but also empathize with. Second, the use of metaphoric language in the narrative clips turned out to be a particularly strong cue for recall in class and latching on to, thereby creating room to construct their own stories of their experience as professional carers. Third, drawing on the images ('the tangled knot of wool') or the implications that were induced (confirming rather than opposing hallucinations) enabled students to bring in their concerns and difficulties as professional carers for people with dementia, as well as discussing their attitudes towards their clients and the solutions they find to deal with these matters (see Extracts 3 and 6).

Other language-based approaches have been developed that aim to foster reflection in group discussions with young people on health and well-being (see Lamerichs, Te Molder, and Koelen, 2009). In this educational setting, however, in which students are taught about aspects of dementia care, the particular content and form of the narratives offers rich grounds to address and stimulate discussion and reflection among students. The fact that identification with the stories offers an 'easy point of entry' to do so might also be particularly useful for this group of students. It was pointed out that VET students sometimes find it difficult to bring in their own experiences (or difficulties) as professional carers back into the classroom setting in college (G. De Boer, personal communication, July 28, 2015).

One of the most important lessons learned was how much fertile ground is offered by introducing these narrative materials in the pilot lessons on dementia care. Although the impact of a teacher who asks questions when working with these narrative clips cannot be underestimated, the pilot lessons showed that narratives proved a highly 'appealing format' for VET students.

The analyses of the pilot lessons show the strength of videotaped narrative accounts of people with dementia as a format that can foster students' empathic response and allow them to acquire a deeper (and sometimes novel) understanding of what it means to live with dementia. The storied accounts of people with dementia and their informal carers also proved an 'easy point of entry' to discuss working practices as professional carers and bring in difficulties that pertain to their professional routines of caring for people with dementia and communicating with their families.

The pilot study also confirmed how rich the videotaped narrative interviews are that were collected for the Dutch DIPEx website project. The selection of rounded-off stories in which people with dementia and their caregivers talk about their experience can be easily linked to students' experiences during their apprenticeships, sometimes even offering them words or images to relate to and use in their subsequent discussions. Especially when metaphors or anecdotes were used, they were readily recalled and used to elaborate on. In this way, not only the content but also the form of the pilot lessons (and the broader thematic content provided in the complete course) fits in nicely with the demands VET colleges are faced with (finding better ways to facilitate learning on the job).

Although there were only two different pilot lessons conducted in the two collaborating colleges, the narrative materials are a promising and fruitful tool to complement existing programmes on dementia care. Future research in this area could consist of enlarging the number of participating VET colleges to further document the value of using narrative interviews in dementia care education. This could include conducting more systematic research to explore the functions of narratives, for example, as a vehicle to induce empathy in students. As the use of anecdotes and metaphorical language worked as a particularly strong stimulus in the pilot lessons, a second area for future research could be to examine in greater detail the characteristics of metaphoric language and detailed anecdotes in stories to see what it is that renders them so appealing, and how this may be beneficial for different learning purposes in education on dementia care.

Acknowledgements

This project was made possible with a grant from The Netherlands Organisation for Health Research and Development (grant number 310200005). We thank Katja van der Linden, who was part of our research team and taught the pilot lessons. We also thank all the students and staff involved at the two collaborating colleges. Without their efforts and enthusiasm, this project would not have been possible.

References

Arntfield, S. L., Slesar, K., Dickson, J., and Charon, R., 2013. Narrative medicine as a means of training medical students towards residency competencies. *Patient Education and Counseling*, **91**, 280–286. DOI: 10.1016/j.pec.2013.01014.

Bruner, J., 1990. *Acts of meaning*. Cambridge, MA: Harvard University Press.

Charon, R., 2006. *Narrative Medicine: honouring the stories of illness*. Oxford: Oxford University Press.

Coulter, A., Locock, L., Ziebland, S., and Calabrese, J., 2014. Collecting data on patient experience is not enough. they must be used to improve care. BMJ 2014, 348:g2225. DOI: 10.1136/bmj.g2225.

Czarniawska, B., 2009. *Narratives in Social Science Research*. London: Sage.

De Boer, G. Personal communication. July 28, 2015.

Green, M. C., 2006. Narratives and cancer communication. *Journal of Communication*, 56(S1), S163–S183.

Hamers, J., Rossum, E., van Peeters, J., Rameckers, V., and Meijs, N., 2012. Ouderenzorg in het middelbaar beroepsonderwijs. Een inventarisatie bij zorgopleidingen (niveau 2 en 3). [Elderly care in Secondary Vocational Education and Training. An inventory in care curricula (level 2 and 3)]. Caphri: Maastricht University Press.

Lamerichs, J., Alma, M., and Van Der Linden, K., 2015. Inventory of Dutch educational programmes in dementia care. Unpublished Working Paper. Groningen: VU University/University Medical Center Groningen.

Lamerichs, J., Koelen, M., and Te Molder, H. F. M., 2009. Turning adolescents into analysts of their own discourse: raising reflexive awareness of everyday talk to develop peer-based health activities. *Qualitative Health Research*, 19(8):1162–1175. DOI: 10.1177/1049732309341655.

Lucius-Hoene, G., Adami, S., and Koschack, J., 2015. Narratives that matter. Illness stories in the 'third' space of qualitative interviewing. In: M. A. Locher and F. Gygax, eds. *Narrative Matters in Medical Contexts across Disciplines*. Amsterdam: John Benjamins. pp. 99–116.

Nordby, H., 2016. The meaning of illness in nursing practice: a philosophical model of communication and concept possession. *Nursing Philosophy*, 17, 103–118. DOI: 10.1111/nup.12111.

VET Board [MBO Raad], 2016. Onderwijsservicedocument Implementatie noodzakelijke onderdelen over ouderen in de opleidingen Helpende zorg & welzijn. [Educational Service Document. Implementation of essential elements about the elderly in professional training of care and well-being assistants, personal health care providers and general nurses]. MBO Raad: Woerden.

Ziebland S (2013). Narrative interviewing. In: S. Ziebland, A. Coulter, J. D. Calabrese, and L. Locock, eds. *Understanding and using health experiences: improving patient care*. Oxford: Oxford University Press. pp.38–48. DOI: 10.1093/acprof:oso/9780199665372.003.0005

Section 6

Narratives in diagnostics

Chapter 17

Using illness narratives in clinical diagnosis

Narrative reconstruction of epileptic and non-epileptic seizures and panic attacks

Elisabeth Gülich

Research background, data, methodology

The research presented in this chapter is a linguist's and narratologist's attempt to make a contribution to medical diagnostics. Its aim is to show how the linguistic analysis of illness narratives which occur in doctor–patient interaction may not only provide important information about the illness itself as well as fruitful insights into how patients live and cope with the illness, but also further contribute to differential diagnostics. Obviously, listening to the patient's history has, and always has had, a central role in doctor–patient talk, but the attention has normally been directed to *what* the patient says about his disorders and *what* symptoms he presents, rather than to *how* he does this. The *manner* in which he describes the development of the illness is usually neglected. The claim is that if the forms of patients' narratives and the narrative techniques they use were analysed in interdisciplinary cooperation by a team of linguists, medical researchers, doctors, and psychotherapists, new approaches, a new diagnostic tool, and ultimately new therapies might be discovered.

The basic idea for the first interdisciplinary project[1] came from practical experience: from treating patients in hospital. Martin Schöndienst, neurologist at the Bethel Epilepsy Centre (Bielefeld), observed noticeable differences between the ways patients suffering from seizure disorders talk about their illnesses. His general assumption was that it should be possible to describe these differentiating features systematically in linguistic or interactive terms and relate them to the different syndromes. Thus, the principal aim for the interdisciplinary research team combining epileptological, psychiatric, linguistic, and narratological competencies was to work out the inter-relationships between the linguistic and the medical dimensions of the illnesses concerned. Since in current classifications of diseases patients' subjective experience of their illness is neglected, from the beginning the team were sure that the findings of the research would have practical implications for diagnosis and therapy.

In order to appreciate the significance of this approach, it is important to realize that there are different types of seizures. The main difference is between epileptic and non-epileptic seizures. A seizure may include falling down, convulsions, trembling, losing consciousness, etc., and yet not be an epileptic one. Epileptic seizures are caused by abnormal electrical activity in the brain, whereas non-epileptic (dissociative/psychogenic) seizures are considered an expression of psychosocial distress. Despite advances in diagnostic techniques, differential diagnosis is often very difficult. It takes on average more than seven years for a patient with dissociative seizures to receive the correct diagnosis (Reuber et al., 2002). The two types of seizure require completely different forms of treatment: patients with epilepsy may need anti-epileptic drugs or an operation, whereas patients with non-epileptic seizures may need psychotherapy. An incorrect diagnosis is obviously followed by inappropriate treatment, sometimes with damaging or dangerous consequences. Developing a new diagnostic instrument is therefore potentially of great value.

So the central question for interdisciplinary research was if it is possible, by analysing the illness narratives and predominantly the seizure narratives of these two types of patients, to discover any clear differentiating features. Can different types of narration be defined which may be related to different types of seizure?

The research was guided by general principles of conversation analysis. One of the best-known quotations from its founder Harvey Sacks is that it is 'possible that detailed study of small phenomena may give an enormous understanding of the way humans do things and the kinds of objects they use to construct and order their affairs' (Sacks, 1984, p. 24). Thus observation is a basic principle: 'We will be using observation as a basis for theorizing' (Sacks, 1984, p. 24). Its empirical basis is 'the use of materials collected from naturally occurring occasions of everyday interaction' (Heritage and Atkinson, 1984, p. 2). In this case that means doctor–patient interactions in ordinary settings. The study collected in-depth interviews conducted with patients as a routine part of the normal clinical treatment in a psychotherapeutically oriented ward. For research purposes, the interviews were audio- or video-recorded and transcribed. A transcription is more than a written version of talk; it takes into account the particular features of spoken language such as hesitations, pauses, repetitions, and self-corrections as well as characteristics of speech delivery and the simultaneity or overlapping of utterances.

Having worked on numerous of these doctor–patient interactions, interview guidelines for doctors were developed in order to improve the comparability of the data (cf. Surmann, 2005, pp. 411–415; Schwabe et al., 2008). These guidelines required the doctor to allow the patient a generous amount of space and aim at highlighting the patient's, rather than the doctor's, relevancies. The doctor opens the interview with a question or a comment encouraging the patient to talk about his/her current situation and expectations. So in this opening sequence, and to a minor extent during the whole encounter, the doctor refrains from any directive questioning in the hope that the patient will build up the conversation from his own perspective and will stress the aspects he himself regards as relevant. Later on in the interview the doctor may ask questions about the seizures, their general development, the pre-sensations or 'auras' which may precede them, and so on. The interviewer may also focus on individual seizure episodes: the first seizure, the last one, the most severe, or the most memorable one. These are questions which positively demand narrative reconstruction.

This way of conducting the interview gives the patients more responsibility than they are used to. The doctor must therefore be prepared for difficulties in formulation, hesitations, frequent pauses, and even long periods of silence. This requires patience but can lead to interesting and revealing narratives.

This practice is in line with the results of research into narrative techniques in a variety of contexts. In order to obtain natural speech for the purposes of sociolinguistic research, Labov tried to record oral 'narratives of personal experience, in which the speaker becomes deeply involved in rehearsing or even reliving events of his past. The 'Danger of Death' question is the prototype (…)' (Labov, 1972, p. 354). When the interviewer asks 'Were you ever in a situation where you were in serious danger of being killed (…)', the interviewee's attention is directed to the narrative reconstruction of the event rather than to the phonetic or grammatical phenomena which were investigated (cf. Labov, 2013, pp. 1–10).

Sociologists also use the technique of the narrative interview as developed by Schütze (e.g., 2016), because this enables them to obtain information which a normal, more or less standardized questionnaire or interview would never produce. The reasons for this are analysed by Kallmeyer and Schütze (1977): a speaker in a narrative is more or less forced to go into detail, to condense, or to expand according to what he regards as relevant, and he has to respect the 'gestalt' he has let himself in for. Conversational narratives almost automatically lead to the speaker saying more than he intended and often giving away things of which he is not aware.

This is particularly true of illness narratives since these are based on extremely personal experiences. These are frequently ignored in the normal doctor–patient situation, which tends to follow the question-and-answer pattern guided by the doctor, leaving little room for the patient to explain how he himself feels about his illness.

One of the main difficulties in conducting our research was the difference in approach of the various disciplines concerned. When conversation analysts start their work, they do not know exactly what they are looking for—in fact, this is the ideal attitude for 'doing conversation analysis'. But it is completely contrary to the procedures medical researchers are familiar with, as they normally formulate theoretical hypotheses and then test them empirically. In conversation analysis, the opposite procedure is preferred: the topics to be investigated should emerge from the data. So the analysis of the interaction does not start with medical categories, but considers the patients' presentation of their own categories and aspects of the disease as relevant. The linguistic analysis aims at finding out the individual participants' recurrent communicative patterns in talking about their seizures. Systematizing these observations allows analysts to discover the conversational methods patients use in describing aspects of a seizure or the event itself. By comparing the methods of different individuals, they can be grouped according to them. This can be achieved by linguists without any medical knowledge. But the last step, which relates the patients' methods to different syndromes, requires medical, and in this case epileptological, expertise. This kind of research can only be done if the approach is an interdisciplinary one.

The following examples of conversational procedures turned out to correspond to different types of seizures (for a more detailed presentation, cf. Schwabe et al., 2008; Surmann, 2005):

- One group of patients typically volunteer information about their seizure symptoms and discuss them in detail. The topic is self-initiated, and the patients have no difficulty in focusing on specific seizure episodes. Another group tends to avoid talking about seizures; the topic is initiated by the interviewer and is discussed sparingly; the patients resist focusing on specific seizure episodes. In comparing these observations to existing diagnoses, it was found that the first group suffered from epileptic, the second group from non-epileptic, seizures.

- Some patients do intensive formulation work, keep stressing the difficulty or even impossibility of describing their sensations and feelings at the beginning of a seizure, but nevertheless try again and again to do so: such patients turned out to be epileptic (Gülich, 2005). Minimal descriptions, pre-patterned speech, negative statements, and silences are characteristic of non-epileptic patients.

- Other differences appeared in the use of metaphorical concepts: epileptic patients typically describe seizures as external and hostile, independent agents; the description of seizures as a space the patient passes through characterizes non-epileptic patients (Surmann, 2005).

This interdisciplinary research was continued by Markus Reuber at Sheffield University,[2] who in 2005 took up this research design and examined whether the interview techniques developed in Bielefeld with German-speaking patients would produce the same results with English-speaking patients. He not only confirmed the Bielefeld findings but was also able to continue the research in a more systematic way and developed a differential diagnosis scoring table (cf. Reuber et al., 2009).

The next project,[3] in which epilepsy data yielded a number of new aspects, was motivated by the discovery of the important role of fear and anxiety. With the main focus on the accounts patients gave of their fear or panic attacks, again it was assumed that the frequent lack of diagnostic information and the unsatisfactory treatment of patients suffering from fear or anxiety disorders are, to a large extent, due to a lack of knowledge about the communicative methods patients use in describing their subjective feelings of fear. Following the guidelines from the first project, new data were collected from patients from an epilepsy hospital and patients from a psychiatric hospital. Both patients with epileptic fear and patients with panic attacks were studied. In these cases an exact diagnosis tends to be very difficult, as they are often mistaken for each other. By tracing the resources patients use to communicate fear, the aim was to see whether certain types of description or narration can be linked to certain types of fear. Thus, the motivation was again the diagnostic use of linguistic analysis.

The following case studies[4] illustrate how the highly subjective sensation and perception of fear is treated in doctor–patient interactions and how these data were analysed. The focus is on the narrative reconstruction of episodes of fear or panic which can be experienced by patients with epileptic (usually temporal lobe) seizures, but can also occur as expressions of psychogenic seizures (cf. Schmitz and Schöndienst, 2006, p. 146).

Case studies

Mrs. Korte

The first case is a patient, 'Mrs. Korte' (cf. Gülich and Lindemann, 2010; Lindemann, 2012, pp. 69–94), a 58-year-old woman from Poland. Having lived in Germany for a long time, she is used to speaking German in the context of her illness. The interviewer is a female doctor from a psychiatric hospital, who has not met the patient before. She begins the interview with an open question to encourage the patient to talk freely and to set her own priorities. The patient speaks of a harmless beginning and a subsequent aggravation of her illness. She then switches to a narrative reconstruction of a seizure episode, during which she suddenly runs out of the house and rings a neighbour's doorbell. In the course of the episode, she is confused and it takes her quite a while to remember where she lives and what her name is. She then reports other episodes of a similar nature, when during a seizure she clearly did not know what she was doing. She places her seizures in the context of her life story and recounts a series of extremely stressful experiences: a business disaster due to fraud committed by an employee, the sudden death of her husband, the death of one of her sons, the protracted dying of her father, for whom she cared. Nevertheless, while all of this can be expected to cause emotional arousal, emotions are hardly ever mentioned during this part of the interview. Yet to her there is a clear link between these unfortunate events and her illness.

Then, after about 30 minutes into the interview, there is a sequence that is essential with respect to communicating the relevance of fear as a factor in her illness. The doctor introduces the topic of fear by asking whether fear plays any part in her life. In a long and complex conversational process the relevance of fear is interactively established and finally becomes the central topic of this part of the interview. This is an impressive example of the difficulties patients experience with regard to speaking about a certain type of fear, namely fear during an epileptic seizure. Initially Mrs. Korte seems not to understand the doctor's question. Then she starts to speak about fear of particular things, such as getting hurt in a seizure, worries about her son not coming home, etc. Finally she starts to talk about the fear or panic she experiences at the onset of her seizures, when she suddenly runs out of the house:

```
(1)    K:      =das is- (1.1) krieg=ich ANGst,
                   that is I get frightened


               (--) [ dass ] GLEICH was pasSIERt,
                   that something is going to happen soon
       I:          [<<p> m=HM,>]


       K:      musst du RAU:S/\/
               you've got to get out
            weil du STERben kannst a=gleich;=NE,
               cos you can die er now.
            .hh und dann:=ä:h (1.4) ENTweder muss=ich AUFstehen,
               and then uh either I have to get up
            (.) und schnell was NEHmen,
               and quickly take something
       I:      m=HM?
       K:      wenn (da da) (.) so (.) nich VIEl (.) von dem angst is,
               if there's not too much fear
            .hh u::nd- oder WEGlaufen;
               and or run away
            (.) <<p> aus=em haus;>
               out of the house
```

This particular episode of running out of the house, which the patient reported at the very beginning of the encounter, is retold here in an entirely new conversational frame: it is explicitly associated with fear of death. This recontextualization (Günthner, 2005) gives the episode a new significance: while in her first narrative reconstruction it appeared in the context of the aggravation of the seizures and inappropriate behaviour resulting from loss of control, it here turns out to be an expression of fear of dying. The doctor reformulates Mrs. Korte's expression of fear and defines it explicitly as fear of dying:

(2)

```
       I:      =also=s=is wie TOdes[angst;]
               so it's it's like fear of dying
       K:                         [ GAN]Z genau.
                                  that's exactly it
       I:      m=HM?=
       K:      =den TOdesangst das=is .hh vielleicht das
               to be afraid of dying maybe that's the


            SCHRECK!lichste <<dim> was sein kann.>
            most awful thing that can happen
```

The patient emphatically agrees, with terminal overlap: 'GANZ geNAU'. ('that's exactly it') and then immediately continues and evaluates the feeling of fear of death as 'the most awful thing that can happen' ('das SCHRECK!lichste <<dim> was sein konn.>') with strong emotional involvement.

This is an important new aspect of this patient's illness: the symptoms she describes might be interpreted, and have been interpreted, by doctors who have seen her previously, as signs of panic attacks. However, the difficulty she has in expressing this kind of fear, the manner in which she speaks about her fear of death, the way she narrates the episode of running out of the house—these, according to systematic analyses—are typical of patients with epileptic seizures. The connection between her fear of death and her running out of the house as an expression of this fear had not been mentioned in the patient's record before. Mrs. Korte's case suggests that the frequently unrecognized psychic triggers of so-called running fits are conditions of intense fear.

Mrs. Wiesinger

'Mrs. Wiesinger' (cf. Gülich, 2007; Knerich, 2013) is an in-patient at a psychiatric clinic. Like Mrs. Korte, she is speaking to a doctor she has not met before. He also starts with an open question to encourage her to report what seems particularly important to her. But in contrast to Mrs. Korte's reaction, it becomes immediately apparent that for Mrs. Wiesinger fear and panic are predominant. While she confirms that she is satisfied with the results of her treatment, she re-emphasises the severity of the panic attacks she used to experience:

(3)

```
W:     das war jetzt SO massiv, äh wie=ich=s (also wirklich)
       noch nich
          it was so strong - like, really, I never
       geHABT habe; u:nd äh:: (--) .hhh mit todesANGST, und
       (1.5)
          had before... and ... . I was scared to death,
       h <<p> ja> .hhh (.) ich konnte nich mehr LAUfen- ich
       konnte nich
          I couldn't walk, I couldn't
       mehr ESSen; (1.5) es ging aso (ne) weile <<f> GAR> nix
       mehr;( ... )
          eat, nothing worked for a while ( ... )
       also das war schon das HEFtigste was ich hatte
          that was the worst I've had
```

The use of intensifiers is a typical element of the 'grammar of panic' described by Capps and Ochs (1995, pp. 72–75).

During the following conversation, Mrs. Wiesinger relates her difficult biographical background and gives detailed narrative reconstructions of her attacks of fear. The doctor tries to differentiate between panic attacks and 'normal' fear, such as anybody else might experience. The patient's reaction is very interesting: although she is narrating episodes of 'normal' fear, she still uses the same techniques as in the narrative reconstruction of panic attacks. An example is provided by a phrase she stereotypically uses when talking about her panic attacks: 'es ging aso (ne) weile <<f> GAR> nix mehr' ('nothing worked for a while') (see the above excerpt, cf. Knerich, 2013, pp. 51–60). This is a good example of the role of negation in the 'grammar of panic'; negation is classified by Capps and Ochs as 'the most obvious grammatical resource for diminishing the role of agent or actor' (1995, p. 71).

In the same context Mrs. Wiesinger relates an example of 'terrible fear' when, long ago, she had a car accident with three children. She sums up the consequence of this experience by saying that since then she has not driven a car, and concludes with a general statement: 'sobald was von RECHTS kommt, äh (--) <<p> geht bei mir NICHTS mehr;>' ('if anything comes from the right, nothing works for me'). Coming back to the narrative of the accident, she confirms that she cannot forget it, being so scared that for a while she was unable to cross the street:

(4)

```
W:      <<p> ja (ich hatte da so) angst, jetz GEHt=s wieder,
             yes I was so scared now it works again
        aber> angst über die STRA::ße zu gehen; ne? (1.5)
            but fear to cross the street
        s war ganz SCHLIMM die die ersten (--) ersten WOCHen;
        ne?
            it was horrible during the first weeks
        (-) i=ich wusste nich wie ich über de STRAße kommen
        sollte;
            I didn't know how to cross the street
I:      nach diesem::[( a::)
            after this
W:                  [ja, jetzt seitDEM ich HIER bin, ne?
            yes now since I am here
        (---)
I:      ach so; ich dachte DAmals seit diesem unfall; mit den
            oh I see; I thought then after the accident with the
        drei [kindern;
            three children
W:           [<<f> DAS war auch erst, aber JETZ auch jetz die
                 that was then too, but now, also now
        letzte ZEIT,> .hh äh ich konnt- ich wusst NICH wie (man
            of late uh I could - I didn't know how
        über die) straße gehen sollte;
            to cross the street
```

There is an interesting misunderstanding on the part of the doctor which can only be discovered by looking closely at the linguistic details of the narration. When the doctor tries to confirm the temporal localization of the fear in the past (i.e., the accident with the three children), the patient initially agrees with him ('ja'), but then immediately shifts to the recent past: 'jetzt seitDEM ich HIER bin,' ('now since I am here'). Thus, it turns out that in fact she is speaking about recent incidents, which led to her being admitted to the hospital. The doctor's change-of-state token (Heritage, 1984) 'ach so; ich dachte' ('oh I see—I thought') shows that he now realizes the misunderstanding. Mrs. Wiesinger then explains that she experienced this fear in both cases: 'DAmals' ('then', after the accident) and 'auch jetzt die letzte ZEIT' ('also now, of late'). This example shows that the fear relating to the accident has become a generalized anxiety, or more precisely, an anxiety disorder.

When we compare the two patients' cases (Table 17.1), we find considerable differences in the narrative reconstruction of fear:

Table 17.1 Two patients: different narrative reconstructions of fear

Mrs. Korte	Mrs. Wiesinger
… comes to speak about fear and to relate episodes of fear only late in the interview and needs intensive support from her interlocutor.	… has no difficulty in talking about fear or panic; her narrations of panic episodes are often self-initiated; she tends to emphasize fervently the relevance of her panic attacks.
… does not only relate fear/panic to particular objects, but also speaks of a general fear which is difficult to explain.	… relates fear to particular objects; panic is triggered by particular objects.
… shows the fundamental difference between epileptic and everyday fear by means of various conversational procedures.	… hardly distinguishes panic attacks from everyday fears; describes episodes in which there is a gradual transition between the two.
… accomplishes intensive formulation work and presents her subjective feelings of fear as difficult to describe.	… tends to construct lists of fears or frightening situations and uses pre-patterned expressions when speaking about panic attacks.
… gives detailed information with emphasis on the nature of the feeling of fear.	… gives detailed information with emphasis on the situation causing the fear.
Diagnosis: epileptic fear	**Diagnosis: panic attacks**

Faced with the same task, the two patients use different conversational procedures—the 'grammar of panic' (Capps and Ochs, 1995) is not the same as the 'grammar' of epileptic seizures (cf. Schöndienst and Lindemann, 2012).

Mrs. Girard

The last case is an interview with a French patient in her late twenties, treated in an epilepsy centre in Germany (cf. Gülich, 2018). 'Mrs. Girard' spoke German fluently and was used to talking about her illness in German, but her doctor hoped that if she had the opportunity to speak about her illness in her native language, this might yield new information relevant to her diagnosis. She might speak differently about her condition, mention other aspects, or use different patterns of narration. At the time of the interview, the differential diagnosis had not been clarified. The person conducting the interview (a linguist) was not aware of any pre-diagnosis.

After the opening sequence, the patient talks about the beginning of her illness, the first severe seizure, and the further development (a seizure every two months for no apparent reason). When the interviewer asks about pre-sensations (auras), the patient replies that they are very difficult to describe, and she repeats or reformulates this frequently. This difficulty also manifests itself in hesitations and all kinds of formulation work (self-corrections, repetitions, reformulations, etc.; cf. Gülich, 2005).

Later on in the interview the patient starts to speak about her very complicated and problematic family situation, especially her fear of her father when she was a child. Whenever he returned from travelling she felt panic, even on hearing the key turning in the lock, and she can still feel this panic as an adult. She describes in detail her feelings of fear at the beginning of a seizure, which seems to be mixed with panic and is characterized as 'indescribable' (cf. Gülich, 2005):

(5)

```
G:      c'est ce angstfühlung je sais même pas si c'est de la
        peur
            it's this feeling of anxiety I even don't know if
            it is fear
        c'est de toute façon un sentiment de panique comme ça
            anyway it is a feeling of panic
        mais il m'arrive de l'avoir sans sans pour autant
        faire une crise
            but I happen to have it without going into a seizure
        ( ... )
I:      qu'est-ce que vous avez senti
            what have you been feeling
G:      <<hörbares Ausatmen>> je sais pas je n'arrive pas à
        expliquer
            <<audible exhale>> I don't know I can't explain
```

In the course of the interview the patient keeps returning to the difficulty of describing this feeling of fear:

(6)

```
G:     oui c'est un c'est un . un pressen c'est euh . une
       congation,
```
   yes it's a presen it's a sensation

```
       hein c'est pas simple ( ) c'est pas palpable, ça se
       touche pas,
```
   that's not simple, that's not palpable, you can't
   touch it

```
       donc euh c'est pas du tout non . et comme je vous dis
       euh (4.0)
```
   so it's not at all - no - and as I told you

```
       quand elle est là, euh quand ce fu euh cette sensation
       est là, oui
```
   when it is present, when this fee this sensation is
   present yes

```
       je peux l'expliquer; je peux l'expliquer pendant pen-
       dant deux
```
   then I'm able to explain it for two

```
       jours, après . parce qu'elle est fraîche,
```
   days, afterwards . because it is fresh

The transcript shows that the 'indescribability' of the patient's feelings is not just stated by means of metadiscursive comments such as 'je n'arrive pas à expliquer' ('I just can`t explain this'), but also demonstrated with many hesitations, self-corrections, incomplete sentences, and false starts.

However, this fear is definitely different from another fear she describes, namely, her fear of spiders:

(7)

```
G:     mhm . mais c'est vraiment plus la même peur? que: euh:;
       euh
```
   but it is really not the same fear as

```
       also j'ai j'ai une peur bleue des araignées?
```
   I'm terribly afraid of spiders

```
I:     hm
G:     mais: ce n'est pas la même peur
```
   but that's not the same kind of fear

```
I:      ouais . oui oui
            yes . yes yes
G:      c'est pas la même chose
            that's not the same
I:      ouais
            yeah
G:      euhm . non . . non non rien à voir
            no no no nothing to do with it
```

The patient emphasizes the completely different nature of this type of fear using numerous nearly identical reformulations.

In the research carried out so far, the conversational procedures used by Mrs. Girard have proved typical of patients with epileptic seizures, especially the degree of detail in the description of subjective feelings, the intensive formulation work, and the clarity with which the types of fear are distinguished. The patient also repeatedly stresses the great difficulty she has in describing the sensation of anxiety, to the extent that she frequently doubts whether 'peur' or 'panique' are the appropriate words.

Therefore, as a differential diagnostic hypothesis on the basis of conversation-analytic work, it is suggested that Mrs. Girard suffers from epileptic seizures. However, as she increasingly mentions a disturbing family situation and also speaks about experiences with panic-type fears, a further hypothesis might be that she also suffers from an anxiety or panic disorder.

In this case the patient's medical records were available for study. After a previous stay in a psychiatric hospital the diagnoses were unclear anxiety attacks, considerable family problems, anxiety and panic disorder, socio-phobia, and dissociative seizures. After her stay in the epilepsy clinic the doctors come to the following conclusion: 'we suspect symptomatic focal epilepsy (…). The paroxysmal anxiety symptoms can certainly be classified as a psychic aura, particularly as the patient described, in her native language, this fear as being different from her fear of anyone or anything, usually manifesting itself without any triggering. In addition there were feelings of anxiety arising from situations where non-epileptic origin is possible. Furthermore, we assume additional dissociative seizures which occur particularly during situations of psychological pressure'.

These diagnoses are in line with the diagnostic hypotheses resulting from the linguistic analysis. This is one of the numerous cases in the research which show the complementarity of the linguistic and the clinical approach (cf. the analyses in Surmann, 2005).

Conclusion

This chapter has presented three cases to show how conversation–analytic research on patients' narratives of their suffering can contribute to differential diagnosis in patients with seizures and/or anxiety disorders. Both of these illnesses are often difficult to diagnose. The example of fear and anxiety was used in order to have a concrete focus for comparing different ways of narrative reconstruction of what from the outside seems to be one and the same phenomenon. Doctors who concentrate exclusively on the *content* of what patients like Mrs. Korte and Mrs. Wiesinger say may come to the conclusion that they are both suffering from panic attacks. By ignoring the *manner* in which patients describe their sensations/feelings or narrate fear or panic episodes, they miss an important source of information. The history of Mrs. Korte's illness and its treatment is long and complicated; it took several years to discover that what seemed to be a sort of panic attack was in fact a specific epileptic aura. Panic and anxiety are among the most frequent psychic disorders, but if they co-occur with another illness, they are often overlooked. For Mrs. Girard's treatment it is important to recognize that she is suffering from epilepsy *as well* as from panic. Doctors should become aware of the importance of the subjective accounts patients give of their illness in narrative reconstructions, and they should know and be able to recognize the characteristic differences in patients' narratives (Jenkins and Reuber, 2014).

There are four main reasons why the *narrative* reconstruction of an illness is such a useful diagnostic tool:

1. To be diagnosed with an illness such as epilepsy, dissociation, or an anxiety disorder is an extremely important and sometimes life-changing event for a patient and those around him/her (cf. Lucius-Hoene, 2008). Such a 'reportable' event naturally lends itself to narrative reconstruction (Labov 2013, pp. 21–23). It is only through narrative reconstruction that it is possible to discover in what way the patient's illness relates to the larger context of his normal life.

2. Narrative reconstruction of seizure or panic episodes requires a number of actions, events, or sensations to be put into some kind of organized sequence; 'any narrative text imposes an order on events and its representation that is never identical with the event it recounts in the case of retellings of an experience' (Gygax and Locher, 2015, p. 2). The importance of discourse structuring is also underlined by Capps and Ochs (1995, pp. 182–185). This aspect of imposing order on chaos can be helpful to the patient.

3. Narrative reconstruction encourages the patient to present his own view of the illness; it allows interpretation and categorization of the event by the patient rather than the result being predetermined by the doctor's questions.

4. Narrative reconstruction and the construction of identity are closely interrelated 'narrative is one of the key constituents of human identity, self-representation and cultural transmission' (Gygax and Locher, 2015, p. 2). Illness is a threat to identity; in narrating the illness the patient may feel he is gaining or regaining control. The activity of telling the story of his illness helps the patient to cope with it (cf. Scheidt and Lucius-Hoene, 2017).

These characteristics of narrative reconstruction become evident in various linguistic details which may seem insignificant at first glance but provide an 'enormous understanding' (Sacks, 1984, p. 24) of the way patients experience their illness and come to terms with it.

The aspect of coping with the illness opens up a new perspective. Studying linguistic details in transcript analyses might not only be useful for differential diagnosis, but can also provide important therapeutic insights. The patient's way of telling typical illness episodes may lead to specific therapeutic interactions. Or the patient's formulation difficulties in describing feelings of fear or panic could lead a psychotherapist to come to his/her aid. In the data are found various examples of co-constructions of 'indescribable' emotions of this kind (Gülich and Krafft, 2015).

As mentioned, understanding the linguistic details in a medical and/or psychotherapeutic context can, of course, only be successful if the approach is an interdisciplinary one. In their 1995 book *Constructing Panic*, Capps, a psychologist, and Ochs, a linguist, provide an impressive example of 'what can be done when psychologists and discourse analysts work together to mine the architecture of sufferers' stories for their understanding of their experiences' (Capps and Ochs, 1995, p. 174). Working on transcripts may be a strange thing to do for medical researchers, doctors, and psychotherapists, just as interpreting the results of transcript analysis in terms of medical or psychological categories is unusual for conversation analysts. But they can learn from each other and the result is worth the effort. Thus this author fully agrees with Capps and Ochs when they continue: 'We encourage psychotherapists to explore linguistic perspectives through cross-disciplinary collaboration and training. At the same time we encourage linguists to work with clinicians to develop more acute understandings of the interface of language and emotion' (Capps and Ochs, 1995, p. 174)

Acknowledgements

This article could not have been written without the long and fruitful co-operation I have had with neurologist Martin Schöndienst, or without my numerous, intensive conversations with Gabriele Lucius-Hoene. I am most grateful to both of them.

Notes

1. *Linguistic differential diagnostics of epileptic and other seizure disorders* (www.uni-bielefeld.de/lili/projekte/epiling); cf. Gülich, 2012, Schwabe et al., 2008.

2. *Listening to people with seizures* (http://listeningseizures.wikidot.com).

3. *Communicative description and clinical representation of fear and anxiety*, a research group at the Centre for Interdisciplinary Research of Bielefeld University in 2004 (www.uni-bielefeld.de/ZIF/KG/2004Angst/index.html); cf. Gülich, 2007, Streeck, 2011.

4. For the transcript notations, see Table 17.2. The names of the patients are pseudonyms.

Table 17.2 Transcript notations (GAT basic transcript)

[]	overlap and simultaneous speech
=	direct tying of two words
(.)	micro pause
(-)	short pause (app. 0.25 sec.)
(--)	medium pause (app. 0.50 sec.)
(---)	longer pause (app. 0.75 sec.)
(2.0)	measured pause in sec.
:;::; ...;	lengthening, depending on duration
beLIEVE	primary- resp. main stress
be!LIEVE!	extra strong stress
!	emphatic exclamation
?	high rising intonation, questioning intonation
,	medium rising intonation
;	medium falling intonation
.	falling intonation
-	level intonation
∧	rising-falling intonation
V	falling-rising intonation
() / (there)	inaudible / suspected wording
<<laughing> oh well>	interpretative commentaries, with given scope
.h;.hh;.hhh	audible inhale, depending on duration
h, hh, hhh	audible exhale, depending on duration

changes in volume and speed of talking with given scope:

<<f> >/<<ff> >	forte, loud/ fortissimo, very loud
<<p> >/<<pp> >	piano, quiet/low/soft/pianissimo, very quiet/low/soft
<<cresc> >	crescendo, gradually becoming louder
<<dim> >	diminuendo, gradually becoming quieter

References

Capps, L. and Ochs, E., 1995. *Constructing panic. The discourse of agoraphobia.* Cambridge, MA: Harvard University Press.

Gülich, E., 2005. Unbeschreibbarkeit: Rhetorischer Topos—Gattungsmerkmal—Formulierungsressource. *Gesprächsforschung—Online-Zeitschrift zur verbalen Interaktion*, **6**, 222–244.

Gülich, E., 2007. 'Volle Palette in Flammen'. Zur Orientierung an vorgeformten Strukturen beim Reden über Angst. *Psychotherapie & Sozialwissenschaft*, 9(1), 59–87.

Gülich, E., 2012. Conversation analysis as a new approach to the differential diagnosis of epileptic and non-epileptic seizure disorders. In: M. Egbert and A. Deppermann, eds. *Hearing aids communication. Integrating social interaction, audiology and user centered design to improve communication with hearing loss and hearing technologies*. Mannheim: Verlag für Gesprächsforschung. pp. 146–156.

Gülich, E., 2018. Analyser la parole pour établir un diagnostic: Perspectives du travail pluridisciplinaire entre médecins et linguistes. In: K. Ploog, S. Mariani-Rousset, and S. Equoy Hutin, eds. *Emmêler & démêler la parole: approche pluridisciplinaire de la relation de soin*. Besancon: Presses Universitaires de Franche-Comté.

Gülich, E. and Krafft, U., 2015. Ko-konstruktion von Anfallsschilderungen in Arzt-Patient-Gesprächen. In: U. Dausendschön-Gay, E. Gülich, and U. Krafft, eds. *Ko-konstruktionen in der Interaktion. Die gemeinsame Arbeit an Äußerungen und anderen sozialen Ereignissen*. Bielefeld: Transkript-Verlag. pp. 373–400.

Gülich, E. and Lindemann, K., 2010. Communicating emotion in doctor-patient interaction. A multidimensional single-case analysis, In: D. Barth-Weingarten, E. Reber, and M. Selting, eds. *Prosody in interaction*. Amsterdam: John Benjamins. pp. 269–294.

Günthner, S., 2005. Narrative reconstructions of past experiences. Ajustments and modifications in the process of recontextualizing a past experience. In: U. M. Quasthoff and T. Becker, eds. *Narrative interaction*. Amsterdam: John Benjamins. pp. 285–301.

Gygax, F. and Locher, M. A., eds, 2015. *Narrative matters in medical contexts across disciplines*. Amsterdam: John Benjamins.

Heritage, J., 1984. A change-of-state token and aspects of its sequential placement. In: J. M. Atkinson and J. Heritage, eds. *Structures of social action. Studies in conversation analysis*. Cambridge: Cambridge University Press. pp. 299–345.

Heritage, J. and Atkinson, J. M., 1984. Introduction. In: J. M. Atkinson and J. Heritage, eds. *Structures of social action. Studies in conversation analysis*. Cambridge: Cambridge University Press. pp. 1–15.

Jenkins, L. and Reuber, M., 2014. A conversation analytic intervention to help neurologists identify diagnostically relevant linguistic features in seizure patients' talk. *Research on language and social interaction*, 47(3), 266–279.

Kallmeyer, W. and Schütze, F., 1977. Zur Konstitution von Kommunikationsschemata der Sachverhaltsdarstellung. In: D. Wegner, ed. *Gesprächsanalysen*. Hamburg: Buske. pp. 159–274.

Knerich, H., 2013. *Vorgeformte Strukturen als Formulierungsressource beim Sprechen über Angst und Anfälle*. Berlin: Logos.

Labov, W., 1972. The transformation of experience in narrative syntax. In: W. Labov, ed. *Language in the inner city. Studies in the Black English vernacular*. Philadelphia, PA: University of Philadelphia Press. pp. 354–396.

Labov, W., 2013. *The language of life and death. The transformation of experience in oral narrative*. Cambridge: Cambridge University Press.

Lindemann, K., 2012. *Angst im Gespräch. Eine gesprächsanalytische Studie zur kommunikativen Darstellung von Angst*. Göttingen: V&R unipress.

Lucius-Hoene, G., 2008. Krankheitserzählungen und die narrative Medizin. *Rehabilitation*, 47, 90–97.

Reuber, M., Fernandez, G., Bauer, J., Singh, D. D., and Elger, C. E., 2002. Diagnostic delay in psychogenic nonepileptic seizures. *Neurology*, 58, 493–495.

Reuber, M., Monzoni, C., Sharrack, B., Plug, L., 2009. Using interactional and linguistic analysis to distinguish between epileptic and psychogenic nonepileptic seizures: A prospective, blinded multirater study. *Epilepsy and Behavior*, 16(1), 139–144.

Sacks, H., 1984. Notes on methodology. In: **J. M. Atkinson** and **J. Heritage**, eds. *Structures of social action. Studies in conversation analysis.* Cambridge: Cambridge University Press. pp. 21–27.

Scheidt, C. E. and **Lucius-Hoene, G.**, 2017. Bewältigen von Erlebnissen. In: **M. Martínez**, ed. *Erzählen: Ein interdisziplinäres Handbuch.* Stuttgart: Metzler, pp. 235–242.

Schmitz, B. and **Schöndienst, M.**, 2006. Anfälle: Epilepsie und Dissoziation. Die Psychosomatik epileptischer und nicht-epileptischer Anfälle. In: **P. Henningsen, H. Gündel**, and **A. Ceballos-Baumann**, eds. *Neuro-Psychosomatik: Grundlagen und Klinik neurologischer Psychosomatik.* Stuttgart: Schattauer. pp.131–175.

Schöndienst, M. and **Lindemann, K.**, 2012. Panic, ictal fear and hyperventilation. In: **M. Reuber** and S. **Schachter**, eds. *Borderland of epilepsy revisited.* Oxford: Oxford University Press. pp. 63–73.

Schütze, F., 2016. Biography analysis on the empirical base of autobiographical narratives: how to analyse autobiographical narrative interviews. In: **F. Schütze**, ed. *Sozialwissenschaftliche Prozessanalyse. Grundlagen der qualitativen Sozialforschung.* Opladen: Barbara Budrich. pp. 75–115.

Schwabe, M., **Reuber, M., Schöndienst, M.**, and **Gülich, E.**, 2008. Listening to people with seizures: how can linguistic analysis help in the differential diagnosis of seizure disorders? *Communication & Medicine,* **5**(1), 59–72.

Streeck, J., 2011. Interaction order and anxiety disorder. A "Batesonian" heuristic of speaking patterns during psychotherapy. *Communication & Medicine,* **8**(3), 261–272.

Surmann, V., 2005. *Anfallsbilder. Metaphorische Konzepte im Sprechen anfallskranker Menschen.* Würzburg: Königshausen & Neumann.

Chapter 18

Structural dream analysis

*A narrative methodology for investigating
the meaning of dream series and their development
in the course of psychotherapy*

Christian Roesler

Introduction

In the psychoanalytic tradition, the work with dreams has always had an important role
in the treatment of psychological disorders and is still considered as the royal road to
the unconscious (Fosshage, 1987). In the psychoanalytic encounter, the patient suffering
from a mental health problem usually presents a dream in the way of telling a story
about what happened during sleep, so dreams in psychotherapy can be seen as narratives
(Boothe, 1994). Even though quite different approaches to the interpretation of dreams
have developed in the different psychoanalytic schools, there is general agreement that
dreams give access to an understanding of the unconscious roots of psychological problems as well as to therapeutic pathways. The dream can be seen as a subtext which points
to the core conflicts underlying neurosis and it also contains constructive impulses for
overcoming the problems. Nevertheless, there is a strong lack of systematic investigations into the meaning of dreams and their connection to process in psychotherapy. This
chapter presents Structural Dream Analysis (SDA) as a narratological method for analysing the meaning of dream series in analytical psychotherapies. For the application of
SDA, dreams are understood as narratives. The dream as an inner world phenomenon—
which is never accessible for research—has to be differentiated from the narrated form: a
text. From a linguistic point of view the genre of this text is a narrative. In narratology,
a narrative is defined as a development from a starting point, which often features a
problem that needs repair or solution; the narrative goes through ups and downs, generally arriving at the solution of the problem or the valued endpoint of the story (Gülich
and Quasthoff, 1985).

Psychoanalytic dream theory and empirical dream research

In the last decades there has been a reconceptualization of psychoanalytic dream theories influenced by insights from empirical dream research. This has led to a convergence of contemporary Freudian theories of the dream towards Jung's understanding

of the dream (e.g. Fosshage, 1987; Levin, 1990). Referring to Barrett and McNamara (2007), the results of empirical dream research can be summarized in the following theory of dreaming: in the dream the brain is in a mode where it does not have to process new input but can use larger capacities for working on problems and finding creative solutions. The dream focuses especially on experiences in waking life that have emotional meaning for the dreamer. The dreaming mind can find solutions for problems more easily compared to waking consciousness because it is able to connect different areas and functions of the brain. This supports the viewpoint taken by C. G. Jung (1925/1971), which sees the psyche as a self-regulating system and the dream as a spontaneously produced picture of the current situation of the psyche in the form of symbols. Jung differentiates between a 'subjective' level and an 'objective' level. In the first perspective, the figures and objects of the dream are interpreted as being representatives for parts or qualities of the dreamer's personality (especially conflictual parts, i.e., complexes), whereas in the objective perspective they are seen as representing persons or entities existing in reality. In dreams the unconscious tries to support ego consciousness by pointing to parts of the psyche not yet integrated into the whole of the personality or to unresolved conflicts. Via dreams the unconscious, because it contains a more holistic knowledge about the development and integration of personality, brings new information to consciousness, which then can be integrated if a conscious understanding of the information is possible. This is the aim of dream interpretation in psychotherapy. As the information in dreams appears in the form of symbols and images it needs translation to be understood by the conscious ego. For this aim Jung developed the method of 'amplification': the symbolic form is enriched with information coming from cultural parallels, the meaning the symbol has in different cultures, mythologies, religious traditions, and spiritual belief systems. Through amplification a network of meaning is constructed around the symbol; the aim is not so much to give a precise interpretation of the symbol but more to stimulate processes in the dreamer to become more conscious of potential solutions offered by the dream.

Many insights from empirical dream research support this view of the dream (for more details see Roesler, 2018). Hall and Van de Castle (1966) argued that it is possible to draw a personality profile based only on dreams of the person. In a study on dreams of persons with multiple personality disorder Barrett (1996) was able to demonstrate that the split-off parts of the personality appeared personified in the dreams. There is a high continuity among the themes in the dreams of a person over a long period of time (Levin, 1990). Cartwright (1977) found that the themes in the dreams change when a person goes through psychotherapy. Greenberg and Pearlman (1978) compared the content of dreams of patients currently in psychoanalysis with the protocols of therapy sessions from the time of the dream and found a strong connection between the themes in the dreams and in psychotherapy. The dream can be read as a report about the current conflictual themes in the waking life of the dreamer. Palombo (1982) could show that analysands reprocess contents from the last analytical session in the following dreams. Popp, Luborsky, and Crits-Christoph (1990) investigated dreams and narratives from therapy sessions with the methodology of the Core Conflictual Relationship Theme. They found that both narratives and dreams were structured by the same unconscious relationship patterns.

So, there is some evidence for psychodynamic theories of dreaming and its role in psychotherapy. Nevertheless, there is a strong need for more systematic studies on the relationship between the content of dreams of a person, namely the development of recurrent themes and figures in a series of dreams, and the course of psychotherapy, namely the development of core conflictual themes of the patient and the overall development of the personality. In Germany there is a certain tradition in psychoanalysis for developing elaborated coding systems for dream content and their use in studies investigating processes in psychotherapy (e.g., Moser and von Zeppelin, 1996). To understand meaning conveyed by the dream, it has to be interpreted. In the psychodynamic schools of psychotherapy this interpretation of dreams takes place in an interaction between therapist and client. For a systematic research on the meaning of dreams it would be necessary to have a method of interpretation which produces more objective and reliable results. The method of SDA presented here is an attempt in this direction.

The method of structural dream analysis

In many psychotherapeutic processes dreams point to the core problems/conflicts, but they also contain elements to solve these problems. During the course of individual psychotherapy treatment, the analyst assumes that the series of dreams follows an inner structure of meaning. SDA aims at identifying this inner structure of meaning from the series of dreams alone without referring to additional information about the dreamer, the psychodynamics, or the course of psychotherapy. The meaning conveyed by the dream is analysed in a systematic series of interpretive steps (see Box 18.1) which makes use of analytic tools developed in narratology; especially two earlier methods of narrative analysis were incorporated:

1. The Russian researcher Vladimir Propp (1975) developed the method of Structural analysis/Functional analysis and applied it to fairy tales. Each fairy tale is divided into its functional parts (e.g., 'The King is ill and needs healing'; 'The hero fights the Dragon') and each functional part receives an abstract symbol, e.g., a letter or number. As a result, each fairy tale can be written as an abstract formula of symbols and then different fairy tales can be compared regarding their structure.

2. Brigitte Boothe and colleagues from the University of Zürich developed the narratological method JAKOB for the analysis of patient narratives from analytical psychotherapies and their development over the course of psychotherapy (Boothe, 1994). An important element in this method is to analyse the role the narrator takes in the narrative regarding activity versus passivity and his/her relation to other protagonists in the narrative.

SDA also makes use of amplification, which was systemized in the form of a manual.

Box 18.1 Overview of the steps of the research

1. Segmentation of the narrative,
2. Episodic models.
3. Fate of the protagonist: the dream narratives are analysed regarding the position of the ego (ego is actively involved, a passive observer, is marginalized, etc.).
4. Functional analysis (following Propp).
5. Integrating the above steps into a structural framework describing the whole dream series.
6. Amplification of core symbols: symbols that appear in several dreams or have a central position to the dream series are analysed using symbol dictionaries and translated into a hypothesis of their psychological meaning.
7. Amplifications are included into the framework of the dream series.
8. Overall interpretation of the meaning of the whole dream series in psychological language.

The interpreters, who are blinded regarding all other information about the case, receive a series of 10 to 20 dreams covering the whole course of a psychotherapy, ideally marking core points and topics. The dreams are provided by practising analysts who also write a case report about the psychopathology and psychodynamics of the patient involved as well as about the development of core conflicts and themes in the course of the therapy.

Exemplary dream series

To illustrate the application of the method, these steps are exemplified by analysing the following dream series (originally written down by the dreamer in German and handed over to the therapist; the translation follows the original style of the client):

1. I walked down the street in the darkness, on both sides small houses behind fences. Lots of barking dogs jumped against the fences. I was frightened but then I became brave. I barked like a dog myself aggressively and the dogs immediately fell silent.
2. I am on my way with my bicycle up a hill. It is demanding. Around me are large trees, it's like in the mountains. Arriving on top there is a little white poodle, it barks, it is on a leash. I'm driving home downhill in sharp curves. Doberman dogs are behind me, I cannot get rid of them because of the curves. They run at my side and bark at me. Then it is light and sunny, arriving on the pass it's beautiful. There is a restaurant, like in Italy, beautiful houses. On top of the pass the black dogs are coming.

3. There is a stillwater, a river? There is a little bridge, somebody on the other side. He falls into the water, he somehow slipped as if under a log. I pull him out, but first I hesitate. He is like dead. But that guy has a sharp knife and he cuts the other helper's throat. I flee.

4. In black and white: at a nearby train station. A girl and another person, who seems to be masochistic, and a very energetic black dog. The dog pulls the other person into the little pond, then pulls the person out of the water and up the hill. The person gives himself a blow job, then to the dog. Then I am at the foot of a tall building. I say: the dog must be put on a leash. The masochistic person says: you have to stroke the dog. I say: no, it must be put on a leash and then removed. The masochistic person is angry and goes into the tall building. The other person says: you have to follow him, he is sad. The dog smells, I put him on a leash but it is disgusting.

5. An elderly, badly smelling dog is with me and my girlfriend in Paris. It just found us. We get on the bus, the badly smelling dog could not go with us, we left it outside. We are already outside of the city limits but will return to the city on the highway. The dog would not have been able to come along behind us.

6. I was the manager of a café in the house. I was promoted like Joseph in the house of Potifar. Everybody says goodbye to a father with his little son, he's in the backyard. There is an elderly man with a Pitbull. He says: I can show you how evil the dog is. But I just had to go. I walked into a vineyard. The dog runs from its leash and goes behind me, but I jump over fences and walls. The path goes uphill through the yard and back down on the other side.

7. In a country restaurant. Two Romanians come in and start begging. I remember: the last time the two of them were masked and committed a robbery. I drive away with the motorcycle. I want to report to the police, because now I know their faces.

8. A little baby is in danger. I cover it with newspaper and carry it with me through a sewerage system. Then I forget about it and leave it somewhere. But then I realize that the baby is missing and go back and find it again. I carry it with me and feed it. I think: the baby is so small, it should get mother's milk, but I can just feed him solid food.

9. I'm sitting on the couch in the garden. A man with two bottles of beer is by my side and offers one to me, maybe my father? I get the feeling of being unfair to the other person. We are having a beer together.

10. My father dies at the age of 49 years. I'm not moved at all. It was strange that he died so young. We don't have such a long life as my grandma with her 102 years of age.

11. I saw a giant toe and found it is my toe. The skin on the nail was grown very wide. I thought: this has to be removed. It could be moved back easily. There was another level of skin below, this one could be taken off easily, too. I was surprised that it did not hurt. Below the skin were very small black worms, everything was rotten, but you could remove it without difficulty. Below that everything was new.

Step 1: segmentation

Each dream is separated into its narrative segments before further steps of analysis are applied (Lucius-Hoene and Deppermann, 2004).

Step 2: episodic models

As described, a narrative consists of a starting point, a development, and a conclusion; this basic structure can be differentiated into different dynamic models. In SDA ten different episodic models (Boothe, 1994) are used to describe the dynamic of the development in the dream narrative.

1. Continuity: a static image, no destabilizing momentum.
2. Climax: a process of growth and optimization.
3. Anticlimax: a process of decline.
4. Restitutio ad integrum (after deintegration): after deintegration a return to normal conditions.
5. Restitutio ad integrum (after climax): after climax a return to normal conditions.
6. Approbation: validation after denigration, by successfully passing an examination or test.
7. Frustration: after a short gradation there is strong degradation.
8. Chance: positive development; the protagonist adapts to conditions and stabilizes.
9. Anti-chance: negative development; the protagonist adapts to negative conditions and stabilizes.
10. Unexplainable changes: the normal course of the narrative is disrupted, something unexpected happens.

Step 3: fate of the protagonist

Analysis of the position the ego takes in the narrative:

1. Only ego initiative: in all phases of the narrative the ego has the initiative; the ego is always in the subject position.
2. Only other's initiative: only other agents have the initiative throughout the narrative; the ego is never in the subject position.
3. Loss of initiative: initially the ego has the initiative, also parallel to other figures, but at the end is in a passive position.
4. Regaining of the initiative: the ego is at the beginning and at the end in the initiating position; during the course of the narrative the ego temporarily loses the initiative to other actors.
5. Embedded in others' initiative: the ego is, from time to time, in the course of the development in the initiative position, but not at the beginning and not at the end.

Applying these systematic steps to the above dream series leads to the following structure (Table 18.1):

Table 18.1 Episodic models and fate of the protagonist for total dream series.

	Episodic model	**Fate of the protagonist**
Dream 1	Restitutio ad integrum (after Deintegration)	Regain of the initiative
Dream 2	Anticlimax	Loss of initiative
Dream 3	Anticlimax	Regain of initiative
Dream 4	Not definable	Embedded in others' initiative
Dream 5	Continuity	Embedded in others' initiative
Dream 6	Frustration	Regain of initiative
Dream 7	Approbation	Regain of initiative
Dream 8	Chance	Only ego initiative
Dream 9	Antichance	Loss of initiative
Dream 10	Continuity	Not definable
Dream 11	Approbation	Only ego initiative

Reproduced courtesy of Christian Roesler.

After this step of analysis an initial summarizing interpretation of the development over the course of the dream series is possible: on both levels of analysis there is a certain development from patterns of decline in the first half of therapy to patterns of approbation or chance which could be called more optimistic; regarding ego initiative there is a development from patterns of loss of initiative or the ego being subjected to others' initiative to patterns dominated by ego initiative. Psychologically speaking, there is a certain development from a situation in which the ego is more of a victim of conditions or others' initiative to a situation where ego consciousness is more capable of taking over initiative and controlling the situation.

Step 4: functional analysis (following Propp)

In this step, each dream is segmented into its functional parts and each part receives an abstract symbol. Here, the interpreter has to decide how far the abstraction of the narrative segment should go. The aim here is to reduce the dream narrative down to its structural elements (see Box 18.2) so that they become comparable. In the current state of the development of SDA the definition of structural elements has to be developed for each new series of dreams—the long-term aim is to build up a corpus of analysed cases which will allow for a generalization of structural elements across cases.

Table 18.2 shows the functional analysis for all the dreams of the above dream series. Recurrent structural elements are marked.

Table 18.2 Functional analysis for total dream series.

	Function I	Function II	Function III	Function IV	Function V	Function VI	Function VII	Function /III
Dream 1	0 Initial situation	**BD** **Threat**	**S** **Constructive strategy**					
Dream 2	0 Initial situation Situation	↑ Way up	**BD** **Threat**	↓ Way down	**V** **Pursue**	**F** **Flight**	↑ Way up	**BD** **Threat**
Dream 3	0 Initial situation	W Water	WT Death /damage	**H** **Help/support**	**BD** **Threat**	**F** **Flight**		
Dream 4	0 Initial situation	VSCH deferrence	& sexual act	KS conflict	KL Conflict solution	**EK** **Disgust**		
Dream 5	0 Initial situation	**V** **Pursue**	**EK** **Disgust**	O Change of place	**V-** **end** **Pursue**			
Dream 6	0 Initial situation	‖ Gradation	VE Goodbye	**BD** **Threat**	**V** **Pursue**	**F** **Flight**	**V-** **end Pursue**	
Dream 7	0 Initial situation	**BH** **Pledge for help/support**	**BD** **Threat**	**S** **Constructive strategy**				
Dream 8	**BH** **Pledge for help/support**	**H** **Help/support**	VG Neglect	HW Taking up action	**IH** **Inadequate measures**			
Dream 9	0 Initial situation	UH Unjust act						
Dream 10	WT Death/Damage							
Dream 11	**GM** **Wish for modification**	**M** **Modification**	**RE** **Renewal/ Regeneration**					

Reproduced courtesy of Christian Roesler.

> **Box 18.2 Repetitive structures that were marked are now extracted**
>
> Dream 1: threat, constructive strategy.
>
> Dream 2: threat, pursue, flight, threat.
>
> Dream 3: help/support, threat, flight.
>
> Dream 4: disgust.
>
> Dream 5: pursue, disgust, pursuit.
>
> Dream 6: threat, pursue, flight, end pursuit.
>
> Dream 7: pledge for help/support, threat, constructive strategy.
>
> Dream 8: pledge for help/support, help/support, inadequate measures.
>
> Dream 11: wish for modification, modification, renewal/regeneration.

Step 6: amplification of major symbols

As to combine the structural elements of the above dreams with content in the next step, the meaning of central symbols of the dreams will be analysed by using Jung's original method of amplification. To arrive at a scientific approach to the interpretation of symbols via amplification in the application of SDA, this step is clearly defined. Amplification of symbols is restricted to the use of a set of symbol dictionaries (e.g., Cooper, 1978) which give information about the cultural background of symbols in the sense of their use and understanding in religious traditions, mythology, cultural beliefs, etc. This is to certify that interpretation of the symbols is done in a way as to be as objective as possible.

This step of interpretation is applied only to a very restricted number of symbols, ideally those which appear repeatedly in the dreams or seem to be especially important to the series of dreams (Table 18.3).

Step 7: translating into psychological language

The above findings just give information about the field or context of meaning of the symbols. In the next step this has to be integrated into the structure of the dream series. This is clearly the more psychological step in the interpretation which makes use of psychological/psychodynamic concepts. Still, this step of interpretation attempts to stay as objective as possible, and therefore the aim here is not to formulate definite interpretations of the dreams, but rather to translate the above structures into a psychological language. As mentioned, dreams do not represent a linear structure of development, but instead usually take up symbols and patterns repeatedly which undergo a process of transformation. In this step of interpretation, it should be attempted to reconstruct this repetitive use of symbols and patterns in the dreams and the transformative process, if there is any. The focus here is on more general topics appearing repetitively in the dreams. This is

Table 18.3 Amplification of symbols

Symbol	Dreams	Amplification
Dog	1, 2, 4, 5, 6	In a number of cultures the dog is related to death. In old Egypt and Greece the dog guards the underworld and is a mediator between the worlds of the living and the dead. Those gods either living in the dark or being ambiguous figures often appear in the form of dogs. The dog clearly has ambiguous meaning: on the one side it is connected with wisdom, grace, and religion, especially the white dog; on the other hand, the dog is connected with primitive affects, impurity, vice, and envy, especially dark dogs. Also, the dog is related to sexuality because dogs in the streets are promiscuous. In some cultures the dog appears as ancestor and creator of man and of civilization because of the wisdom and the sexual power that is related to it.
Child	8	The child is a symbol for impeccably clean purity and innocence because it is so close to birth. It also represents the original and therefore is related to an abundance of possibilities.
Foot/toe	11	The foot/toe is that part of the body which is closest to the earth. Therefore, symbolically as an organ of movement it is in a strong relation to the will. In the context of psychoanalysis the foot is also seen as phallic. Related to this aspect of the symbol naked feet can have a decisive role in rituals of initiation and generativity.
Worm	11	The worm is a being that lives below the earth and in the dirt. Therefore, in several cultures this animal is connected with the snake and the devil. Also, the worm is related to darkness and death and the rebirth of life from death.

Reproduced courtesy of Christian Roesler.

illustrated in Table 18.4 below where the structural elements are combined with a psychological interpretation of symbols and their meanings and included in an overall description of the dreams series.

Step 8: Integrating and summarizing the dreams

Lastly, all the findings from the above steps are integrated into a general description or summary of the series of dreams from a psychological point of view.

In the first half of the process the ego is confronted with threatening aspects. By analysing the symbol of the dog these aspects can be characterized as having an aggressive and destructive, even murderous, character. They also seem to be connected with sexuality. Finally, they carry a certain ambiguity, changing between aggressiveness and helpless neediness. At the start of the dream the ego is threatened and experiences strong fear. It is not capable of coping with these aspects but flees from them. In the beginning even flight is not always successful as the ego gets caught and is overwhelmed by these destructive aspects. In the further course of the dream series the shadow aspects begin to lose their threatening character. The ego now experiences disgust regarding these parts of the psyche and rejects them. Now a new thematic field is introduced. It is centred on

Table 18.4 Integration of amplification into dream structure.

Nr				
1	Threat *The ego is threatened by shadow aspects.*	Constructive strategy *The ego takes over forms of expression of shadow aspects and by doing that, succeeds in making these aspects give up their threatening position.*		
1	The ego is threatened by shadow aspects in the form of dogs. By taking over the act of barking from the shadow aspects, the ego succeeds in making the shadow aspects stopping their threatening behaviour.			
2	Threat *The ego is threatened by shadow aspects,*	Pursue *and pursued by them,*	Flight *and flees from them,*	Threat *but the threat persists.*
2	In reaction to the confrontation and pursue by shadow aspects in form of dogs, the ego flees. But the ego does not succeed and gets caught by the shadow aspects.			
3	Help/support *The ego starts actions to give help/ support to other aspects of the psyche.*	Threat *The ego is threatened by shadow aspects.*	Flight *The ego flees from threatening shadow aspects.*	
3	The ego tries to take a supportive stance towards a helpless aspect of the psyche. But this part of the psyche comes out to be threatening and destructive. In reaction to the threat, the ego flees into an area in which it is not longer threatened by shadow aspects.			
4	Disgust *The ego feels disgust towards shadow aspects,*			
4	The ego is confronted with shadow aspects in the form of dogs. The ego denies and pushes away these aspects out of disgust.			
5	Pursue *The ego is pursued by shadow aspects,*	Disgust *The ego feels disgusted by shadow aspects,*	End Pursue *The pursuit is successfully brought to an end,*	
5	The ego tries to flee from the confrontation with shadow aspects in the form of dogs. This is because the ego feels strong denial and disgust towards the shadow aspects. The ego succeeds in getting away from the confrontation.			

#			
6	**Threat** — *The ego is threatened by shadow aspects.*	**Pursue** — *The ego is pursued by shadow aspects.*	**Flight** — *The ego flees from threatening shadow aspects.*	**Interruption Pursue** — *A pursuit through shadow aspects is interrupted.*
6	In reaction to being threatened by shadow aspects in the form of dogs, the ego flees. The ego succeeds in getting away from the shadow aspects.			
7	**Pledge for help/support** — *The ego becomes aware of aspects of the psyche that need help/support.*	**Threat** — *The ego is threatened by shadow aspects.*		**Constructive strategy** — *The ego is able to recognize in time a danger that comes from shadow aspects. It begins to activate forces of order and security.*
7	The ego tries to give support to a part of the psyche that needs help. But this part of the psyche comes out to be threatening and destructive. The ego is able to recognize the approaching danger in time and activates components of the psyche that are able to re-establish order and security.			
8	**Pledge for help/support** — *The ego recognizes aspects of the psyche that need help/support.*	**Help/support** — *The ego goes into action to give help/support to other parts of the psyche.*		**Inadequate forms of help** — *The ego is missing adequate forms to give help to other parts of the psyche.*
8	The ego recognizes a part of the psyche in form of an infant which needs help and support. The ego already has an idea how to give support. But still it is missing the adequate measures to realize this support.			
11	**Wish for modification** — *The ego realizes the necessity to modify a part of the psyche.*	**Modification** — *The ego begins to modify a part of the psyche.*		**Renewal/regeneration** — *Through activity of the ego a process of regeneration and renewal becomes visible on a part of the psyche.*
11	The ego realizes the necessity to modify a part of the psyche. This is a part connected with willpower and movement. Through activity of the ego a process of renewal and regeneration on this part of the psyche comes about.			

Reproduced courtesy of Christian Roesler.

situations where the ego is asked to act in a helpful and supportive way and to be active. Some pledges for help appear to be dangerous because these parts of the psyche that ask for help are also destructive powers. The ego therefore is in the danger of supporting destructive energies and being destroyed itself in the process. It can be assumed that in this change the original ambiguity of the shadow aspects are contained and they move towards the helpless and needy side. In the image of the infant needing help, these parts have finally lost their destructive aspects and the ego meets a pure, positive part of the psyche which points to a new beginning. These parts of the psyche need support but the ego has some difficulty in overcoming disgust and rejection and finding a supportive attitude towards these parts. Then the ego increasingly realizes how these parts have to be cared for, even though some of the necessary means and strategies are still missing. Towards the end of the dream series the ego actively takes part in a process where some parts of the psyche experience a process of death and renewal. These aspects of the psyche can be associated with willpower and intention.

Case description (delivered by the analyst)

The client is a young man (30 years). Before starting psychotherapy, the client was imprisoned having committed physical violence in more than 100 cases. No longer openly violent after imprisonment, he suffered from feelings of strong tension, unrest, and emptiness that were almost unbearable against the background of a severe depression. The only means to deal with these depressive states was a strong compulsion to consume pornographic media, especially those scenes containing physical violence towards women.

The client comes from a broken home. His father suffered from severe alcoholism and tended to be violent towards his wife and children. On several occasions the client experienced fear of death and was almost killed by his father. The father also seems to have suffered from a sexual obsession: he collected pornographic videos in large numbers and stored them in his bedroom. This aspect of the father's life was always fascinating for the client. His mother grew up in former Yugoslavia and was never able to speak German properly; it might be that the mother was mildly mentally disabled. The client stated that 'she was too dumb to understand what I needed'. In adolescence the client was taken out of his family by the welfare authorities because of the difficult situation and was placed in protective custody. Later, he joined a group of hooligans and committed a large number of violent crimes. In prison the client experienced a religious conversion and became member of a fundamentalist Christian sect. He came into psychotherapy with the explicit intention of overcoming his aggressive impulses. His intimate relationships often followed a sado-masochistic pattern.

Psychodynamics

The client seems to have experienced severe abandonment, helplessness, and anxiety in childhood. The frustration of basic needs in the client has led to compensatory aggression. From the psychodynamic viewpoint the client suffers from severe depression based on a narcissistic disorder connected with a strong sexual drivenness towards violent contact with women. There is a deep contempt in the client towards women, originating on the one hand from the frustration experienced with the mother, but also influenced by the father's sexual obsession. The denigration of women also seems to have the function of a defence against depression. The religious conversion has equipped the client with a strong superego which helps him to control himself in social life; nevertheless, this does not solve his inner conflicts. There is a very strong and violent destructive complex in the psyche which was formerly dealt with by directing it outwards to other people, but now it goes against the ego.

Course of therapy

In the first years of therapy the focus was on helping the client to formulate his needs and feelings and communicate them in social relationships, which helped to decrease the pressure of frustration and aggression. In the transference, the therapist came to carry the position of the threatening father. The experience of security in the therapeutic relationship which also included a certain control over the analyst helped to integrate these experiences and strengthen ego functions. In the course of therapy, the relationships with women changed and the client became capable of building a marriage and family. When his first son was born, the client experienced panic as he felt aggressive impulses towards the infant. By working through these impulses and their connection to early experiences in life, the inner pressure of frustration and aggression slowly receded. By the end of therapy, the client was living in a very solid social, family, and job situation. From time to time the client still needs to use violent pornographic videos to control his inner states of emptiness and frustration. In social life the client is now fully adapted. This low-frequency therapy took six years, with two minor interruptions, and 206 hours.

Comparison between the results of structural dream analysis and the course of therapy

The parallels between the structure of the dream series and the psychodynamics and course of therapy are apparent. The negative complex leading to aggression and sexual compulsiveness can easily be identified in the symbol of the threatening dogs, also because the dog symbolically is connected with sexuality; on the other hand, the image of the pursuing dogs is a very direct expression of the experience of the violent father. In the course of therapy, the dreamer becomes increasingly conscious of the neediness and helplessness behind the destructive complex, which culminates in the image of the helpless infant. To the extent that the client can accept these needs and take care of them the ego gains control over the complex and the destructive aspects become integrated. In the end, with a symbol of renewal, a new state of ego strength and wilful control over the personality has been established.

SDA is currently applied by research teams in Switzerland, Germany, Japan, and the United States. The aim of the joint international project is to build up a corpus of at least 30 cases which will allow for identifying structures across cases. Here the following questions will be investigated: are generalized structures to be found in the development of dreams in successful psychotherapies compared to failed ones? Are there connections between the type of psychopathology, e.g., depression, and the symbols and structures in the dreams?

An interesting preliminary result is that in successfully completed therapies a general structure can be found. Initially the dream ego is threatened by a dream figure representing a complex—the ego applies inadequate measures (flight, paralysis) and the threat persists. This pattern changes over the course of therapy to a pattern where the dream ego can manage the threatening figure with a constructive strategy and the threat vanishes or is incorporated; threatening animal figures become human (like in the exemplary case above). In all cases, strong parallels between symbolism of the dreams and the themes in therapy were found. The overall aim is to formulate an empirically grounded theory of the meaning of dreams and their development in the course of psychotherapies.

A general problem in the application of SDA is the risk that the interpretation is overly influenced by psychoanalytic concepts. One way to control for this influence is to engage interpreters not trained in psychoanalytic thinking. The advantage of SDA as an interpretive method is in its narratological orientation and exclusive focus on the text of the dreams. A future aim would be to cross-validate the results of this kind of analysis of psychotherapy processes with other process and outcome data in a multimethod psychotherapy process study.

References

Barrett, D., 1996. Dreams in multiple personality. In: **D. Barrett**, ed. *Trauma and dreams*. Cambridge, MA: Harvard University Press.

Barrett, D and **McNamara, P.**, eds., 2007. *The new science of dreaming. Vol. 2: Content, recall and personality correlates*. Westport: Praeger.

Boothe, B., 1994. *Der Patient als Erzähler in der Psychotherapie*. Göttingen: Vandenhoek & Ruprecht.

Cartwright, R. D., 1977. *Night life*. Englewood Cliffs: Prentice-Hall.

Cooper, J. C., 1978. *Dictionary of traditional symbols*. London: Thames and Hudson.

Fosshage, J. L., 1987. New vistas on dream interpretation. In: **M. Glucksman**, ed. *Dreams in new perspective. The royal road revisited*. New York: Human Sciences Press. pp. 23–43.

Greenberg, R. and **Pearlman, C.**, 1978. If Freud only knew: A reconsideration of psychoanalytic dream theory. *International Review of Psycho-Analysis*, **5**, 71–75.

Gülich, E. and **Quasthoff, U.**, 1985. Narrative analysis. In: **T. A. Van Dijk**, ed. *Handbook of discourse analysis, Vol. II*. London: Academic Press. pp. 169–19.

Hall, C. S. and **Van de Castle, R.**, 1966. *The Content Analysis of Dreams*. New York: Appleton-Century-Crofts.

Jung, C. G., 1925/1971. *Allgemeine Gesichtspunkte zur Psychologie des Traumes*. GW Bd. 8. Olten: Walter.

Levin, R., 1990. Psychoanalytic theories on the function of dreaming: a review of the empirical dream research. In: **J. M. Masling**, ed. *Empirical studies of psychoanalytic theories*. Hillsdale, NJ: Lawrence Erlbaum.

Lucius-Hoene, G. and **Deppermann, A.**, 2004. *Rekonstruktion narrativer Identität: ein Arbeitsbuch zur Analyse narrativer Interviews.* Wiesbaden: VS Verl. für Sozialwiss.

Moser, U. and von Zeppelin, I., 1996. *Der geträumte Traum. Wie Träume entstehen und sich verändern.* Stuttgart: Kohlhammer.

Palombo, S. R., 1982. How the dream works: the role of dreaming in the psychotherapeutic process. In: **S. Slipp**, ed. *Curative factors in dynamic psychotherapy.* New York: McGraw Hill. pp. 223–242.

Popp, C., Luborsky L., and Crits-Christoph, P., 1990. The parallel of the CCRT from therapy narratives with the CCRT from dreams. In: **L. Luborsky** and **P. Crits-Christoph**, eds. *Understanding transference. The CCRT method.* New York: Basic Books. pp. 158–172.

Propp, V., 1975. *Morphologie des Märchens.* Frankfurt a.M: Surkamp.

Roesler, R., 2018. *Research in Analytical Psychology. Empirical Research.* London: Routledge.

Narratives in decision making

Chapter 19

What's in a name?

Anecdotes, experience, and the meaning of stories

Christine Holmberg

Anecdotes

When it comes to complex medical decisions, cold hard statistics may hold little sway over patients in the face of a single, compelling anecdote.

(Szalavitz, 2012)

An anecdote is a literary genre defined as a short story that poignantly characterizes a situation, person, or event of general interest to an audience. It could, for instance, be a telling story about a famous person or an episode within an important historical event. It often has a funny twist or a surprising ending. Anecdotes may include societal critique or are an insightful description of existing moral orders and values, and thus provide a rich source for social and cultural analysis.

The term 'anecdote' has gained momentum in evidence-based medicine and decision-making research. Here, the term anecdote denotes a truncated story, often reported in the media, of a person's illness experience and particular treatment decisions, which may unduly skew other individuals' healthcare decision making. Examples of such celebrity stories include Warren Buffet's decision to go public about his experience with prostate cancer and Angelina Jolie discussing her decision to undergo an elective double mastectomy and elective oophorectomy (Garnick, 2012, Jolie Pitt, 2015). Such stories clearly influence other people's decisions to seek out medical care and/or diagnostic tests (Desai and Jena, 2016).

This influence of media stories on healthcare decision making is problematic, particularly because such stories often talk about medical diagnoses and practices that are surrounded by significant scientific debate, such as prostate-specific antigen (PSA) screening for prostate cancer risk or treatment choices for prostate cancer, and mammography screening for breast cancer. They often also present a single dominant storyline (see also Grob and Schlesinger, Chapter 23 in this volume).

Evidence-based medicine aims to inform medical care so that for treatment decisions the results of valid epidemiological study findings should be taken into account (Sackett et al., 1996), rather than individual stories. The prominent slogan 'from eminence to

evidence' (Bhandari, Zlowodzki, and Cole, 2004) highlights the aspiration to make medical treatment decisions more transparent and independent of an individual physician's
preferences or knowledge. An important driver of such approaches was, and is, the aim to
restrict or tame the pharmaceutical industry's influence on treatment choices in medical
care. To do so, a range of scientific research approaches, such as the randomized controlled trial, have been developed (Marks, 1997). However, evidence-based medicine is
not only about changing or making more transparent the knowledge base according to
which treatment decisions are made; it is predominantly a part of standardization procedures that coordinate and transform clinical work, and structure the involved actors and
situations in particular ways (Timmermans and Berg, 2003).

In Sackett and colleagues' (1996) ground-breaking work conceptualizing evidence-
based medicine, the authors constructed a triad of (i) epidemiological study findings (evidence); (ii) physicians' clinical expertise; and (iii) patients' choices; where all three should
be taken into consideration in healthcare decision making. In this model, patient choice
became a relevant factor in the conceptualization of healthcare provision for the first time.
Patients have likely always made their own decisions in the healthcare process, but they
did so perhaps more hidden from the physician's notice. Until the advent of Sackett et al.'s
paper, patient involvement played little role in the theoretical concepts of the medical
profession in terms of how healthcare delivery should take place. With this conceptualization, the idea of what a patient ought to be and how a patient should behave unfolded in
new ways (Cribb and Entwistle, 2011). From the perspective of proponents of evidence-
based medicine, this meant that patients needed to gain medical knowledge as well as
basic statistical understandings in order to understand the knowledge base of medical decision making and be able to engage in the decision-making process appropriately. From
this perspective, patients needed to understand their own values and preferences, as these
were considered an important part of decision making (Nelson et al., 2007).

Assigning a patient such an explicit role in terms of weighing his or her preferences
and choices in healthcare decision making has the implication that there is a 'right'
choice to be made (Landmark, Svennevig, and Gulbrandsen, 2016). It also assumes a
patient has a clear set of values and preferences. The ensuing research on how best to
present medical information and the available epidemiological information on patient-
friendly approaches within healthcare have led to a new field of decision research that
is concerned both with the presentation of information (Fagerlin et al., 2007, Fagerlin,
Zikmund-Fisher, and Ubel, 2011) as well as with what good decision making is (Vickers,
2017). Decision making is then conceptualized as a formal strategy, often following
algorithmic decision-trees (Samerski, 2002). To enable patients to follow such formal
and more deliberative decision-making approaches, the development of decision aids
to guide patients through their healthcare decision making and help them clarify their
values and preferences have become an important part of the provision of evidence-
based medicine (Coulter et al., 2013, Nelson et al., 2007). Shaffer and Zikmund-Fisher
(Chapter 20 in this volume) illustrate the scientific challenges and uncertainties faced in
the creation of such decision aids.

The endeavour to bring the patient formally into healthcare decision making, which aims to base decision making on epidemiological study findings, rather than on intuitive and implicit considerations, implies a substantial conflict with which proponents of evidence-based medicine must struggle: research shows that, by and large, individuals make decisions based on their own and others' experiences (Holmberg et al., 2017, Holmberg et al., 2015, Ziebland and Herxheimer, 2008), and more often than not, no explicit 'decision points' exist in the delivery of healthcare so that much of 'real life' decision making is not the deliberate process envisioned (Ziebland, Chapple, and Evans, 2015).

In the world of evidence-based medicine basing a decision on the experiences of others presents a problem, as these experiences may or may not be in line with what the 'scientific evidence' postulates. In the language of evidence-based medicine, such individual experiences are sometimes tagged as 'anecdotal evidence', in contrast to 'scientific evidence'. Anecdotal basically means that the information is based on an individual's story or stories, which may or may not be true, in contrast to the scientific evidence that is based on statistical analysis and reasoning. Sometimes the development of information sheets and decision aids to improve patients' knowledge of the medical and epidemiological aspects of their illness is tested with respect to how successful the information provision is towards minimizing the effects of anecdotes and skewing individual decision making so that it is based more on the provided medical and epidemiological information (Arkes and Gaissmaier, 2012).

The complexity of most healthcare decisions, with the ever-increasing influence of a wide variety of financial interests and players, make such a transparent presentation of information both highly desirable and necessary. However, there is a severe problem in the approach of judging people's experiences in comparison to epidemiological study findings or 'scientific evidence'. The two are different forms of knowledge, which cannot be compared or weighed against one another as if they were similar. Each presents epistemologically different forms of knowledge. The use of the term 'anecdote' or 'anecdotal evidence' for an individual's experiences devalues and misunderstands his/her stance and knowledge in comparison to statistically derived scientific evidence produced through epidemiological studies. To tease out this epistemological juxtaposition of experience and epidemiological evidence, and the profound differences between these different forms of knowledge, this chapter investigates the nature of what experience consists of based on scholars working from a phenomenological tradition.

Experience

What is experience? What does it mean when we speak of people making decisions based on experiences that they or others have had? How are experiences made? Throop (2003) provides a comprehensive answer based on phenomenological philosophers such as Dilthey, Merleau-Ponty, Husserl, Schutz, Heidegger, and James, as well as anthropological investigations into the nature of experiencing. Experiencing is understood as the process whereby the consciousness of an individual or a group of people comes into being, and social relations, modes of perception, things, and events are integrated to become our lived experiences. From a phenomenological perspective, experiencing the world begins prior to an organization of the stimuli encountered in forms and structures (James, 1996). James calls this 'pure experience',

> which he understood to be a non-reflexive, non-verbal, preconceptual 'feeling' that grasps the 'immediate flux of life' in terms of its undifferentiated unfolding in the field of sensory immediacy, prior to its organization into distinctive contents, forms, and structures (Throop, 2003, p. 229).

In this view, the medium and grounding of experience lies in the 'lived body' and is reflected in the concept of 'embodiment', which enables experiential engagements with the world in a pre-reflective space (Fuchs, Sattel, and Henningsen, 2010, Merleau-Ponty, 2012). Through the lived body, experiencing is always grounded in the materiality of the world and the sensual nature of the human body. It is from this basis of pure experience that forms of conceptualization, verbalization, narration, and understanding of 'experience' are derived. Through such reflective forms of experience, the objectification of the world comes into being. Thus, from a phenomenological perspective, differentiating between an outer (objective) and an inner (subjective) world does not make sense, as everything is mediated through modes of perception and becoming.

Such a perspective allows for an analysis and an understanding of what underlies processes of differentiation such as inner and outer world, e.g., the understanding and perception of things (Merleau-Ponty, 2012). These processes are structured by the historical and cultural conditions that inform the values, assumptions, ideals, and norms embedded within the lifeworld, which is what is perceived to be the pre-theoretical and familiar world in which people live (Desjarlais and Throop, 2011; Holmberg, 2005; Schütz and Luckmann, 2003). It is the lifeworld that provides the structures within which experiences may take on conscious form.

Experience always fluctuates between the unstructured and unreflected 'struggling along', a term coined by Desjarlais (1994, 1997) to describe a mode of being-in-the-world of inhabitants of a homeless shelter, and the effort of occupational therapists to create order in the midst of action, as Mattingly (1998) investigated in her ethnographic study on occupational therapy. As Throop (2003, p. 233) states:

> In the writings of James, Husserl and Schutz, I believe that we find a basis for outlining a model of experience that works to integrate the immediacy of temporal flux and the mediacy of reflective assessment. We find that for all three thinkers it is never simply an 'either/or', but a 'both/and' perspective that best characterizes the structure of experience. From the perspective of this model we can see that Mattingly is correct in her position that there is an important structural homology between narrative and experience. However, this model also incorporates those varieties of experience, significantly highlighted by Desjarlais, that even in their temporal structure, do not simply conform to the ordered coherence that is often implied in emplotted narrativity, a point that Mattingly (1998, p. 154) also recognizes in her assertion that it is perhaps not coherence but drama that serves as the pivotal link between narrative and experience.

Thus, to be human means that not all experience is narratively structured, although temporality does play a central role in the realm of experience and being-in-the-world.

Experience is temporally structured in that past experiences are always in the present moment and feed towards anticipated futures. At the same time, all experiencing includes gaps, discontinuities, and disjunctions of temporal movements, and presents important 'potential constituents of the structure of experience' (Mattingly, 1998). Such experiences feed into some of the heuristics, which have been identified as driving decision-making approaches of individuals (Finucane et al., 2000).

To further understand the relationship between experience and decision making in healthcare, it is important to recognize the temporal movement of experience in which a future orientation is already implicated. According to Throop, James argues that past experiences are part of each moment of our stream of consciousness as humans, and this 'feeds forward to anticipate the horizon of future perceptions, feelings, sensations, motivations, and actions' (Throop, 2003, p. 229). Thus, in the cognized present, we continually and unconsciously look backwards and forwards in time simultaneously with our lived body, and the cognized present therefore always includes encountered sensations of the past. Experiencing entails possibilities that are embedded in the temporal structuring of experience, with both cognized and pre-phenomenal behaviours structuring social action.

Such structuring requires culturally elaborated systems of significant symbols, 'webs of significance' (Geertz, 1973; Throop, 2003). Experiences become interpretable through such webs of significance, which help humans to structure their experiences into meaningful temporal sequences and order what might otherwise seem to be a dissolution of their everyday lifeworld; something that, according to Geertz, would lead to anxiety, angst, and disquiet (Geertz, 1973). Folktales, master narratives, or anecdotes are important vectors for such webs of significance and important sources out of which experiential structures are formed. Through them, moral values and understandings of the world are reflected and perpetuated and being-in-the world becomes palpable and meaningful.

In this reading, anecdotes present a powerful tool and point of reference with which to negotiate and order experience. Changing the webs of significance in healthcare is, of course, in part what proponents of evidence-based medicine approaches envision when they work against the stories of individual celebrities in the media. It becomes problematic when such representations become synonymous for individuals' experiences more generally. When the stories of actual patients are at stake, the use of the term 'anecdote' is a de facto devaluation of a particular experience since the usage of this language implies that it may simply not be a true and valid experience. Such a perspective does not help the aim of assisting patients in decision making. It not only devalues the patient's stance, but worse, hides the richness of information that personal stories can provide when it comes to understanding healthcare decision making and healthcare delivery (Kleinman, 1988).

Stories

Mulligan and Brunson (2017) have critiqued the way in which mainstream health policy researchers decry personal stories as 'incapable of providing the "evidence" necessary to develop and assess health policies'. In their analysis, they argue that according to such an understanding of how to create scientific evidence, stories become data points to be plotted on a graph, a process that makes those data points (stories) that are closer to the regression line 'truer' than the outliers. The web of significance that some proponents of evidence-based medicine wish for patients then comes down to a regression line. According to such a view, only many stories can give meaningful information since any individual story may always be an outlier and thus less true. Mulligan and Brunson (2017) contend that:

> stories represent a different kind of truth than survey responses or other types of measured behaviors that can be aggregated into a quantitative data set. At their heart, stories are an act of self-representation that tell us how someone makes sense of and understands their world. Stories issue from a particular person's perspective, and who the person is telling their story to can make a difference. Anthropologists and other researchers collect stories because we are interested in how people present and talk about themselves, make sense of their worlds, and decide about their health care. Stories can also provide important counterpoints and context that can reveal the blindspots of policymakers and researchers.

Thinking of other experiences based on a plot as more or less true is also a misrepresentation and misunderstanding of how others' experiences factor into healthcare decision making. For example, in risk contexts one's own and others' experiences are carefully compared and evaluated in order to come to a conclusion regarding how one's own risk may play out (Blakeslee, McCaskill-Stevens, and Parker, 2017; Gunn et al., 2017; Holmberg et al., 2015). Mattingly (1998) has argued that humans, in the midst of the messiness of life, try to work towards a narrative structuring of their doings. People's behaviours and interactions may provide a glimpse of their engagement with an ongoing temporal structuring of their actions, as they organize their action towards an intended future.

Mattingly has developed this idea in her observations of occupational therapists, where she developed the notion of 'therapeutical emplotment' (Mattingly, 1998), which describes the narrative structuring of therapeutic interactions with patients. According to Mattingly, in order to engage patients in therapy, a narrative plot structure is necessary. This means that single therapeutic activities are placed within a larger therapeutic story or story of healing. Therapeutic emplotment then means invoking hope by linking the therapeutic activity to a desired future, and thus hope and meaning are created and embedded within the therapeutic engagement. This process of emplotment and meaning-making is not done retrospectively and linguistically but is an ongoing process in which individuals work towards a narrative structure in their actions. Other people's experiences that are witnessed, experienced, or heard of can be seen as 'data points' that help structuring in the midst of action, sometimes by providing role models in terms of where one wants to be, at other times acting as companions (Caren Schnur, 2013) as one struggles along (Desjarlais, 1994).

But there is more to say about the more general view on storytelling and narration as one that brings coherence and order to the stream of consciousness that constitutes life in retrospect, rather than in the midst of it. There are two layers here that are of interest when looking at healthcare decision making and the role of other people's experiences in it. One is the story and its creation, and the other is the process of creation, and the activity of storytelling. It is necessary to elucidate both what a story may be and what storytelling may do in order to better understand the devaluation and misunderstanding of experience that occurs in some approaches to evidence-based healthcare decision making, as well as to appreciate more fully the value of individuals' stories.

In the process of storytelling, particular events become poignant and are ordered into a temporal sequence of meaningful events that highlight or explain things that have happened to oneself or others. However, as Jackson (2013, p. 21) has noted, 'Everything can be a story, if only because everything is the outcome of a process; although not everything is "sayable"'. Thus, stories are but one means through which experience acquires meaning (Jackson, 2013), or indeed may acquire many different meanings, all of which include some pattern of or orientation towards temporality. Throop (2003, p. 234) differentiates four temporal orientations that structure the experience of self and world:

> (1)an orientation to the present moment that consists of unfulfilled protentions as open anticipations toward an indeterminate future; (2) an explicit future orientation that consists of imaginal anticipations of a determinate future that are predicated upon residues of past experiences […]; (3) a retrospective glance that entails the plotting of beginnings, middles, and ends over the already elapsed span of a delimited field of experience; and (4) the subjunctive casting of possible futures and even possible pasts across the 'fluid space between a past and a future.'

Depending on when, where, and at what time of a process a story is told, this temporal orientation may lead to a different story than if it was told at another time and place. This means that meaning-making through temporal ordering, as one possible shaping of experience through narration, is a necessarily ever-changing activity and one that mainly captures those experiences that present a reflective stance (Desjarlais, 1994). The conditions of late modernity are particularly conducive to treating such individual stories as meaning-making and identity-shaping (Beck, Giddens, and Lash, 1994; Giddens, 1991; Taylor, 1989), since the telling of individual stories presents a crucial way of becoming aware of oneself and of creating self and identity. The story needs a listener to exist, and the storyteller needs a listener in order to receive the significance and acknowledgement for herself through which storytelling can become an act on the world (Maggio, 2014).

A story creates and shapes relationships between teller and listener. Stories need to be understood and analysed through the 'processual and contextual dynamics of storytelling' (Maggio, 2014, p. 91). In telling, stories 'rearrange and transform our experiences' (Jackson, 2013, p. 14). Stories are meaning-making devices that help those telling the story to acquire significance through the ear of the listener. Storytelling must be understood not only as one means to grasp the experiences of others but also as a crucial way of creating community and a 'sharable world' in which one can truly walk in the shoes of the other and recognize him or her. Through storytelling, the teller acts on the world and works towards shaping it to his liking (if a listener is present). The telling of stories thus changes the storyteller as much as listening to a story changes the listener (Frank, 1997).

Storytelling provides a unique space in which the teller and listener become immersed in an 'ethnographic present' (Hastrup, 1990); it is an intersubjective creation of experience (Maggio, 2014). The process of storytelling is therefore a means to enter the space of the other and reshape the distinction between the inner and outer world. Husserl understood intersubjectivity as the possibility to be 'in the place where the Other is' (Duranti, 2010, p. 16). Storytelling creates this space—one that may open up also the messy and discontinuous aspects of streams of consciousness, as postulated by James in terms of pure empiricism. Storytelling is about creating community and a shared lifeworld. In this view, storytelling becomes a 'vital human strategy for sustaining a sense of agency in the face of disempowering circumstances. To reconstitute events in a story is no longer to live those events in passivity, but to actively rework them, both in dialogue with others and within one's own imagination' (Jackson, 2013, p. 15). The manipulation of stories is thus different from a mere 'lie'; it presents a coping strategy through which the patient may change how they experience what is going on. Because storytelling creates an intersubjective space, it allows emotions to be transported from teller to listener, and a shared understanding and feeling becomes possible. This is a fundamental pre-requisite for social life.

> The facts that the world before us is held to be the same sharable world that we mutually inhabit, that others are recognized as experiencing beings who orient to and abide by the same sharable world as we do, that the bodies of others, which are objects and subjects for us, are often the zero point of their experiential fields and vice versa, are all deemed by phenomenologists to be necessary intersubjective building blocks to the very possibility and constitution of social life (Desjarlais and Throop, 2011, p. 91).

While in some aspects experiencing comes *before* storytelling, in other aspects it comes *during* storytelling. Experiencing is a deeply engrained sensual being-in-the-world with more or less structured parts. To grasp the profoundness of experience as human condition, not only retrospective forms such as storytelling need to be considered, but also forms of capturing the sensual and observational aspects of experience (Stroeken, 2010; Throop, 2003). On the one hand, this profoundness and nature of experience beyond storytelling and its inscription into the human body has yet to be integrated into the efforts of proponents of evidence-based medicine to make epidemiological study findings a meaningful ground for individual healthcare decision making. On the other hand, acts of storytelling are fundamental social acts that are central to enabling social life, social recognition, and healing. In this sense, stories are less important for their factual contents than for their meaning-making capacities and their ability to change the world and experience of both teller and listener. Storytelling itself shapes experience and is a form of acting on the world. The process of storytelling, together with past experience, constitutes the present and, more importantly, the subjunctive mode of the future (Good, 1994).

What's in a name?

Anecdotes, as a literary genre and trope that floats through societies, present the possibility to give cultural significance to things that happen to a person. As such, they present an important influence on individuals' lives, understandings, and experiences. Labelling media representations of individuals' experiences 'anecdotes' may be a valid assessment considering the literary genre and the importance of such representations as cultural tropes. What one often reads about, however, in evidence-based medicine approaches is an equation between 'anecdote', 'anecdotal evidence', and 'individual experience'. The use of such language and the equation of anecdote with what individuals experience and talk about presents a devaluation of experience, as well as a profound misunderstanding of what experience is, and even worse, of the importance for social life of shared experiences through storytelling. Calling such media stories and individual's experiences and individuals' sharing of healthcare and illness stories both as anecdotes is a misnomer.

Storytelling and the shaping of meaning is much more than a cultural trope. It is an embodied, intersubjective reality, which at the same time is radically subjective and world-making (Scarry, 1985). Experience is world-making and community-building because it is 'mediated through culturally shaped systems of linguistic, symbolic and representational forms' (Throop, 2003, p. 226). For this reason, as Troop (2003) highlights, both Geertz and Turner stress the 'suprapersonal, external, collective, shared and public nature of "experience" '. As relational anthropology has it today, being-in-the-world as 'dividuals' shapes and creates meaningful relationships (Niewöhner et al., 2016). Experience thus ties sensory, emotional, and bodily dimensions together with cognitive processes to shape human existence and being-in-the-world. Storytelling in part represents the cognitive processes in which the cultural and social structures can be discerned. It is, however, only one part of what experience consists of, as it fluctuates between messiness and coherence, as Husserl contends.

When people's healthcare decision making is influenced by experiences of self and other, this is a deeply embodied endeavour, and much more than listening to a story. Decrying lived experiences as false or anecdotal misses the significance of these fundamental aspects of the human condition, something that Arendt (1958) alluded to. Lived experiences are necessarily shaped by the experiential structures in which economic, scientific, social, cultural, and biological structures are enmeshed. They may therefore be considered 'false' from a scientific stance, but they are real, nonetheless (Stroeken, 2010, p. 40).

To change cultural practice, as evidence-based medicine sets out to do, the profoundness of experience should be taken seriously as an important signpost of how to enable and structure the envisioned and necessary changes. A regression line is unlikely to ever present the webs of significance that make life meaningful and create community and sociality. Considering the importance of anecdotes as cultural trope, new anecdotes need to be created which allow for an understanding of how social experiences may differ depending on how an individual goes about making healthcare decisions in the contemporary clinical setting.

Healthcare decision making has many of the elements as well as uncertainties involved in narrative emplotments. Treatment decisions are often characterized by different choices, of which one is not necessarily superior to another, but rather all are characterized by different risks and benefits. They work in the subjunctive mode in that they present possibilities and open ends and require patients to imaginatively evaluate the potential outcomes of treatment options. Healthcare decision making means imagining one's body as it might be in the future by relating it to one's own and others' experiences (Blakeslee, et al., 2017). Healthcare decision making is about finding a plot, which is inherently narratively structured. Helping patients to make 'better' decisions may thus necessitate presenting storylines in which future outcomes are envisioned that take both the intersubjective knowledge of patients and the scientific knowledge of epidemiology into account.

References

Arendt, H., 1958. *The human condition*. Chicago, IL: University of Chicago Press.

Arkes, H. R. and Gaissmaier, W., 2012. Psychological research and the prostate-cancer screening controversy. *Psychological Science*, **23**(6), 547–553.

Beck, U., Giddens, A., and Lash, S., 1994. *Reflexive modernization: politics, tradition and aethetics in the modern social order*. Stanford, CA: Stanford University Press.

Bhandari, M., Zlowodzki, M., and Cole, P. A., 2004. From eminence-based practice to evidence-based practice: a paradigm shift. *Minnesota Medicine Magazine*, **87**(4), 51–54.

Blakeslee, S. B., McCaskill-Stevens, W., and Parker, P. A., Gunn, C. M., Bandos, H., Bevers, T. B., Baggaglia, T. A., Fagerlin, A., Müller-Nordhorn, J., and Holmberg, C., 2017. Deciding on breast cancer risk reduction: the role of counseling in individual decision-making—a qualitative study. *Patient Education and Counseling*, **100**(12), 2346–2354.

Caren Schnur, N., 2013. Our stories, our companions: a conversation with Arthur W. Frank. *Storytelling, self, society*, **9**(2), 261–276.

Coulter, A., Stilwell, D., Kryworuchko, J., Mullen, P. D., Ng, C. J., and van der Weijden, T. 2013. A systematic development process for patient decision aids. *BMC Medical Informatics and Decision Making*, **13**(Suppl 2), S2.

Cribb, A. and Entwistle, V. A., 2011. Shared decision making: trade-offs between narrower and broader conceptions. *Health Expectations*, **14**(2), 210–219.

Desai, S. and Jena, A. B., 2016. Do celebrity endorsements matter? Observational study of BRCA gene testing and mastectomy rates after Angelina Jolie's *New York Times* editorial. *BMJ*, 355.

Desjarlais, R., 1994. Struggling along: the possibilities for experience among the homeless mentally Ill. *American Anthropologist*, **96**(4), 886–901.

Desjarlais, R., 1997. *Shelter blues. Sanity and selfhood among the homeless*. Philadelphia: University of Pennsylvania Press.

Desjarlais, R. and Throop, C. J., 2011. Phenomenological approaches in anthropology. *Annual Review of Anthropology*, **40**(1), 87–102.

Duranti, A., 2010. Husserl, intersubjectivity and anthropology. *Anthropological Theory*, **10**(1-2), 16–35.

Fagerlin, A., Ubel, P. A., Smith, D. M., and Zikmund-Fisher, B. J., 2007. Making numbers matter: present and future research in risk communication. *American Journal of Health Behavior*, 31(Suppl 1), S47–56.

Fagerlin, A., Zikmund-Fisher, B. J., and Ubel, P. A., 2011. Helping patients decide: ten steps to better risk communication. *Journal of the National Cancer Institute*, **103**(19), 1436–1443.

Finucane, M. L., Alhakami, A., Slovic, P., and Johnson, S. M., 2000. The affect heuristic in judgments of risks and benefits. *Journal of Behavioral Decision Making*, **13**(1), 1–17.

Frank, A. W., 1997. *The wounded storyteller: body, illness, and ethics*. Chicago, IL: University of Chigago Press.

Fuchs, T., Sattel, H. C., and Henningsen, P., 2010. *The embodied self. Dimensions, coherence and disorders.* Stuttgart: Schattauer.

Garnick, M. B., 2012. Buffett's prostate cancer: poor decisions, *Harvard Health Blog*, 23 April. Available at: <https://www.health.harvard.edu/blog/buffetts-prostate-cancer-poor-decisions-201204234621> (Accessed 27 October 2017)

Geertz, C., 1973. *The interpretation of cultures.* New York: Basic Books.

Giddens, A., 1991. *Modernity and self-identity: self and society in the late modern age.* Stanford: Stanford University Press.

Good, B., 1994. *Medicine, rationality and experience: an anthropological perspective.* Cambridge: Cambridge University Press.

Gunn, C. M., Bokhour, B., Parker, V. A., Parker, P. A., Blakeslee, S., Bandos, H., and Holmberg, C., 2017. Exploring explanatory models of risk in breast cancer risk counseling discussions: NSABP/NRG oncology decision-making project 1. *Cancer Nursing.* doi: 10.1097/NCC.0000000000000517.

Hastrup, K., 1990. The ethnographic present: a reinvention. *Cultural Anthropology*, 5(1), 45–61.

Holmberg, C., 2005. *Diagnose Brustkrebs. Eine ethnografische Studie über Krankheit und Krankheitserleben.* Frankfurt: Campus-Verlag.

Holmberg, C., Bandos, H., Fagerlin, A., Bevers, T.B., Battaglia, T. A., Wickerham, D. L., and McCaskill-Stevens, W. J., 2017. NRG oncology/national surgical adjuvant breast and bowel project decision-making project-1 results: decision making in breast cancer risk reduction. *Cancer Prevention Research.* doi: 10.1158/1940-6207.CAPR-17-0076.

Holmberg, C., Waters, E. A., Whitehouse, K., Daly, M., and McCaskill-Stevens, W., 2015. My lived experiences are more important than your probabilities: the role of individualized risk estimates for decision making about participation in the study of tamoxifen and raloxifene (STAR). *Medical Decision Making*, 35(8), 1010–1022.

Jackson, M., 2013. *The politics of storytelling: variations on a theme by Hannah Arendt.* 2nd edn. Copenhagen: Museum Tusculanum Press.

James, W., 1996. *Essays in radical empiricism.* Lincoln, NE: University of Nebraska Press.

Jolie Pitt, A., 2015. Angelina Jolie Pitt: diary of a surgery, *The New York Times*, 24 March. Available at: https://www.nytimes.com/2015/03/24/opinion/angelina-jolie-pitt-diary-of-a-surgery.html (Accessed 27 October 2017)

Kleinman, A., 1988. *The illness narratives: suffering, healing, and the human condition.* New York: Basic Books.

Landmark, A. M., Svennevig, J., and Gulbrandsen, P., 2016. Negotiating treatment preferences: physicians' formulations of patients' stance. *Social Science & Medicine*, 149, 26–36.

Maggio, R., 2014. The anthropology of storytelling and the storytelling of anthropology. *Journal of Comparative Research in Anthropology and Sociology*, 5(2), 89–106.

Marks, H. M., 1997. *The progress of experiment. Science and therapeutic reform in the United States, 1900-1990.* Cambridge: Cambridge University Press.

Mattingly, C., 1998. *Healing dramas and clinical plots: the narrative structure of experience.* Cambridge: Cambridge University Press.

Merleau-Ponty, M., 2012. *Phenomenology of perception*: London: Routledge.

Mulligan, J. and Brunson, E. K., 2017. The 'anecdote' insult, or, why health policy needs stories. *Medical Anthropology Quarterly*, 4 March. Available at: <http://medanthroquarterly.org/2017/03/07/the-anecdote-insult-or-why-health-policy-needs-stories/> (Accessed 24 October 2017)

Nelson, W. L., Han, P. K., Fagerlin, A., Stefanek, M., and Ubel, P. A., 2007. Rethinking the objectives of decision aids: a call for conceptual clarity. *Medical Decision Making*, 27(5), 609–618.

Niewöhner, J., Bieler, P., Heibges, M., and Klausner, M., 2016. Phenomenography. relational investigations into modes of being-in-the-world. *The Cyprus Review*, 28(1), 67–84.

Sackett, D. L., Rosenberg, W. M., Gray, J. A., Haynes, R. B., and Richardson, W. S., 1996. Evidence based medicine: what it is and what it isn't. *BMJ*, **312**(7023), 71–72.

Samerski, S., 2002. *Die verrechnete Hoffnung. Von der selbstbestimmten Entscheidung durch genetische Beratung*. Münster: Westfälisches Dampfboot.

Scarry, E., 1985. *The body in pain: the making and unmaking of the world*. New York: Oxford University Press.

Schütz A, Luckmann T (2003). *Strukturen der Lebenswelt*. Constance: UVK Verlagsgesellschaft mbH.

Stroeken, K., 2010. *Moral power: the magic of witchcraft*. New York: Berghahn Books.

Szalavitz, M., 2012. Why people stick with cancer screening, even when it causes harm, *Time*, 25 May. Available at: <http://healthland.time.com/2012/05/25/why-people-cling-to-cancer-screening-and-other-questionable-medical-interventions-even-when-they-cause-harm/> (Accessed 27 October 2017)

Taylor, C., 1989. *Sources of the self: the making of the nodern identity*. Cambridge: Cambridge University Press.

Throop, C. J., 2003. Articulating experience. *Anthropological Theory*, **3**(2), 219–241.

Timmermans, S. and Berg, M., 2003. *The gold standard. The challenge of evidence-based medicine*. Philadelphia, PA: Temple University Press.

Vickers, A. J., 2017. Decisional conflict, regret, and the burden of rational decision making. *Medical Decision Making*, **37**(1), 3–5.

Ziebland, S., Chapple, A., and Evans, J., 2015. Barriers to shared decisions in the most serious of cancers: a qualitative study of patients with pancreatic cancer treated in the UK. *Health Expectations*, **18**(6), 3302–3312.

Ziebland, S. and Herxheimer, A., 2008. How patients' experiences contribute to decision making: illustrations from DIPEx (personal experiences of health and illness). *Journal of Nursing Management*, **16**(4), 433–439.

Chapter 20

Narratives in decision aids
A controversy

Victoria A. Shaffer and Brian J. Zikmund-Fisher

Personal stories

Imagine Dana, a new mother anxiously awaiting the birth of her first child. She knows that the arrival of her child will result in many changes in her life. She is very much looking forward to being a mother, but she still feels unsure about exactly what this will mean in her life. She is aware that a baby will mean many sleepless nights, but how will the rhythms of her life change as the result of becoming a parent? As she prepares for her new role, she tries to gather as much information as possible about the experience of parenting an infant.

Dana could try doing this in several different ways. First, she might try to gather relevant facts about newborns. For example, she could try finding information from respected organizations, like the American Academy of Pediatrics, on the Internet. Using this method, she might find facts about parenting newborns like: a newborn baby eats approximately every three hours, sleeps one to three hours between feedings, and requires eight to twelve diaper changes per day. Such information may help if they correct factual misconceptions (e.g., that newborns tend to sleep longer than that amount of time).

Alternatively, Dana could rely on stories from friends, family, or other new mothers online to learn about life with a newborn. Using this approach, she may hear the following types of stories:

> My goal each day was just to shower, but I wasn't always successful. There is always something to do every hour or two. There is never a minute to sit and put my feet up and just relax. My daughter ate so frequently; it felt like having a job where I was working 24 hours a day, 7 days a week. The naps in between the feeding were often so short that by the time I did even one task, like folding the never-ending laundry, the nap was over. As a result, you will be so exhausted that basic tasks like eating or getting dressed will require too much effort. You will probably wear the same clothes all day and night and eat peanut butter directly from the jar instead of expending the energy to make a whole sandwich.

Narratives as texture

The story of Dana illustrates how information learned from narratives differs from didactic or fact-based forms of information. Specifically, the primary advantage of narrative information is that it can provide texture or context for the factual information (Heath and Heath, 2013).

In the case of parenting a newborn, the experiential information present in the narrative, but absent in the didactic information, can provide a richer, more complete description that can allow new mothers to be more adequately prepared for this next phase of their life. While searching for information about newborn schedules on reputable websites will provide useful and accurate information, the reader will struggle to apply this information and understand how these schedule disruptions might make them feel. For example, there is a difference between knowing that a new-born baby will need to eat every two to three hours, which will make you tired from having interrupted sleep, and hearing about how these frequent day and night wakings can make new parent feel so bone tired that they cannot muster up the cognitive energy to put together a complete sentence. That difference between knowing how something will affect your life and feeling how something will affect your life can help patients cope, prepare for the future, and have realistic expectations about their experiences (Focella, Zikmund-Fisher, and Shaffer, 2016).

Patient narratives (i.e., stories about health-related experiences that others have personally lived through) would therefore seem to have inherent value whenever someone is facing an unfamiliar situation. The textual information they provide complements, but does not replace, the role of didactic information. Yet, their use in patient decision aids—tools designed to help patients make decisions in cases of clinical equipoise—is a controversial practice (Holmes-Rovner et al., 2007; Bekker et al., 2013; Shaffer and Zikmund-Fisher, 2013).

This chapter first presents the case against using narratives in health communication materials, outlining three main concerns by decision psychologists and health services researchers. Taking these points into account, it then offers a rationale for including narratives in decision aids, despite the risks, because the balance of evidence suggests that the benefits outweigh the risks. Finally, it offers a method for developing evidence-based narratives, which will allow the experiential information of narratives to improve the decision process and will minimize the biases associated with individual stories.

Concerns about narratives

Why are narratives so controversial in this context? First, theoretical and empirical work in cognitive and social psychology suggests that narratives may be more powerful than other message formats. Broadly, research has suggested that narratives will have a stronger influence on decision making than didactic or statistical information. Narratives accomplish this by being more engaging (Cox and Cox, 2001; Volk et al., 2008) and more memorable than other message formats (Graesser, Olde, and Klettke, 2002; Kilaru et al., 2014), while being less likely to develop resistance to the message through the generation of counter arguments (Slater and Rouner, 1996; Green, 2006). In short, narratives can be much more persuasive.

Second, there is great concern among decision psychologists, physicians, and health services researchers that, because of their powerful influence, narratives can bias decision making. Although the impact of narratives on decision making can vary (e.g., Winterbottom et al., 2008; Shaffer and Zikmund-Fisher, 2013), several well-known studies have demonstrated that the use of narratives can significantly alter preferences for medical treatment. For example, Ubel and colleagues (2001) showed that participants responding to a hypothetical scenario about chest pain had significantly different preferences for treatment when provided with narratives and statistical data about the efficacy of the two treatments than when given statistical information only. Specifically, they preferred the less invasive treatment when provided with narratives but the more invasive treatment when only statistical data was provided. Additionally, Volandes and colleagues reported that participants had different preferences for end-of-life care for patients with dementia when provided with a video narrative about life with dementia compared with a verbal description of advanced dementia (Volandes et al., 2009; Volandes, Barry, and Chang, 2010). More participants who viewed the video narrative expressed a preference for comfort care over limited care or life-prolonging care (Volandes et al., 2009).

The use of narratives by health professionals is also considered controversial because the narratives themselves are not typically subject to scientific scrutiny; therefore, patient narratives provide an opportunity to pass on misinformation. For example, stories about vaccines causing autism exist and are shared despite evidence to the contrary (Witteman and Zikmund-Fisher, 2012; Doucleff, 2014; Cawkwell and Oshinsky, 2016; Hiltzik, 2015), and have had a significant influence on vaccination behaviour in the United States (Betsch et al., 2011; Brown and Sevdalis, 2011; Larson et al., 2011; Doucleff, 2014). Work by Betsch and colleagues (2011) reported a negative correlation between the number of anti-vaccine narratives read and vaccination intentions, with the influence of the narratives being stronger than the statistical information provided about vaccine risk. Further, the emotionality of the narratives also influenced the perceived risk of vaccines, where narratives that were more emotional resulted in greater perceived riskiness of vaccines. More recent work demonstrated that reading cases that were collected as part of the Vaccine Adverse Event Recording System (VAERS) in the US for the human papilloma virus (HPV) vaccine reduced interest in the HPV vaccine despite the fact that the VAERS data overwhelmingly supported the safety of the vaccine (Scherer et al., 2016). This suggests that even a single story about a person who believed their loved one was harmed by the vaccine can overpower data to the contrary from millions of patients.

Similarly, Arkes and Gaissmaier (2012) have argued that outrage over the recommendation against the use of the prostate specific antigen (PSA) test for prostate cancer screening by the US Preventative Services Task Force (USPSTF) is caused, at least in part, by the proliferation of narratives about how the PSA test saves lives. Despite the fact that the evidence reviewed by the USPSTF suggests that using the PSA test for early detection of prostate cancer does not provide a benefit to the population, public comment on the USPSTF recommendation reveals that people are more persuaded about the benefits of the PSA test from stories of people in their lives than from the epidemiological data

(Arkes and Gaissmaier, 2012). This common experience is frustrating to public health experts, whose data from thousands of patients is trumped by a single story.

A related criticism about the use of narratives in patient decision aids is that when narratives and statistical information are presented together, narratives can overshadow the statistical information (Ubel, Jepson, and Baron, 2001). For example, research in decision psychology has shown that when presented together, many people ignore statistical information and overweight individual stories in their decision making (Taylor and Thompson, 1982). More specifically, the use of narratives causes what decision psychologists refer to as 'base rate neglect', where people are more influenced by the vividness of the event than its likelihood of occurrence (Bar-Hillel, 1980; Bar-Hillel and Fischhoff, 1981). Returning to Betsch and colleagues' (2011) work on vaccination, the narratives about adverse events provided in these studies were more influential than base rate information about the frequency of these adverse events. Therefore, even when narratives appear alongside relevant statistics about risk information, the risk data is down-weighted relative to the narrative information, increasing perceived likelihood. This can have the consequence of making rare outcomes appear equally as likely as common ones. While this distortion of the information is not the same as narratives providing misinformation, the end result, where health behaviours are disproportionately influenced by narrative information, continues to frustrate public health experts and health professionals. In the case of PSA testing for prostate cancer, stories about lives saved are outweighing the population-level data that shows no difference in the number of deaths from prostate cancer between men who have been screened and men who have not. Here, the general public is underweighting what experts believe is the important information and not behaving in accordance with the epidemiological evidence.

Taken together, the controversy about using narratives in patient decision aids stems from their persuasive power, ability to bias medical decisions, and tendency to proliferate the spread of misinformation. As a result, practitioners of patient education are reluctant to use them in decision aids and other health communication interventions for fear of causing undue harm to the decision process.

Reasons in favour of using narratives

While there are reasons to be cautious about the potential for bias when using patient narratives in healthcare materials, the use of narratives in health communication should not be rejected outright. Rather, there are several reasons why narratives should instead be embraced as a powerful tool in our health communication toolbox.

The first reason to support the use of narratives in decision aids is that it is impossible to keep narratives out of the decision-making process. Narratives about healthcare experiences already exist, and they are competing with the evidence-based communications produced. Patients will hear them whether they actively seek them out or friends and family passively provide them. This 'one-sided use of narratives' has been observed in several debates about public health issues, including mammography screening and the use of vaccines (Meisel and Karlawish, 2011). Further, these one-sided stories are controlling the debate, and healthcare practitioners and public health experts who only bring facts and figures to the table lose the argument (Witteman and Zikmund-Fisher, 2012). Therefore, instead of constantly fighting narratives with more data, it makes more sense to use narratives in ways that harness their powerful influence to improve communication efforts. In fact, there are an increasing number of narratives available on the web that are curated either by patients themselves or by various health organizations, such as the DIPEx (database of patient experiences) project available at www.healthtalk.org (Herxheimer et al., 2000; Chou et al., 2011; Haigh and Hardy, 2011; Shaffer et al., 2016).

Second, other informational tools in the health communication toolbox have potential for bias, as do narratives. Standard didactic, plain-language descriptions about treatments and their risks and benefits are the hallmark of good risk communication and are used in almost all health communication tools. However, even the way this information is presented is rife with bias. For example, which treatment should be described first? Should benefits or risks be discussed first? It turns out that these choices matter (Fagerlin, Zikmund-Fisher, and Ubel, 2011). For example, Ubel and colleagues (2010) demonstrated that perceptions of a chemoprevention drug, tamoxifen, were more favourable when the risks of the drug were presented first as compared to presenting the benefits of the drug first.

Nor are there unbiased ways of presenting numerical information. The way that data are described significantly impacts risk perception (Fagerlin, Ubel, et al., 2007; Zikmund-Fisher, Fagerlin, and Ubel, 2010). Risks are perceived to be greater when numbers are displayed as frequencies as compared to percentages, e.g. '10/100' feels more likely than '10 percent' (Peters, 2012). Additionally, changes in risk that are described in terms of relative risks are perceived to be much larger than changes described in terms of absolute risks, e.g., difference between an absolute risk of 3% and 1.5% represents a 50% relative risk reduction (Malenka et al., 1993; Fagerlin, Zikmund-Fisher, and Ubel, 2007).

Reactions to less-familiar types of quantitative data can also be influenced by presenting the data in side-by-side comparisons rather than in isolation (Hsee, 1996; Zikmund-Fisher et al., 2004). The reason is that the interpretation of a number is heavily influenced by any available anchors or reference points (Tversky and Kahneman, 1974; Tversky and Kahneman, 1975). A known health application of this effect is that presenting comparative information can substantially alter risk perception, even at equivalent absolute levels of risk (e.g., 'Is my risk above or below the base rate?'). Fagerlin and colleagues (2007) demonstrated that being at greater than average risk increased the likelihood that people would elect to take a chemoprevention drug, while having a lower than average risk decreased interest in preventative treatment (Fagerlin, Zikmund-Fisher, and Ubel, 2007). Different ways of visually representing risk information (e.g., bar graph, pie chart, pictograph) also affect risk perception and comprehension (Fagerlin, Zikmund-Fisher, and Ubel, 2011).

Third, didactic and statistical information alone are not enough to combat major public health issues (Meisel and Karlawish, 2011), and hence narratives are necessary for effective health communications. When put in a head-to-head competition, narratives will generally be more influential than data (e.g., Betsch et al., 2011; Arkes and Gaissmaier, 2012). Therefore, our data-based communications will likely never be enough to motivate people to action or to counteract anecdotes that run counter to the evidence (Saffran, 2014). Further, beyond fighting stories with stories, narratives are also an important way the people make sense of data (Meisel and Karlawish, 2011; Saffran, 2014). In fact, we may be preprogrammed to need stories to understand quantitative evidence. Information is more easily processed in story form than in an abstract, statistical form (Borgida and Nisbett, 1977). Therefore, narratives can actually be used to improve health communication by illustrating the meaning of the scientific evidence and facilitating the translation and dissemination of research to the public.

In sum, narratives may be the most powerful tool we have in the health communication toolbox. As a result, it would put scientific progress at a disadvantage if narrative communication techniques are not employed. Patients will always be exposed to anecdotes and stories, whether intentionally or unintentionally. And, narratives do not introduce more bias than other tools in the toolbox; even standard approaches to health communication need to be carefully considered and are prone to bias. Narrative techniques can actually improve comprehension of evidence-based medicine and move patients to action (Meisel and Karlawish, 2011; Saffran, 2014). Therefore, researchers and practitioners should choose to deliberately bring narratives into the health communication toolbox. If not, the cycle will remain where stories outside of expert control counteract data-based health communications, and stories will continually be fought with more data.

How should narratives be used?

If narratives are treated as an important and useful tool in the health communication toolbox, the question remains of how narratives should be used? Meisel and Karlawish (2011) have argued that there are two important ways that narrative techniques can be utilized in health communication.

First, counter-narratives can be employed to 'neutralize' other stories that promote misinformation or conflict with existing scientific evidence. For example, the common narrative about PSA screening providing successful early detection for prostate cancer can be combatted with a counter-narrative describing decreased quality of life after receiving unnecessary treatment for prostate cancer.

Second, narratives can help the public understand the scientific process and improve translation of research findings. For example, when important guidelines change, the academic bodies responsible for the generation of new guidelines could craft a narrative illustrating their evidence-review and decision-making process, which could increase the transparency of the decision-making process associated with guideline development and increase understanding about the process of scientific inquiry. Using narratives for this purpose also takes advantage of their ability to reduce counterarguments (Slater and Rouner, 1996; Green, 2006). Narratives used in this way could either tell the story about how researchers reached these new conclusions or find patients whose stories illustrate the need for a change in the guidelines (e.g., a patient with ductal carcinoma *in situ* whose cancer was treated unnecessarily and resulted in side effects that reduced her quality of life). Further, narratives in this context will increase information recall (Graesser et al., 2002; Kilaru et al., 2014), by making the message 'more sticky' (Heath and Heath, 2008).

Which narratives should be used?

When narratives are used to inform audience perceptions of outcomes or experiences, a key consideration becomes the selection of which narratives to provide. Narratives, by definition, represent the experience or outcome of a single case—a very different type of information than population rates or distributions. In every communication, the narratives told are drawn from a distribution of all possible stories. As a result, a critical element of evidence-based storytelling is to clearly communicate where a given story falls on that distribution (Steiner, 2007).

One way that narratives can be misused or misunderstood is when stories that represent rare, or uncommon experiences, are assumed to illustrate a modal or common experience. Therefore, when choosing stories to tell under an evidence-based communication model, it will be important to be intentional about the selection of specific stories and consider which elements of the distribution are most important to highlight. For one health condition, this may mean selecting stories that emphasize experiences that are most representative of the population of experiences. If it is only possible to tell a single story in this case, then the storyteller must be explicit about where this narrative falls on the distribution (Steiner, 2005). For example, when sharing a story about a patient who experienced lymphoedema after undergoing radiation treatment for breast cancer, it is important to be clear that this side effect develops in a minority of patients who have this treatment; approximately one in five people treated with radiation will develop lymphedema. When possible, consider using multiple stories that can illustrate the range of possible experiences in the distribution, illustrating different themes and important variations (Steiner, 2005, 2007).

However, there will be other cases where it is more important to emphasize extreme values in the range of possible experiences. For some health conditions, patients typically overestimate or underestimate the pain or discomfort associated with a particular experience. For example, people often overestimate the negative impact of an ostomy on the quality of daily life (Angott, Comerford, and Ubel, 2013). In these cases, narratives representative of the modal experience will not improve affective forecasting errors, or biases in predictions of future experiences (Focella, Zikmund-Fisher, and Shaffer, 2016); Shaffer et al., 2016). Instead, presenting more extreme experiences (or targeted narratives) can help debias the general tendency to underestimate or overestimate the discomfort of an experience and provide more realistic expectations (Shaffer et al., 2016).

Narratives and data

This chapter maintains that while narratives should be used carefully in health communication, arguments in favour of their use outweigh concerns. It is hoped that the evidence and arguments herein have disabused readers (and other health services researchers and health communication practitioners) of the notion that narrative techniques should be automatically rejected from use in decision aids and other communications about healthcare.

Instead, the chapter argues for a new, integrative model that respects the complementary roles of both data and narrative communications in communications design. The question is not whether data-based communications OR narrative techniques should be employed; this is an artificial dichotomy that leaves some of the most effective communication tools unused in different situations. Instead, models of health communications should focus on how data-based communications *and* narrative techniques can routinely be used in complementary ways (c.f. Meisel and Karlawish, 2011).

This kind of approach is not trivial to implement. Instead, it will require research to create an evidence-based model of narrative communication that reflects up-to-date scientific evidence about how narratives can be used to improve comprehension of complex medical information. However, investing in this type of dual approach to health communication has the potential to yield significant benefits. In particular, selective, intentional use of narratives holds the potential to reduce public misunderstandings about the gap between evidence-based medicine and the patient experience.

References

Angott, A. M., Comerford, D. A., and Ubel, P. A., 2013. Imagining life with an ostomy: does a video intervention improve quality-of-life predictions for a medical condition that may elicit disgust? *Patient Education and Counseling*, **91**(1), 113–119.

Arkes, H. R. and Gaissmaier, W., 2012. Psychological research and the prostate-cancer screening controversy. *Psychological Science*, **23**(6), 547–553.

Bar-Hillel, M., 1980. The base-rate fallacy in probability judgments. *Acta Psychologica*, **44**(3), 211–233.

Bar-Hillel, M. and Fischhoff, B., 1981. *When do base rates affect predictions?* Perceptronics Descision Research, Eugene, OR. Available at: <http://www.dtic.mil/dtic/tr/fulltext/u2/a099491.pdf > (Accessed 10 May 2017).

Bekker, H. L., Winterbottom, A., Butow, P., Dillard, A. J., Feldman-Stewart, D., Fowler, F. J., Jibaja-Weiss, M. L., Shaffer, V. A., and Volk, R. J., 2013. Do personal stories make patient decision aids more effective? A critical review of theory and evidence. *BMC Medical Informatics and Decision Making*, **13**(S2), S9.

Betsch, C., Ulshöfer, C., Renkewitz, F., and Betsch, T., 2011. The influence of narrative v. statistical information on perceiving vaccination risks. *Medical Decision Making*, **31**(5), 742–753.

Borgida, E. and Nisbett, R. E., 1977. The differential impact of abstract vs. concrete information on decisions. *Journal of Applied Social Psychology*, **7**(3), 258–271.

Brown, K. and Sevdalis, N., 2011. Lay vaccination narratives on the web: are they worth worrying about? *Medical Decision Making*, **31**(5), 707–709.

Cawkwell, P. B. and Oshinsky, D., 2016. Storytelling in the context of vaccine refusal: a strategy to improve communication and immunisation. *Medical Humanities*, **42**(1), 31–35.

Chou, W. Y. S., Hunt, Y., Folkers, A., and Augustson, E., 2011. Cancer survivorship in the age of YouTube and social media: a narrative analysis. *Journal of Medical Internet Research*, **13**(1), e7.

Cox, D. and Cox, A. D., 2001. Communicating the consequences of early detection: the role of evidence and framing. *Journal of Marketing*, **65**(3), 91–103.

Doucleff, M., 2014. *How vaccine fears fueled the resurgence of preventable diseases*. Available at: <http://www.npr.org/sections/health-shots/2014/01/25/265750719/how-vaccine-fears-fueled-the-resurgence-of-preventable-diseases>. (Accessed 5 January 2016).

Fagerlin, A., Ubel P. A., Smith, D. M., and Zikmund-Fisher, B. J., 2007. Making numbers matter: present and future research in risk communication. *American Journal of Health Behavior*, **31**(S1), S47–S56.

Fagerlin, A., Zikmund-Fisher, B. J., and Ubel, P. A., 2007. 'If I'm better than average, then I'm ok?': comparative information influences beliefs about risk and benefits. *Patient Education and Counseling*, **69**(1–3), 140–144.

Fagerlin, A., Zikmund-Fisher, B. J., and Ubel, P. A., 2011. Helping patients decide: ten steps to better risk communication. *Journal of the National Cancer Institute*, **103**(19), 1436–1443.

Focella, E. S., Zikmund-Fisher, B. J., and Shaffer, V. A., 2016. Could physician use of realistic previews increase treatment adherence and patient satisfaction? *Medical Decision Making*, **36**(6), 683–685.

Graesser AC, Olde B, Klettke B (2002). How does the mind construct and represent stories? In: **M. C. Green**, J. J. Strange, and T. C. Brock, eds. *Narrative impact: social and cognitive foundations*. Mahwah, NJ: Lawerence Erlbaum Associates, Inc. pp. 229–262.

Green, M. C., 2006. Narratives and cancer communication. *Journal of Communication*, **56**(S1), S163–S183.

Haigh, C. and Hardy, P., 2011. Tell me a story—a conceptual exploration of storytelling in healthcare education. *Nurse Education Today*, **31**(4), 408–411.

Heath, C. and Heath, D., 2008. *Made to stick: why some ideas die and others survive*. 2nd edn. New York: Random House.

Heath, C. and Heath, D., 2013. *Decisive: how to make better choices in life and work*. New York: Random House.

Herxheimer, A., McPherson, A., Miller, R., Shepperd, S., Yaphe, J., and Ziebland, S., 2000. Database of patients' experiences (DIPEx): a multi-media approach to sharing experiences and information. *Lancet*, **355**(9214), 1540–1543.

Hiltzik, M., 2015. *Jenny McCarthy: anti-vaxxer, public menace*. Available at: http://www.latimes.com/business/hiltzik/la-fi-mh-jenny-mccarthy-antivaxxer-public-menace-20150127-column.html (Accessed 6 January 2016).

Holmes-Rovner, M., Nelson, W. L., Pignone, M., Elwyn, G., Rovner, D. R., O'Connor, A. M., Coulter, A., and Correa-de-Araujo, R., 2007. Are patient decision aids the best way to improve clinical decision making? Report of the IPDAS Symposium. *Medical Decision Making*, **27**(5), 599–608.

Hsee, C. K., 1996. The evaluability hypothesis: an explanation for preference reversals between joint and separate evaluations of alternatives. *Organizational Behavior and Human Decision Processes*, **67**(3), 247–257.

Kilaru, A. S., Perrone, J., Auriemma, C. L., Shofer, F. S., Barg, F. K., Meisel, Z. F., 2014. Evidence-based narratives to improve recall of opioid prescribing guidelines: a randomized experiment. *Academic Emergency Medicine*, **21**(3), 244–249.

Larson, H. J., Cooper, L. Z., Eskola, J., Katz, S. L., and Ratzan, S., 2011. Addressing the vaccine confidence gap. *Lancet*, **378**(9790), 526–535.

Malenka, D. J., Baron, J. A., Johansen, S., Wahrenberger, J. W., Ross, J. M., 1993. The framing effect of relative and absolute risk. *Journal of General Internal Medicine*, **8**(10), 543–548.

Meisel, Z.F. and Karlawish, J., 2011. Narrative vs evidence-based medicine—and, not or. *JAMA*, **306**(18), 2022–2023.

Peters, E., 2012. Beyond comprehension: the role of numeracy in judgments and decisions. *Current Directions in Psychological Science*, **21**(1), 31–35.

Saffran, L., 2014. 'Only connect': the case for public health humanities. *Medical Humanities*, **40**(2), 105–110.

Scherer, L. D., Shaffer, V. A., Patel, N., and Zikmund-Fisher, B. J., 2016. Can the vaccine adverse event reporting system be used to increase vaccine acceptance and trust? *Vaccine*, **34**(21), 2424–2429.

Shaffer, V. A., Focella, E. S., Scherer, L. D., Zikmund-Fisher, B. J., 2016. Debiasing affective forecasting errors with targeted, but not representative, experience narratives. *Patient Education and Counseling*, **99**(10), 1611–1619.

Shaffer, V. A. and Zikmund-Fisher, B. J., 2013. All stories are not alike: a purpose-, content-, and valence-based taxonomy of patient narratives in decision aids. *Medical Decision Making*, **33**(1), 4–13.

Slater, M. D. and Rouner, D., 1996. Value-affirmative and value-protective processing of alcohol education messages that include statistical evidence or anecdotes. *Communication Research*, **23**(2), 210–235.

Steiner, J. F., 2005. The use of stories in clinical research and health policy. *JAMA*, **294**(22), 2901–2904.

Steiner, J. F., 2007. Using stories to disseminate research: the attributes of representative stories. *J Gen Intern Med*, **22**(11), 1603–1607.

Taylor, S. E. and Thompson, S. C., 1982. Stalking the elusive 'vividness' effect. *Psychological Review*, **89**(2), 155–181.

Tversky, A. and Kahneman, D., 1974. Judgement under uncertainty: heuristics and biases. *Science*, **185**(4157), 1124–1131.

Tversky, A. and Kahneman, D., 1975. Judgment under uncertainty: heuristics and biases. In: **D. Wendt** and C. Vlek, eds. *Utility, probability, and human decision making. Selected proceedings on an interdisciplinary research conference, Rome, 3–6 September, 1973*. Dordrecht: D. Reidel Publishing Company. pp. 141–162.

Ubel, P. A., Jepson, C., and Baron, J., 2001. The inclusion of patient testimonials in decision aids: effects on treatment choices. *Medical Decision Making*, **21**(1), 60–68.

Ubel, P. A., Smith, D. M., Zikmund-Fisher, B. J., Derry, H. A., McClure, J., Stark, A., Wiese, C., Greene, S., Jankovic A., and Fagerlin A., 2010. Testing whether decision aids introduce cognitive biases: results of a randomized trial. *Patient Education and Counseling*, **80**(2), 158–163.

Volandes, A. E., Barry, M. J., Chang, Y., and Paasche-Orlow, M. K., 2010. Improving decision making at the end of life with video images. *Medical Decision Making*, **30**(1), 29–34.

Volandes, A. E., Paasche-Orlow, M. K., Barry, M. J., Gillick, M. R., Minaker, K. L., Chang, Y., Cook, E. F., Abbo, E. D., El-Jawahri, A., and Mitchell, S. L., 2009. Video decision support tool for advance care planning in dementia: randomised controlled trial. *BMJ*, **338**, b2159.

Volk, R. J., Jibaja-Weiss, M. L., Hawley, S. T., Kneuper, S., Spann, S. J., Miles, B. J., and Hyman, D. J., 2008. Entertainment education for prostate cancer screening: a randomized trial among primary care patients with low health literacy. *Patient Education and Counseling*, **73**(3), 482–489.

Winterbottom, A., Bekker, H. L., Conner, M., and Mooney, A., 2008. Does narrative information bias individual's decision making? A systematic review. *Social Science & Medicine*, **67**(12), 2079–2088.

Witteman, H. O. and Zikmund-Fisher, B. J., 2012. The defining characteristics of Web 2.0 and their potential influence in the online vaccination debate. *Vaccine*, **30**(25), 3734–3740.

Zikmund-Fisher, B. J., Fagerlin, A., and Ubel, P. A., 2004. 'Is 28% good or bad?' Evaluability and preference reversals in health care decisions. *Medical Decision Making*, **24**(2), 142–148.

Zikmund-Fisher, B. J., Fagerlin, A., and Ubel, P. A., 2010. Risky feelings: why a 6% risk of cancer does not always feel like 6%. *Patient Education and Counseling*, **81**, S87–S93.

Section 8

Narratives in healthcare

Chapter 21

Understanding and using health experiences to improve healthcare— examples from the United Kingdom

Lisa Hinton, Louise Locock, and Sue Ziebland

Introduction

This chapter explores the variety of ways in which people's narrative accounts of their health experiences can be harnessed to inform practice, service development, and health policy as well as a more traditional research agenda. Collecting data on patient experience as an activity in isolation is not enough. There is a strong case for health experiences to be used to improve care (Ziebland et al., 2013, Coulter et al., 2014). This chapter presents examples of projects conducted in the United Kingdom where patient narratives collected as part of the Healthtalk project (www.healthtalk.org) for health service improvement have been used.

How do we know what matters to patients?

The endeavour of collecting and understanding patient experiences has expanded and matured in recent years. Patient experiences can be gathered through many routes: unsolicited sources, such as complaints direct to hospitals and also a wide variety of research and audit methods including questionnaire surveys (either national, local, or hospital specific), in video feedback kiosks in hospitals where patients can leave feedback messages, in focus groups (run face-to-face or online), and in research interviews in various forms (structured, semi-structured, or narrative). These sources are varied in the kinds of data they can give, and in the Internet age, they are diversifying rapidly. Similarly, what matters to patients can be captured through a range of sources such as ratings websites (e.g., Patient Opinion, or service-specific ones) as well as less-direct sources, such as YouTube videos, Twitter, social media sites, personal blogs, and online patient forums, see Box 21.1.

There are strengths and limitations to all sources of patient experience data. The detail (richness) of the experience is to a large degree dependent on the source—a narrative interview will potentially give richer insights into a patient's experiences of healthcare (e.g., an outpatient hospital appointment, inpatient care) than responses given to a patient satisfaction questionnaire. The insights from an interview may also uncover unanticipated

> **Box 21.1 Examples of online sources of patients' views**
>
> 1. Patient Opinion
> 2. You Tube video channel for patient feedback
> 3. Twitter handles
> 4. Social media
> 5. Blogs/vlogs
> 6. Patient forums

details of care that would be glossed over by patients in questionnaire responses that are often overly positive (Ziebland, Evans, and Toynbee, 2011). But conversely, constrained by time and money, researchers may be able to collect questionnaire responses from hundreds of patients, but narrative interviews with only a few.

The Health Experiences Research Group (HERG) in the University of Oxford's Nuffield Department of Primary Care Health Sciences has conducted over 100 narrative studies of health experiences since 1999 that form an archive of interviews with more than 4,000 patients. Since 2001, analytic summaries of key themes in these patient experiences, illustrated with video and audio excerpts from the interviews, have been published on the website Healthtalk.org (formerly known as DIPEx and Healthtalkonline), designed as a resource for patients, relatives, and carers, the general public, policy makers, and health professionals in practice and training. HERG researchers have also published over 180 peer-reviewed papers in clinical and social science journals and the interview archive has been used for numerous secondary analyses, reports, and papers.

The value of narrative

Narratives engage hearts as well as minds, conveying a message 'under the radar' and bypassing rational objections. Psychological approaches, such as transportation theory and the concept of narrative persuasion (Cin et al,. 2004; Green and Brock, 2000), suggest that narratives are a credible, powerful, and persuasive way of accessing human experience, transporting us directly into another's perspective. This can encourage care providers to rethink attitudes and motivate them to reflect on how services could be improved (Greenhalgh, Russell, and Swinglehurst, 2005; Bate and Robert, 2007). Authors in the Journal of the American Medical Association (JAMA) argued that 'although narrative is often maligned as anecdote and thus scrubbed from the toolbox of guideline developers, epidemiologists and regulatory scientists, these experts should consider narrative to develop and translate evidence-based policies'(Zachary and Karlawish, 2011).

Box 21.2 provides examples of where a secondary analysis of illness narratives, originally collected for use on the Healthtalk.org website and now stored in the Health Experiences Research Group (HERG) archive, has been used. Each study here has used transcripts of interviews previously collected for other projects for a re-analysis to inform new research studies

Box 21.2 Studies using transcripts of interviews previously collected for other projects for a re-analysis to inform new research studies

- 'Information for Choice' project included secondary analysis of five collections from the HERG archive (Hunt et al., 2009)

- Identifying item pools for questionnaire development e.g., e-Health Impact Questionnaire (Kelly et al., 2013)

- Analysis of 80 + narrative interviews to inform General Medical Council 'end of life' guidelines for doctors (GMC, 2010)

- Redesigning the medical curriculum on autism for family doctors (Soar et al., 2014)

- Gathering treatment uncertainties from patient/carers using different methods: evaluation report for the Oxford Biomedical Research Centre with the James Lind Alliance Hip and Knee Replacement for Osteoarthritis Priority Setting Partnership (Crowe and Regan, 2014)

- Service improvement 'trigger films' for co-design workshops (Locock et al., 2014)

- Informing NICE Guideline and Quality standards (Ziebland et al., 2014)

Secondary analysis

Patient experiences can inform health policy across areas wider than the single health conditions. These activities can take place as part of the primary research project, or through secondary analysis projects (Heaton, 2004). One example was a 2014 study funded by the National Institute of Health Research (NIHR) to use a secondary analysis of a purposive sample of HERG narrative interviews (on experiences of autism, rheumatoid arthritis, cancer, and infertility) to identify core components of what 'good healthcare' looks like. Initial analyses were tested in focus groups with hard-to-reach populations (e.g., travellers, migrant workers, people with a long-term condition). A scientific summary was published in the NIHR publications library and illustrative clips were included on Healthtalk. org (Ziebland et al., 2014). See Box 21.3.

Service improvement 'trigger films' for experience-based co-design

Another avenue for making use of patient narratives for service improvement is through an approach called experience-based co-design (EBCD), a participatory action research approach in which patients and staff work together to improve quality. In its pure form (Bate and Robert, 2007, The King's Fund, 2013) it is based on narratives collected via local interviews with patients and staff about their experiences of a particular service (the discovery phase). Interviews with patients are recorded on video, and short trigger films of their experiences are produced to show to staff and patients working together as equal partners. Agreed priorities for change are taken forward to staff and patient/carer groups to plan and implement improvements together (the co-design phase). Evaluations suggest

> **Box 21.3 What does good healthcare look like to patients?**
>
> 1. Having a friendly and caring attitude.
> 2. Having some understanding of how my life is affected.
> 3. Letting me see the same health professional.
> 4. Guiding me through difficult conversations.
> 5. Taking time to answer my questions and explain things well.
> 6. Pointing me towards further support.
> 7. Efficient sharing of my health information across services.
> 8. Involving me in decisions about my care.

that this approach is highly effective (Piper et al., 2012, Donetto et al., 2015), but also time and resource intensive. This led to a project testing whether the national narrative studies in the HERG/Healthtalk archive could be used to contribute to service improvement.

'Accelerated' experience-based co-design (AEBCD)

In this accelerated form of EBCD, trigger films on lung cancer and intensive care were produced from a secondary analysis of the HERG archive instead of conducting local interviews in the discovery phase. These were used in two trusts as the first step in the process, enabling the trusts to move swiftly to the co-design phase. Both staff and patients engaged positively with the material, and similar results to a traditional EBCD project were achieved (Locock et al., 2014).[1] Importantly this study demonstrated that existing narrative data could be re-used to stimulate change across multiple sites, without the need to repeat interviews in each new location.

Having demonstrated proof of concept in this initial study, the same material from Healthtalk has been further re-used in the SILENCE study aimed at lowering elements of noise in the critical care environment.[2] The intensive care unit (ICU) is a specialist hospital ward where the most critically ill or unstable patients are cared for. A patient in ICU usually has one-to-one nursing care, as they require constant medical attention and support to keep their body functioning. They may be unable to breathe and have multiple organ failure. Patients are often sedated or unconscious. The units tend to be small, highly technical environments with several monitors at each bedside. They are also noisy. Although the World Health Organization (WHO) recommends that the average hospital sound levels should not exceed an average of 35dBA with peak sounds no lounder than 40dBA (Berglund et al., 1999). But in reality a typical ICU is about as loud as a busy restaurant or the traffic on a main road (around 60dB) (Darbyshire and Young, 2013). This cacophony of unfamiliar noises can be terrifying to vulnerable patients, and high background noise is likely to contribute to abnormal sleep and ICU-acquired delirium, which can in turn lead to longer hospital stays and more health problems after discharge (Darbyshire et al., 2016).

The overall aim of the SILENCE study was to design an intervention to reduce noise levels in the ICU. In addition to technical changes, a practical behaviour change was attempted, informed by patient narratives.[3] In the summer 2015 a joint staff and patient workshop used the AEBCD framework and showed trigger films produced from the narratives of patient and relative experiences of ICU in the HERG archive. Sixteen people, including three patients, two patient advocates, ICU nurses, doctors and a manager, were shown trigger films themed around 'alarms', 'lights', 'being disturbed by equipment', 'being disturbed by people', and 'feeling overwhelmed'. The group agreed a cohesive package of changes required to enable the ICU to become 'quiet'.

Developing training materials based on patient narratives

Individuals prefer to learn in different ways. This must be accounted for when designing an educational intervention to ensure that all learners have a productive experience. Honey and Mumford (1986) describe four stereotypes. These are reflectors (those who when provided with new information prefer to consider this thoroughly before acting), activists (who prefer to learn by experimentation), theorists (integrate information into a coherent and rational scheme), and pragmatists (keen to receive concepts directly applicable to them and less interested in abstract theory).

Taking account of this variation, the findings from the secondary analysis of narratives and the AEBCD event were used to inform the development of a teaching package for ICU staff in a UK hospital. This was designed to raise awareness of the effect high noise levels can have on the patient experience of intensive care and had something to offer for all learning styles. It incorporated an e-learning module that included information presented in a variety of formats, as well as self-assessment questionnaires. It also included an experiential aspect, a critical part of the adult learning processes. Adults learn very differently from children and are motivated by perceived personal need. Kolb and Fry (1975) describes a cycle by which adults reflect upon experiences and adapt their behaviours based on this reflection. Therefore, experiential learning is a powerful tool in adult education (Kolb and Kolb, 2005).

During the experiential session staff were asked to lie on a hospital bed, as if a patient. They were played simulated ICU sounds, given poor vision (with an eye mask) and subjected to 'live activities' going on around them. This live action was based on activities witnessed during ethnographic observation sessions undertaken earlier in the SILENCE project and included having their blood pressure and oxygen saturation measured (with altered alerting parameters to induce an unexpected alarm), drawers and doors being opened, apron rollers spinning, bin lids crashing, and trolleys being pushed by.

An assessment tool was also designed to test knowledge and attitudes post-training. Nurses, doctors, and physiotherapists took part. When asked to describe the immersive experience staff identified words such as 'uncomfortable', 'watched', 'alone', 'frightening',

'confused', and 'worrying'. Staff found the experience useful and felt it re-created the patient experience well. They described various changes to their own practice including
reassuring patients and reducing noise through lowering verbal volume and attending
to equipment noise and alarms more swiftly. The combination of environmental changes
and awareness teaching successfully reduced noise levels by about 4dB with before and
after median (inter quartile range) 24-hour levels of 57.0 (3.2) and 53.2 (5.1) respectively.
Sound level 'signatures' were also altered after the intervention suggesting that a reduction in peak values may be the 'driver' for the change.

Potential drawbacks to using health narratives to guide healthcare improvements

Patients' narratives about their experiences can be powerful, invoking a strong emotional
response from those who engage with them. They can also be memorable, shaping staff
practices in subtle as well as overt ways. These characteristics mean that they have the
potential to do harm as well as good, especially if the members of staff close ranks de-
fensively, or suspect that the narratives have been chosen to criticize practice or reflect
minority interests.

Any improvement work may divert staff from usual patient care, adding strain to the
delivery of the service—it is therefore imperative that the narratives are chosen carefully,
that they provide balanced reflections on care and (as far as can be ascertained) do not
serve as a vehicle for vested interests.

Patients' narratives are nowadays also freely available online through blogs and social media as well as feedback sites. To date, there has been little examination of the
individual and organizational responses to the use of online feedback in the NHS. The
diffusion of innovations in healthcare, especially information technology-based innovation, is complex and influenced by multiple individual and organizational factors. For
example, many clinicians appear resistant to the idea of online feedback, worrying about
selection bias, vulnerability to 'gaming' or malice, and concerned that there is no fundamental relationship between subjective patient experience and objective care quality
(Greenhalgh et al., 2004, Greenhalgh et al., 2008, Ward et al., 2008, McCartney, 2009).
A pilot review of Patient Opinion in Scotland suggests that some organizations regarded
patients' comments as 'unreasonable' (Better Together, 2012). While there is no representative data on the attitudes and behaviour of health professionals to online feedback,
and no in-depth analysis of the barriers and facilitators to guide its use in NHS organizations, a multi-discliplinary study was underway in 2016 to explore these issues in English
hospitals.[4]

While narrative has the potential to be persuasive and memorable, there are some
drawbacks. Firstly, in the context of a medical culture of evidence-based medicine, evidence derived from narrative may be resisted as less 'valid' than quantitative studies.
Experience suggests that once people are exposed to narrative its importance becomes
obvious, but getting them in the room in the first place may be difficult. In particular,

engaging doctors in quality improvement remains a challenge (Davies et al., 2007). Secondly, narrative research is time and resource intensive and requires particular skills to collect and analyse data in a rigorous and theoretically informed way. This is where re-use of existing research, through secondary analysis and through re-use of existing narrative materials, can help.

Notes

1. The project *Testing accelerated experience-based co-design: a qualitative study of using a national archive of patient experience narrative interviews to promote rapid patient-centred service improvement* was funded by the National Institute of Health Research (NIHR) Health Service & Delivery Research (HS&DR) scheme (10/1009/14). The views expressed are those of the authors and not necessarily those of the NHS, the NIHR or the Department of Health.

2. The project *Sleep in the Intensive Care Unit: lowering elements of noise in the critical care environment (SILENCE)* was funded by the NIHR Research for Patient Benefit (RfPB) scheme (PB-PG-0613-31034). The views expressed are those of the authors and not necessarily those of the NHS, the NIHR or the Department of Health.

3. http://www.healthtalk.org/peoples-experiences/intensive-care/intensive-care-patients-experiences/topics. Module funded by Intensive Care National Audit and Research Centre (ICNARC)

4. The project *Improving NHS quality using internet ratings and experiences (INQUIRE)* was funded by the National Institute of Health Research (NIHR) Health Service & Delivery Research (HS&DR) scheme (14/04/48). The views expressed are those of the authors and not necessarily those of the NHS, the NIHR, or the Department of Health.
https://www.phc.ox.ac.uk/research/health-experiences/research-projects/improving-nhs-quality-using-internet-ratings-and-experiences-inquire

References

Bate, P. and Robert, G., 2007. *Bringing user experience to healthcare improvement: the concepts, methods and practices of experience-based design*. Oxford: Radcliffe Publishing.

Berglund, B., Lindvall, T., and Schwela, D., 1999. *Guidelines for community noise*. Geneva: World Health Organization.

Better Together, 2012. Patient Opinion evaluation. *Twintangibles.* Available at: https://www.patientopinion.org.uk/resources/poscotland-eval-final.doc (Accessed 20 October 2017).

Coulter, A., Locock, L., Ziebland, S., and Calabrese, J., 2014. Collecting data on patient experience is not enough: they must be used to improve care. *BMJ*, **348**, g2225.

Crowe, S. and Regan, S., 2014. James Lind Alliance. Gathering treatment uncertainties from patients/carers using different methods: Evaluation Report for Oxford Biomedical Research Centre. Oxford Health Experiences Research Group and the JLA Hip and Knee Replacement for Osteoarthritis Priority Setting Partnership. Available at: <http://www.jla.nihr.ac.uk/news-and-publications/downloads/Different%20methods%20of%20gathering%20treatment%20uncertainties%20final-evaluation-report.pdf>. (Accessed 16 October 2017).

Dal Cin, S., Zanna, M. P., and Fong, G. T., 2004. Narrative persuasion and overcoming resistance. In: E. S. Knowles and J. A. Linn, eds. *Resistance and persuasion*. Mahwah, NJ: Lawrence Erlbaum Associates. pp. 175–91.

Darbyshire, J. L., Greig, P. R., Vollam, S., Young, J. D., and Hinton, L., 2016. 'I can remember sort of vivid people ... but to me they were plasticine.' Delusions on the intensive care unit: what do patients think is going on? *PloS ONE*, **11**(4), e0153775.

Darbyshire, J. L. and Young, J. D., 2013. An investigation of sound levels on intensive care units with reference to the WHO guidelines. *Critical Care*, 17(5), R187.

Davies, H. A., Powell, A., and Rushmer, R., 2007. Why don't clinicians engage with quality improvement? *Journal of Health Services Research & Policy*, 12(3), 129–130.

Donetto, S., Pierri, P., Tsianakas, V., and Robert, G., 2015. Experience-based co-design and healthcare improvement: realizing participatory design in the public sector. *The Design Journal*, 18(2), 227–248.

General Medical Council, 2010. *The development of treatment and care towards the end of life: good practice in decision making*. Available at: <http://www.gmcuk.org/Story_of_the_EoL_guidance2. pdf_32510823.pdf>. (Accessed 18 February 2014).

Green, M. C. and Brock, T. C., 2000. The role of transportation in the persuasiveness of public narratives. *Journal of Personality and Social Psychology*, 79(5), 701–21.

Greenhalgh, T., Robert, G., Macfarlane, F., Bate, P., and Kyriakidou, O., 2004. Diffusion of innovations in service organizations: systematic review and recommendations. *Milbank Q* 82(4), 581–629.

Greenhalgh, T., Russell, J., and Swinglehurst, D., 2005. Narrative methods in quality improvement research. *Quality and Safety in Health Care*, 14(6), 443–449.

Greenhalgh, T., Stramer, K., Bratan, T., Byrne, E., Mohammad, Y., and Russell, J., 2008. Introduction of shared electronic records: multi-site case study using diffusion of innovation theory. *BMJ*, 337, a1786.

Heaton, J., 2004. *Reworking qualitative data*. London: Sage.

Honey, P. and Mumford, A., 1986. *Using your learning styles*. 2nd ed. Maidenhead: Peter Honey.

Hunt, K., France, E., Ziebland, S., Field, K., and Wyke, S., 2009. 'My brain couldn't move from planning a birth to planning a funeral': a qualitative study of parents' experiences of decisions after ending a pregnancy for fetal abnormality. *International Journal of Nursing Studies*, 46(8), 1111–1121.

Kelly, L., Jenkinson, C., and Ziebland, S., 2013. Measuring the effects of online health information for patients: item generation for an e-health impact questionnaire. *Patient Education and Counseling*, 93(3), 433–438.

The King's Fund, 2013. *Experience-based co-design toolkit*. Available at: <https://www.kingsfund.org.uk/projects/ebcd>. (Accessed 2 June 2017)

Kolb, A. Y. and Kolb, D. A., 2005. Learning styles and learning spaces: enhancing experiential learning in higher education. *Academy of Management Learning & Education*, 4(2), 193–212.

Kolb, D. A. and Fry, R., 1975. Toward an applied theory of experiential learning. In: C. L. Cooper, ed. *Theories of group processes*. London: Wiley. pp. 33–58.

Locock, L., Robert, G., Boaz, A., Vougioukalou, S., Shuldham, C., Fielden, J., Ziebland, S., Gager, M., Tollyfield, R., and Pearcey, J., 2014. Testing accelerated experience-based co-design: a qualitative study of using a national archive of patient experience narrative interviews to promote rapid patient-centred service improvement. *Health Services and Delivery Research*, 2(4).

McCartney, M., 2009. Will doctor rating sites improve the quality of care? No. *BMJ* 338(b1033).

Piper, D., Iedema, R., Gray, J., Verma, R., Holmes, L., and Manning, N., 2012. Utilizing experience-based co-design to improve the experience of patients accessing emergency departments in New South Wales public hospitals: an evaluation study. *Health Services Management Research*, 25(4), 162–172.

Soar, S., Ryan, S., and Salisbury, H., 2014. Using patients' experiences in e-learning design. *The Clinical Teacher*, 11(2), 80–83.

Ward, R., Stevens, C., Brentnall, P., Briddon, J., 2008. The attitudes of health care staff to information technology: a comprehensive review of the research literature. *Health Information & Libraries Journal*, 25(2), 81–97.

Zachary, M. and **Karlawish, J.**, 2011. Narrative vs evidence-based medicine—and, not or. *JAMA*, **306**(18), 2022–2023.

Ziebland, S., Evans, J., and **Toynbee, P.**, 2011. Exceptionally good? Positive experiences of NHS care and treatment surprises lymphoma patients: a qualitative interview study. *Health Expectations*, **14**(1), 21–8.

Ziebland, S., Coulter, A., Calabrese, J. D., Locock, L., 2013. *Understanding and using health experiences: improving patient care*. Oxford: Oxford University Press.

Ziebland, S., Locock, L., Fitzpatrick, R., Stokes, T., Robert, G., O'Flynn, N., Bennert, K., Ryan, S., Thomas, V., and **Martin, A.**, 2014. *Informing the development of NICE (National Institute for Health and Care Excellence) quality standards through secondary analysis of qualitative narrative interviews on patients' experiences. Health Services and Delivery Research*, **2**(45). DOI: 10.3310/hsdr02450.

Chapter 22

Illness narratives as evidence for healthcare policy

Susan Law, Ilja Ormel, David Loutfi, and John Lavis

Introduction

> *Collecting data on patient experience is not enough: they must be used to improve care ...*

> *(Coulter et al., 2014)*

Collecting and using information about patient preferences and experiences of illness has become a growth industry around the globe over the past decade—for both the scientific and decision-making communities engaged in promoting evidence-informed health service delivery. This trend has been fuelled by system-wide policies and programmes for greater patient and public engagement and patient-centred care, research funding opportunities from national granting agencies that require patient partnerships and knowledge translation strategies to improve care, the emergence of training programmes for patients and public, and demand from patients and family members themselves. The most potent arguments in bringing patient voices to the fore, however, come from the emerging evidence about impact—e.g., improvements in quality of care (effectiveness and efficiency gains), patient and professional experiences, and health outcomes (Coulter, 2012; Hibbard and Green, 2017). On the research side, there has been rapid growth in the science of collecting qualitative and quantitative information about patient experience, and, to some extent (as noted in the epigraph), there have been efforts to apply this knowledge in quality improvement processes, largely at the institutional and clinical levels of care within the healthcare system (Coulter et al., 2014). One of the areas deserving of further attention, however, is the integration of patient experience 'data' as evidence within healthcare policy.

This chapter addresses how patient narratives about experiences of illness, including their needs for information and support, can inform health policy processes that aim to improve health and healthcare. It considers the challenges and opportunities for qualitative researchers and for policy makers (including elected officials, political advisors, and public/civil servants) in bridging these different worlds to support the integration of narrative evidence into policy structures and processes. It focuses on the potential value and use of evidence-based collections of narratives or stories (as told by patients, family, and/

or caregivers) that feature a diverse range of individuals and types of experiences to influence political and public opinion, and eventually shift policy. It argues for the cultivation of a deliberate and bi-directional link between the scientific production of this particular type of evidence and the messy, real world of policy making to promote change that is both evidence-based and that matters to patients and families.

First, it explores the different worlds of narrative research and policy making, and then considers mechanisms to bridge the gap between these worlds through effective knowledge translation, with some examples of success. Finally, it offers advice for policy makers and for researchers regarding communication and engagement to promote more effective and efficient exchanges where the need for narrative evidence and its supply might intersect.

Policy and research: different worlds

Policy and the aspiration of *evidence*-informed decision making for patient-centred care

The world inhabited by policy makers is typically characterized as quite distant from that of researchers and knowledge generation, where scientific information is but one type of input to decision-making processes that combine evidence, values, and external factors through some form of collective deliberation, and within a set of institutional constraints, to formulate policy (Lomas et al., 2005; Black, 2001; Lavis et al., 2002; Greenhalgh and Russell, 2009). Nonetheless, inspired by the evidence-based medicine movement, there has been growing support from health systems (see, for instance, the UK Best Research for Better Health Strategy, 2006), and from research granting agencies (see, for instance, the Strategy for Patient-Oriented Research, Canadian Institutes for Health Research, 2011) to strengthen structures and processes that privilege the use of evidence in policy and practice (Lomas, 1997). Such knowledge translation strategies to facilitate evidence-informed decision-making have been characterized as efforts by researchers to 'push' evidence to knowledge users, approaches by healthcare organizations to 'pull' evidence from decision making, or strategies that promote means of 'exchange' or engagement between researchers and decision makers (Ellen et al., 2013). Yet the policy domain presents unique challenges to the notion of evidence-informed decision making for many reasons, including: those related to the nature, availability, and value of evidence; the human and behavioural limitations associated with decision making in policy contexts— e.g., bounded rationality and tendencies towards satisficing; the structures and processes for policy development and implementation; and the more pragmatic constraints imposed in policy settings (McCaughey and Bruning, 2010; Oliver et al., 2014). It is for these reasons that the policy world is described as inherently 'messy', with decision-making processes that defy the more 'naïve rationalism' tenants of the evidence-based medicine movement, and where policy-making processes are construed as 'the struggle over ideas and values' involving rhetoric and argument that set the path to decisions (Russell et al., 2008). Processes to define questions and answers in policy regarding what should be done to achieve particular social objectives, do indeed exist in a different world involving a different type of discourse and process, than the world where questions and answers are addressed through the scientific process.

The more recent shift in health policy worldwide to promote patient-centred healthcare has brought expectations for new types of evidence, related to patient and family experience, to be factored into decision making at clinical, organizational, and systems/policy levels. There has been encouragement from government, healthcare organizations, and health research agencies alike to invest in a deeper understanding of the lived experiences of patients and family members with respect to their illness and interactions with the healthcare system, followed by strategies to apply this learning in policy and practice to improve health and healthcare (World Health Organization, 2000; US Department of Health and Human Services, 2008; Ontario Legislature, 2016). The focus on patient and family-centred care also inspired new mechanisms of engaging patients and families in research and in the application of results for service, organizational, and/or health system redesign—with patient, research, and health system-led initiatives. 'No decision about us without us' was the influential phrase adopted by a UK government policy white paper to stimulate a shift to a more patient and public-focused National Health Service (Secretary of State for Health, 2010, p. 13). There has been a consequent rise in 'co-design' approaches applied to policy and practice where patients, families, and professionals are engaged with researchers in processes of 'discovery' (knowledge creation) and 'design' (knowledge use)—as an extension of the 'exchange' mechanism towards integrated knowledge translation (Bate and Robert, 2006).

The rationale for policies and practice to promote patient-centred care and engagement is wide ranging and includes evidence related to cost-effectiveness, enhanced experiences of care, and better health (Coulter, 2012)—consistent with Triple Aim objectives for health reform (Berwick et al., 2008). There are current efforts around the globe to improve the measurement, collection, and reporting of quantitative and qualitative evidence of patient experience, and in particular, to understand experience in relation to other measures of clinical outcomes and quality (see, for instance, Black et al., 2014; Manary et al., 2013). Overall, the theoretical and practical issues around collecting and applying evidence about patient experience to inform policy have very much turned to questions of 'how' rather than 'why'. On the quantitative side, there are now validated, and in several cases mandated, tools to capture the more meaningful notion of patient and family 'experience' in place of 'satisfaction', such as the Hospital Consumer Assessment of Healthcare Providers and Systems (HCAHPS) survey tools developed in the United States and adapted in Canada as the Canadian Patient Experience Survey (CPES). This was developed by the Canadian Institute for Health and Information and endorsed by Accreditation Canada (Canadian Institute for Health Information, 2015). A relatively simple evaluation tool was developed in the United Kingdom—the Friends and Family Test (FFT)—now mandated throughout the National Health Service as a measure of experience. Furthermore, there is a growing literature on the effectiveness of collecting and using patient and family experiences to support shared decision making in clinical settings (Barry and Edgman-Levitan, 2012), patient-reported outcome and experience measures (Black, 2013), experience-based co-design initiatives (Boyd et al., 2012), and deliberative processes to engage patients in the development of recommendations for policy or systems guidance (Boivin et al., 2014).

In summary, there are broad policy initiatives and a growing body of evidence in support of patient-centred care, yet there are attributes of the world of policy making that create challenges for evidence-informed decision making. Next, we consider the challenges and opportunities related to the type of research that aims to gather patient experience as evidence, and the goal of applying this evidence to healthcare policy. The subsequent section argues that there are mechanisms to bring these worlds closer together through strategies for integrated knowledge translation. Furthermore, as Flyvbjerg (2001) suggests, in studying this dynamic between the experiences of patients as actors in the healthcare system and policy making as an integral component of the structure of healthcare systems, there are analytic opportunities for advancing social science for greater social relevance—in consideration of the factors at individual versus programme, organizational, or system/policy levels that lead to actions and consequences for the other, what he terms 'actor/structure' connections.

Narrative research and the aspiration of *experience*-informed policy making for patient-centred care

There are many examples of national efforts to promote programmes of research dedicated to understanding patient experiences, promoting patient engagement in research, and to understand the impact of experience and engagement on practice and policy, such as the Patient-Centered Outcomes Research Initiative (PCORI) in the United States (Frank et al., 2015) and the Strategy for Patient-Oriented Research (SPOR) in Canada (Canadian Institutes for Health Research, 2011). These initiatives have contributed to new methods for gathering this type of evidence, and a growing body of evidence (both qualitative and quantitative) as a potential source of information available to decision-making processes at practice and policy levels. This chapter focuses on the value and contribution of qualitative research to produce evidence about patient experience.

According to Pope and Mays (1995), qualitative research reaches 'the parts other methods cannot reach' and there are established methods for gathering evidence about people's experiences and perspectives, such as through focus groups, deliberative processes, and individual narrative interviews (open and in-depth) with a diverse sample of participants (Ziebland, 2013). This type of evidence may then be available as an input or sources of information for decision-making processes alongside other types and sources of information, providing ideas for policy development and/or insights, and feedback regarding existing policies and practices. Yet, given limitations related to the production and use of narrative evidence for health system improvement (Greenhalgh et al., 2005), as well as uncertainties regarding the notion of patient-centred care in health policy (Kitson et al., 2013), it is not surprising that there will be both challenges and opportunities related to aspirational goals set for experiential evidence to inform policy (see also Meyer and Xyländer (Chapter 5) as well as Grob and Schlesinger (Chapter 23) this volume).

The Database of Individual Patient Experience (DIPEx) initiative is an example of national-level efforts, now established using standardized methods in 13 countries (see: http://www.dipexinternational.org), to produce and share experiential evidence through collections of narratives about health and illness. This initiative was launched in 2001 at the University of Oxford (Ziebland and McPherson, 2006) with the explicit purpose of enhancing public and professional understanding of patient and family experiences. The approach involves a two-stage interview with the first as an open narrative question 'Tell me about your experience in living with xx from the beginning when you noticed something had changed' followed by semi-structured questions to address issues relevant to illness experiences as documented in the literature or raised by clinical and patient advisors. In the qualitative analysis of the transcripts, the research team (that typically includes patients, family, and community members) identifies topics of greatest importance to the participants, and the data is summarized under these topics or themes and presented on the web site with illustrative audio, video, or text clips from the original interviews. Participants sign a copyright form for use of their material on the web, in teaching, and for future research and other non-commercial applications. The intent with each module is to highlight the diversity of lived experience and range of perspectives that are balanced and supported with best available evidence; indeed, the substantial contribution and strength of this approach is in the representation of diversity of voices and varied experiences in the results. This is in contrast to the use of individual testimonials such as presented in the media or for marketing purposes. The impact of the UK healthtalk.org resource (with over 100 health and illness topics, and more than 30,000 voices represented, featured in the online collection) has been overwhelmingly positive as a public health information web resource, in teaching (Field and Ziebland, 2008), further research, the redesign of health services (Locock et al., 2014), and, in policy although with fewer examples to date (discussed more further on).

Here, this section offers a brief overview of some of the challenges associated with the nature and valuation of narrative evidence as a source of evidence in decision making. These types of considerations may help to inform efforts to bridge these two worlds, as discussed in the subsequent section with regards to opportunities provided through the principles and practice of integrated knowledge translation.

Key challenges in the production of experiential evidence relate to issues that are first, more generally associated with qualitative research, such as the perceived lack of value for this work, in combination with the lack of training and skill in conducting and appraising qualitative studies—leading to noted problems of publication bias, discounting of relevance and significance for theory or practice, and lower success rates in research granting cycles (Greenhalgh et al., 2016). These problems contribute to the lack of available evidence in the public domain, and generally lower proximity of qualitative researchers to policy makers. Second, are challenges related specifically to the DIPEx approach, such as:

◆ sampling—e.g., What is a 'national' sample? What is success with respect to maximum variation in terms of experiences and personal attributes?

◆ recruitment—how to ensure inclusion of marginal or vulnerable groups? Given the departure from usual assurances of confidentiality and anonymity in research, and online presentation of results, who is not represented in the sample?

◆ curated collection—the need to curate and update collections to adjust for temporal changes in health service interventions, context, and/or patient preferences.

◆ how to accommodate context and culture in cross-country comparisons of findings from DIPEx collections.

Nonetheless, there are considerable strengths to be acknowledged in this approach that uses rigorous scientific methods to generate evidence in the form of insights about the lived experiences and information needs of people with particular illnesses relevant to questions about health system improvement. Yet, in considering the path to policy influence, several challenges arise related to how policy agendas are set, when and how evidence contributes to decision making in policy development, and how policy is implemented and monitored.

Public policy is 'a set of interrelated decisions taken by a political actor or group of actors concerning the selection of goals and means of achieving them within a specified situation where these decisions should, in principle, be within the power of these actors to achieve' (Jenkins, 1978). The goals of health policy development and implementation are typically concerned with maximizing health and optimizing the delivery of healthcare and are largely the domain of governments in setting guidance for structures and actors in the system (Doern and Phidd, 1992). Policy development in healthcare, as in other areas, is considered primarily a decision-making *process*, but health policy itself should also be viewed, as argued by Malone (1999), as a *product* with important implications for people and society on moral and economic dimensions. Policy makers at the level of government, and other decision-making organizations with policy authority, typically have a limited range of instruments through which to exert their power, such as those that are legal (e.g., regulations, acts, or the creation of agencies), economic (e.g., taxes, fees, or insurance schemes), voluntary (e.g., standards, guidelines, partnerships, and networks), and information and educational by nature (Lavis and Hammill, 2016).

The opportunity to influence the policy process, as proposed by Kingdon (1984), begins with the convergence of three separate 'streams' or sets of factors related to problems and possible solutions: the *problem* stream (e.g., changes in national indicators for a programme or comparison of performance between jurisdictions); the *policy* stream (e.g., assessment of possible solutions given technical feasibility, public acceptability, etc.), and the *political* stream (e.g., public opinion, interest groups, changes in authority or governance). In this model, a 'policy window' opens to permit change or modification of the policy agenda when these three streams come together. Experiential evidence could contribute information in any one of these streams, as a source of feedback about a problem or a particular policy introduced to address a problem. People who can effectively bring these factors together, as a 'policy entrepreneur', may help to move an issue onto the government's agenda. Subsequent phases of policy development and implementation, are influenced by *institutions* (e.g., government structures, policy legacies, and networks), *interests* (e.g., patient groups, industry groups, elected officials, etc.), and *ideas* about *what is* and *what ought to be* (e.g., from sources such as research evidence, tacit knowledge, mass opinion, etc.), and contextual or external factors (e.g., political change, new disease, technological change)—known as the 3-i framework (Hall, 1997; Gauvin, 2014). Experiential evidence fits within this framework as a source of ideas, but can be mobilized by interests, such as patient groups, and research networks, and its use can be institutionalized—to feature in structures and processes related to policy formulation and implementation.

Enabling strategies to bridge narrative evidence and policy

This section briefly outlines five areas where there may be important opportunities for creating better bridges or connectivity between narrative evidence and policy—within each there are different strategies that may be deployed by researchers and/or policy makers as key actors in the system to bring experiential evidence closer to consideration in policy. These areas constitute a framework that can be used to assess progress in the adoption of strategies to support evidence-informed decision making (Moat and Lavis, 2012).

Creating a climate for research use

The extent to which, in a given jurisdiction, health and social policy agendas and health system actors value the use of research evidence to inform policy, organize, and advocate for evidence-informed decision making can be assessed, in part, by considering a broad range of contextual factors related to the integration of research evidence in policy. These factors and activities, such as support for knowledge syntheses and the creation of KT resources, contribute to a 'climate' for evidence-informed policy making within a jurisdiction (see, for example, Ongolo-Zogo et al., 2014). Contributions to shifting the climate or culture within any particular jurisdiction can be supported by actions on either side—by government to invest in functions, organizations, and resources that support research production and use, or by researchers who can produce the sorts of evidence that are relevant to policy problems.

Prioritization and co-production

Likely among the strongest strategies for bridging the worlds of policy and research involve collaboration among policy makers and scientists to set priorities for research based on health system and policy needs, such as the 'listening' initiatives in Canada and the United Kingdom (Lomas et al., 2003), and/or to engage in the co-production of new knowledge (Lomas, 2000). The James Lind initiative offers a patient-led model for priority-setting that engages patients and clinicians in a deliberative process to define the top research questions to fill knowledge gaps regarding clinical uncertainties

(Petit-Zeman et al., 2010). The literature on public and patient engagement in healthcare policy and priority-setting indicates substantial opportunity for the field of narrative research to contribute both content regarding patient perspectives and methods expertise to these tables (see, for instance: Mitton et al., 2009; Conklin et al., 2012).

The adoption of approaches that involve the co-production of knowledge via collaboration between decision makers and researchers, such as in participatory research (Green et al., 1995) and integrated knowledge translation (Kohtari, McCutcheon, and Graham, 2017), are more likely to yield greater value for health and healthcare in comparison to research that does not involve knowledge users (Jagosh et al., 2012; Canadian Institutes for Health Research, 2013). Experience-based co-design (EBCD) is another such model, though rarely tested in the policy context, that involves the engagement of qualitative researchers, patients, and healthcare professionals in a process of 'discovery' to identify patient and family experiences of care, and then 'design' to implement change to improve the quality of care (Bate and Robert, 2006; King's Fund, 2013).

Enhancing packaging and push

On the research side, a substantial array of resources and tools now exists, largely from academic centres and health research funders, to support researchers' ability to package research results in ways relevant and useful to decision makers and policy. For example, the Health Systems Learning initiative at the McMaster Health Forum builds on the above frameworks to provide practical resources and tools for researchers to help identify the multiple factors that influence policy processes and provide examples of potential interventions to promote the uptake of evidence in agenda setting, and policy development and implementation (Lavis, 2015; see: https://www.mcmasterhealthforum.org/about-us/our-resources). Lavis and colleagues also include considerations of external factors, such as changes in technologies or new investment opportunities, consistent with other models of policy analysis that consider more explicitly the context for policy development and change (see, for example, Walt and Gilson, 1994). Researchers are encouraged to review the SUPPORT series and tools developed by this group, which also features resources for policy makers regarding how to find and use research evidence (Lavis, 2016) as well as how to make use of the best-available evidence (Lavis, 2013). In the United Kingdom, narrative evidence produced by the Health Experiences Research Group (HERG) at Oxford University and published on www.healthtalk.org has explicitly contributed (alongside other types and sources of evidence) to national policy guidance. Examples include health system policy guidance for improving the experiences of users of adult mental health services (National Institute for Health and Care Excellence, 2011) and a government-funded report on young people's views on obesity and body size, shape, and weight (Rees et al., 2013) to inform the development of policy for this group. Furthermore, this research group has illustrated the potential value in conducting secondary analysis of such collections to expedite the production of policy-relevant evidence, with examples of applications in accelerated co-design and in the development of national guidelines on end of life care (Ziebland and Hunt, 2014).

Facilitating pull

Strategies for facilitating the 'pull' of evidence into policymaking are more the domain of governments and research funders, and include mechanisms to co-locate or embed researchers within decision-making or policy organizations (see, for example, the recent launch of Health System Impact Fellowships sponsored by the Canadian Institutes for Health Research to provide training opportunities for graduate students within health system organizations), the direct commissioning or co-sponsorship of research by government, and creating opportunities to showcase the best available research in response to identified policy problems (e.g., the 'Best Brains' initiative funded by Canadian Institutes for Health Research in Canada that brings experts together in closed sessions to meet with government decision makers to develop solutions to priority problems). An example of an innovative practice in this area has been developed by the provincial Ministry of Health in British Columbia (BC), Canada. The Patient-Centred Performance Measurement and Improvement team designed a programme for routine comprehensive reporting that now includes qualitative data alongside routinely collected quantitative data 'to give life to the numerical data', using quotes and narrative evidence in text boxes alongside tables and charts of performance measures (Cuthbertson, 2015). Their aim is to humanize the measurement data to engage clinicians and healthcare leaders in quality improvement with respect to provincial standards. Evaluation of this initiative has indicated that the inclusion of qualitative data in combination with quantitative data contributes to clinical perception of validity of the data, and that the real transformational value of these reports lies in stimulating local conversations about quality between health system leaders and clinical teams (Cuthbertson and Parsons, 2016). Finally, health system and policy organizations can facilitate pull by building 'receptor' capacity among decision makers for finding and using the results of research (Denis et al., 2008).

Enabling exchange

Strategies that facilitate formal and informal opportunities for enhanced exchange or connectivity between policy actors and researchers will contribute to enhanced relevance of research activities in response to policy priorities, and enhanced use of the results and products of research (Lomas, 2000). Exchange is a key element of knowledge translation that often 'takes place within a complex system of interactions between researchers and knowledge users which may vary in intensity, complexity, and level of engagement depending on the nature of the research and the findings, as well as the needs of the particular knowledge user' (Canadian Institutes for Health Research, 2000; Graham et al., 2006). Deliberative dialogues are one example that brings together decision makers and researchers to consider the best available evidence in the context of a particular need for actionable solutions or health system guidance (Boyko et al., 2012). Lomas (2006) preferred the idea that 'knowledge transfer and exchange is a contact sport and team game'—i.e., for producers and users of research evidence, there needs to be regular and meaningful interactions to have impact.

Conclusions and considerations for policy makers and narrative researchers

This chapter has outlined the challenges and strategies related to the contribution of narrative evidence to healthcare policy. The development, implementation, and evaluation of policy at a health systems level is a relatively 'messy' business in comparison to the processes and expectations for research production. Strategies for bridging these worlds may be found in the science and practice of integrated knowledge translation that may contribute to an enabling context for experiential research use and evidence-informed policy in accordance with values, beliefs, and opportunities for change.

Scientifically produced evidence of any sort is but one of several types of inputs to healthcare policy, although consideration of the best available evidence is more likely with dedicated investment in proven mechanisms, such as health system investment in longer-term researcher–policy partnerships to enhance 'connectivity', building capacity among policy 'receptors' for understanding the value and use of research, and a deeper grasp of the principles and practice of effective knowledge translation. Approaches to policy development and analysis that incorporate principles and practices of co-design (among different actors—e.g., researchers, patients, and public) may enhance the efficiency and effectiveness with which experiential evidence is valued and integrated in the processes of agenda-setting, policy development, and implementation, as well as monitoring. In this scenario, the connections between structure and actors are more closely situated (even if not aligned), creating opportunities for policy makers to communicate, in a timely manner, the need for experiential evidence. Finally, beyond the inclusion of evidence *about* patient experience in policy development, if patients and caregivers could be more engaged as partners in decision-making processes, our health systems and policies are more likely to define and achieve targets for patient-centred care.

In studies of the use of research in policy, it is clear that some policies and processes are more amenable to influence than others, and that citable research and engagement with policy makers is important (Lavis et al., 2005). Advice for researchers to maximize the potential contributions of evidence to policy was succinctly captured by an Assistant Deputy Minister for the province of Ontario, Canada, in stating that researchers need to have (Kennedy, 2015):

- The right *focus*—in terms of being strategically aligned with government priorities, is scalable, and engages the necessary stakeholders in a collaborative approach;
- The right *format*—in terms of clarity of results and real-world implications; and,
- The right *timing*—in that researchers need to become knowledgeable partners in the policy production process, with an understanding of 'policy windows' and timelines, and willing to invest in building relationships with decision makers.

Mechanisms to facilitate routine connections between decision makers and researchers adopted by this Ministry (encouraging research 'pull') include focused exchanges (policy roundtables and monthly 'research to policy' dialogues), dissemination events (research 'showcases' for decision makers), and activities to foster collaboration and co-design of evidence-informed policy (e.g., funding for projects to respond to the Ministry's applied health research questions). The government of Ontario recently introduced The Patients First Act—legislation to support the implementation of the action plan to create a more patient-centred healthcare system, improving experiences and outcomes (Ontario Legislature, 2016). It includes objectives to improve access for patients and families, improve coordination and integration, provide better information and support, and enhance 'protection' through public health services. In such types of decision-making contexts, with research-savvy decision makers as well as leadership for improving patient experience and outcomes, there is good potential for considering and integrating evidence about patient experience within policy development and implementation processes.

References

Barry, M. J. and Edgman-Levitan, P. A., 2012. Shared decision-making—the pinnacle of patient-centered care. *New England Journal of Medicine*, **366**(9), 780–781.

Bate, P. and Robert, G., 2006. Experience-based design: from redesigning the system around the patient to co-designing services with the patient. *Quality & Safety in Health Care*, 15, 307–310.

Berwick, D. M., Nolan, T. W., and Whittington, J., (2008). The Triple Aim: care, health, and cost. *Health Affairs*, **27**(3), 759–769.

Black, N., 2001. Evidence-based policy: proceed with care. *BMJ*, **323**, 275–279.

Black, N., 2013. Patient reported outcome measures could transform healthcare. *BMJ (Clinical Research Edition)*, **346**, f1167. doi:10.1136/bmj.f167.

Black, N., Varaganum, M., and Hutchings, A., 2014. Relationship between patient reported experience (PREMs) and patient reported outcomes (PROMs) in elective surgery. *BMJ Quality & Safety*, **23**(7), 534–542.

Boivin, A., Lehoux, P., Burgers, J., and Grol, R., 2014. What are the key ingredients for effective public involvement in healthcare improvement and policy decisions? A randomized trial process evaluation. *The Milbank Quarterly*, **92**(2), 319–350.

Boyd, H., McKernon, S., Mullin, B., and Old, A., 2012. Improving healthcare through the use of co-design. *The New Zealand Medical Journal (Online)*, **125**(1357), 76–87.

Boyko, J. A., Lavis, J. N., Abelson, J., Dobbins, M., and Carter, N., 2012. Deliberative dialogues as a mechanism for knowledge translation and exchange in health systems decision-making. *Social Science and Medicine*, **75**(11), 1938–1945.

Canadian Institute for Health Information, 2015. *Canadian preliminary core patient experience measures*. Available at: https://www.cihi.ca/en/patient-experience (Accessed 22 October 2017).

Canadian Institutes for Health Research, 2000. *Knowledge Translation*. Available at: <http://www.cihr-irsc.gc.ca/e/29418.html> (Accessed 10 September 2017).

Canadian Institutes for Health Research, 2011. *Canada's strategy for patient-oriented research: improving health outcomes through evidence-informed care*. Ottawa: Canadian Institutes for Health Research.

Canadian Institutes for Health Research, 2013. *Evaluation of CIHR's Knowledge Translation Funding Program*. Available at: <http://www.cihr-irsc.gc.ca/e/47332.html> (Accessed 15 August 2017).

Conklin, A., Morris, Z., and Nolte, E., 2012. What is the evidence-based for public involvement in health-care policy? Results of a systematic scoping review. *Health Expectations*, **18**, 153–165.

Coulter, A., 2012. Patient engagement—what works? *Journal of Ambulatory Care Management*, **35**(2), 80–89.

Coulter, A., Locock, L., Ziebland, S., and Calabrese, J., 2014. Collecting data on patient experience is not enough: they must be used to improve care. *BMJ*, **348**, g2225. doi: 10.1136/bmj.g2225.

Cuthbertson, L., 2015. Patient-centered measurement in British Columbia: statistics without the tears wiped off. *Healthcare Papers*, **14**(4), 46–54. doi:10.12927/hcpap.2015.24345.

Cuthbertson, L. N. and Parsons, L., 2016. *Patient-centred measurement of experiences and outcomes of care in British Columbia, Canada: statistics without the tears wiped off*. Conference abstract: ISQUA 16-1473, 59.

Denis, J. L., Lomas, J., and Stipich, N., 2008. Creating receptor capacity for research in the health system: the Executive Training for Research Application (EXTRA) Program in Canada. *Journal of Health Services Research & Policy*, **13**(1 Suppl), 1–7.

Doern, G. B. and Phidd, R., 1992. *Canadian public policy: ideas, structure, process*. 2nd edn. Toronto: Nelson Canada.

Ellen, M. E., Leon, G., Bouchard, G., Lavis, J. N., Ouimet, M., and Grimshaw, J. M., 2013. What supports do health services organizations have in place to facilitate evidence-informed decision-making? A qualitative study. *Implementation Science*, **8**, 84. doi: 10.1186/1748-5908-8-84.

Field, K. and Ziebland, S., 2008. *'Beyond the textbook': a preliminary survey of the uses made of the DIPEx website (www.dipex.org) in healthcare education*. Oxford: DIPEx Research Group.

Flyvbjerg, B., 2001. *Making social science matter*. Cambridge: Cambridge University Press.

Frank, L., Forsythe, L., Ellis, L., Schrandt, S., Sheridan, S., Gerson, J., Konopka, K., and Daugherty, S., 2015. Conceptual and practical foundations of patient engagement in research at the patient-centered outcomes research institute. *Quality of Life Research*, **24**(5), 1033–1041.

Gauvin, F-P., 2014. *Understanding Policy Developments and Choices Through the 3-i Framework: Interests, Ideas and Institutions*. Briefing Note. Montreal, Quebec: National Collaborating Centre for Healthy Public Policy. Available at: <http://www.ncchpp.ca/docs/2014_ ProcPP_3iFramework_EN.pdf>. (Accessed 13 January 2017).

Graham, I. D., Logan, J., Harrison, M. B., Straus, S. E., Tetroe, J., Caswell, W., and Robinson, N., 2006. Lost in knowledge translation: time for a map? *The Journal of Continuing Education in the Health Professions*, **26**(1): 13–24.

Green, L., George, M. A., Daniel, M., Frankish, C. J., Herbert, C. P., Bowie, W. R., and O'Neill, M., 1995. *Review and recommendations for the development of participatory research in health promotion in Canada*. Ottawa: The Royal Society of Canada.

Greenhalgh, T., Annandale, E., Ashcroft, R., et al., 2016. An open letter to the BMJ editors on qualitative research. *BMJ (Clinical Research Edition)*, **352**, i563.

Greenhalgh, T. and Russell, J., 2009. Evidence-based policymaking: a critique. *Perspectives in Biology and Medicine*, **52**(2), 304–318.

Greenhalgh, T., Russell, J., and Swinglehurst, D., 2005. Narrative methods in quality improvement research. *Quality & Safety in Health Care*, **14**, 443–449.

Hall, P. A., 1997. The role of interests, institutions, and ideas in the comparative political economy of the industrialized nations. In: M. I. Lichbach and A. S. Zuckerman, eds. *Comparative politics: Rationality, culture, and structure*, Cambridge: Cambridge University Press. pp. 174–207.

Hibbard, J. and Greene, J., 2017. What the evidence show about patient activation: better health outcomes and care experiences; fewer data on costs. *Health Affairs*, **32**(2), 207–214.

Jagosh J, Macaulay A, Pluye P, Salsberg, J., Bush, P. L., Henderson, J., Sirett, E., Wong, G., Cargo, M., Herbert, C. P., Seifer, S. D., Green, L. W., and Greenhalgh, T., 2012. Uncovering the benefits of participatory research: implications of a realist review for health research and practice. *The Milbank Quarterly*, **90**(2), 311–346.

Jenkins, W. I., 1978. *Policy analysis: a political and organizational perspective*. New York: St. Martin's Press.

Kennedy, N., 2015. Ontario Ministry of Health and Long-term Care: knowledge transfer and exchange. Annual Conference of the Canadian Association for Health Services and Policy Research, 25–28 May 2015, Toronto, Canada. Available at: https://www.cahspr.ca/en/presentation/5574fafe37dee83819501953 (Accessed 15 January 2017).

The King's Fund, 2013. Experience based co-design toolkit. King's Fund, London UK, Available at: <https://www.pointofcarefoundation.org.uk/resource/experience-based-co-design-ebcd-toolkit/>. (Accessed 20 October 2017).

Kingdon, J. W., 1984. *Agendas, alternatives, and public policies.* Boston, MA: Little, Brown.

Kitson, A., Marshall, A., Bassett, K., and Zeitz, K., 2013. What are the core elements of patient-centred care? A narrative review and synthesis of the literature from health policy, medicine and nursing. *Journal of Advanced Nursing,* **69**(1): 4–15.

Kohtari, A., McCutcheon, C., and Graham, I., 2017. Defining integrated knowledge translation and moving forward: a response to recent commentaries. *International Journal of Health Policy and Management,* **6**(5): 299–300.

Lavis, J. N. and Hammill, A. C., 2016. Governance arrangements, in: J. N. Lavis, ed. *Ontario's health system: Key insights for engaged citizens, professionals and policymakers.* Hamilton: McMaster Health Forum. pp. 45–71.

Lavis, J. N., Hammill, A., Gildiner, A., McDonagh, R. J., Wilson, M. G., Ross, S. E., Ouimet, M., and Stoddart, G. L., 2005. A systematic review of the factors that influence the use of research evidence by public policymakers. *Final Report Submitted to the Canadian Population Health Initiative.* Hamilton, Canada: McMaster University Program in Policy Decision-Making.

Lavis, J. N., 2013. *SUPPORT Tools for evidence-informed health policymaking.* Hamilton, Canada: McMaster Health Forum.

Lavis, J. N., 2015. *Setting agendas and developing and implementing policies.* Hamilton, Canada: McMaster Health Forum.

Lavis, J. N., 2016. *Finding and using research evidence.* Hamilton, Canada: McMaster Health Forum.

Lavis, J. N., Ross, S. E., and Hurley, J. E., 2002. Examining the role of health services research in public policymaking. *The Milbank Quarterly,* **80**(1), 125–154.

Locock, L., Bate, R., Boaz, A., Vougioukalou, S., Shuldham, C., Fielden, J., Ziebland, S., Gager, M., Tollyfield, R., Pearcey, J., 2014. Using a national archive of patient experience narratives to promote local patient-centred quality improvement: an ethnographic process evaluation of 'accelerated' experience-based co-design. *Journal of Health Services Research & Policy,* **19**(4), 200–207.

Lomas J (1997). *Improving research dissemination and uptake in the health sector: beyond the sound of one hand clapping. Commentary C97-1.* McMaster University Centre for Health Economics and Policy Analysis, Hamilton Ontario.

Lomas, J., 2000. Using 'linkage and exchange' to move research into policy at a Canadian foundation. *Health Affairs,* **9**(3), 236–240.

Lomas, J., 2006. Knowledge transfer and exchange [Le transfert des connaissances]. In: Prévenir l'incapacité au travail: un symposium pour favoriser l'action concertée. *Program of the 10th Journées annuelles de santé publique.* Montreal, Québec, Canada. 23–27 October 2006.

Lomas, J., Culyer, T., McCutcheon, C., McAuley, L., and Law, S., 2005. *Conceptualizing and combining evidence for health system guidance.* Ottawa: Canadian Health Services Research Foundation. Available at: <http://www.chsrf.ca/migrated/pdf/insightAction/evidence_e.pdf>. (Accessed 13 August 2017).

Lomas, J., Fulop, N., Gagnon, D., and Allen, P., 2003. On being a good listener: setting priorities for applied health services research. *The Milbank Quarterly,* **81**(3), 363–388.

Malone, R. E., 1999. Policy as product: morality and metaphor in health policy discourse. *Hastings Center Report 29,* 3, 16–22.

Manary MP, Boulding W, Staelin R, Glickman S (2013). The patient experience and health outcomes. *The New England Journal of Medicine*, **368**(3), 201–203.

McCaughey D, Bruning N (2010). Rationality versus reality: the challenges of evidence-based decision making for health policy makers. *Implementation Science*, **5**, 39. doi: 10.1186/1748-5908-5-39.

Mitton, C., Smith, N., Peacock, S., Evoy, B., and Abelson, J., 2009. Public participation in healthcare priority-setting: a scoping review. *Health Policy*, **91**(3): 219–228.

Moat, K.A. and Lavis, J. N., 2012. 10 best resources for … evidence-informed health policy making. *Health Policy and Planning*, **28**, 215–218.

National Institute for Health and Care Excellence, 2011. *Service user experience in adult mental health. NICE guidance on improving the experience of care for people using adult NHS mental health services.* London: National Institute for Health and Care Excellence.

Oliver, K., Innvar, S., Lorenc, T., Woodman, J., and Thomas, J., 2014. A systematic review of barriers to and facilitators of the use of evidence by policymakers. *BMC Health Services Research*, **14**, 2. Available at: http://www.biomedcentral.com/1472-6963/14/2 (Accessed 7 January 2017).

Ongolo-Zogo, P., Lavis, J. N., Tomson, G., and Sewankambo, N. K., 2014. Climate for evidence informed health system policymaking in Cameroon and Uganda before and after the introduction of knowledge translation platforms: a structured review of governmental policy documents. *Health Research Policy and Systems*, **13**:2.

Ontario Legislature, 2016. Bill 41, Patients First Act, 2016. The Legislative Assembly of Ontario. Available at: http://www.ontla.on.ca/web/bills/bills_detail.do?locale=en&BillID=4215 (Accessed 15 January 2017).

Petit-Zeman, S., Firkins, L., Scadding, J. W., 2010. The James Lind Alliance: tackling research mismatches. *Lancet*, **376**, 667–669.

Pope C, Mays N (1995). Qualitative research: reaching the parts that other methods cannot reach: an introduction to qualitative methods for health and health services research. *BMJ*, **311**, 42–45

Rees, R., Caird, J., Dickson, K., Vigurs, C., and Thomas, J., 2013. *The views of young people in the UK about obesity, body size, shape and weight: a systematic review.* London: EPPI-Centre, Social Science Research Unit, Institute of Education, University of London.

Russell, J., Greenhalgh, T., Byrne, E., and McDonnell, J., 2008. Recognizing rhetoric in health care policy analysis. *Journal of Health Services Research & Policy*, **13**(1), 40–46.

Secretary of State for Health, 2010. *Equity and excellence: liberating the NHS.* Richmond: Her Majesty's Stationery Office.

US Department of Health and Human Services, 2008. *Personalized health care: pioneers, partnerships, progress.* Washington, DC: US Department of Health and Human Services.

Walt, G. and Gilson, L., 1994. Reforming the health sector in developing countries: the central role of policy analysis. *Health Policy and Planning*, **9**, 353–370.

World Health Organization (2000). *The world health report 2000—health systems: improving performance.* Geneva: World Health Organization.

Ziebland, S., 2013. Narrative interviewing. In: S. Ziebland, A. Coulter, J. Calabrese, and L. Locock, eds. *Understanding and using health experiences: improving patient care*, pp.38–48. Oxford: Oxford University Press.

Ziebland, S. and Hunt, K., 2014. Using secondary analysis of qualitative data of patient experiences of health care to inform health services research and policy. *Journal of Health Services Research & Policy*, **19**(3), 177–182.

Ziebland, S. and McPherson, A., 2006. Making sense of qualitative data analysis: an introduction with illustrations from DIPEx (personal experiences of health and illness). *Medical Education*, **40**(5), 405–414.

Chapter 23

When public and private narratives diverge

Media, policy advocacy, and the paradoxes of newborn screening policy

Rachel Grob and Mark Schlesinger

Introduction

Illness narratives are compelling because they give disease a face. They turn abstractions into stories. Make statistics come alive. Humanize suffering. Highlight resilience.

In the United States (US), individuals' health experiences are as varied as the diverse culture which has always been the country's defining characteristic. Yet in the public domain, the rich chorus of patients' voices (that is audible if we listen closely) is often drowned out by a crafted monologue which conveys a simplified, compelling, and actionable message. This chapter explores how and why public narratives can come to diverge from aggregated private ones. It also describes the influence that a single kind of patient experience, told and re-told, can have on policy discourse and action.

To examine how illness narratives can be used to craft messages which telescope the breadth of human experiences down to a focal point then leveraged for policy change, this study focuses on the role of the news media and employs an illustrative case study: narratives about newborn screening for heritable disorders (NBS). It argues that forces aligned in the US to promote rapid expansion of NBS around the turn of the twenty-first century created an opening for public and private narratives to diverge in consequential ways. This chapter describes the intersection of a single 'urgency narrative' used by advocates to promote expanded screening with state-level policy-making and news media coverage. It concludes with reflections on the value of maximally diverse stories as a public good.

The media as a prism for public narratives

Personal accounts bring media stories to life. This is especially true for media coverage of health and healthcare, where individual narratives can feel extremely personal. When journalists want to convey news about emerging health threats, advances in medical knowledge, or the arcane workings of medical care or health policy, they seek out individual vignettes designed to render reporting more meaningful for readers (Seale, 2003).

Personal narratives are integral to most media coverage of health matters, and thus profoundly shape how and what the public learns about policy issues in this significant domain (Jamison and Hardy, 2011).

Not all personal narratives are equally compelling, however. Reporters strive to find individual accounts that will best grab and hold their audiences' attention—thereby garnering for their stories more air time, front page placements, or voluminous hits on the internet (Deyo and Patrick, 2005). For decades, the most appealing plot lines for health stories in the US have been poignant tales of illness, suffering, and death that could have been avoided, if only medical providers, patients, or health systems had acted differently (Rachul and Caulfield, 2015). These poignant narratives comport both with journalists' professional edict to convey truth in compelling ways, and with commercial pressures increasingly shaping media practices (Deyo and Patrick, 2005).

But the media's reliance on personal narratives can also induce public misperceptions. Because individual narratives are so common in news coverage, the public regularly views personal choices as a disproportionate cause of health problems and underestimates the importance of social determinants such as poverty (Kim et al., 2015; Barry, Brescoll, and Gollust, 2013). Because journalists accord poignant narratives special primacy, news coverage often singles out unrepresentative images of patient suffering. For example, as breast cancer gained the US media spotlight in the 1990s, coverage over-represented narratives of women diagnosed under the age of 40—mothers whose tragically untimely deaths would leave young children behind (Burke et al., 2001). But the fact that almost half of all magazine stories focused on this subset of affected women obscured the reality that they represent less than 5% of people with breast cancer.

Biases can also emerge from deliberate efforts to manipulate media coverage. For advocates concerned about particular medical conditions and treatments, more favourable coverage is expected to translate into more medical research funding and improved insurance coverage (Rose, 2013). These are big stakes—and more than sufficient motivation for advocates to reinforce the media's hunger for compelling narratives by selectively conveying vignettes that promote their objectives (Dresser, 1999).

NBS's policy expansion around the turn of the twenty-first century, before the significant rise of social media, presents an apt case study for exploring the influence of a crafted public narrative in the media.

The changing technological and normative foundations for newborn screening

Newborn screening began in the US with a test developed by the physician Robert Guthrie in the mid-1960s to identify babies with phenylketonuria (PKU), a metabolic disorder that causes disability or death if left untreated. A diet without phenylalanine, however, can significantly mitigate the disease's impact. Within a decade, Guthrie's screening test became mandated under public health law in all 50 states, and 'the heel stick' became standard practice for collecting newborns' blood for screening.

Over the next several decades, screening techniques were slowly developed for several additional congenital conditions. Each of these required a separate procedure—but all could be conducted using the blood already being collected for PKU. Norms for judging what additional conditions should be screened at birth were based on criteria developed by the World Health Organization (WHO) for population-based disease screening in the early 1960s. According to these principles, mandatory NBS was ethically defensible only if: (1) the condition in question could be effectively treated, (2) screening methods were sufficiently reliable, (3) the condition had early age of onset, and (4) the public accepted mandatory screening as a legitimate exercise of government authority.

Changing technology at the turn of the century

Beginning in the 1990s, a new technology called tandem mass spectrometry (MS/MS) radically altered the NBS terrain. MS/MS's automated process made it possible to simultaneously screen an infant's blood for the spectral 'signatures' of a large number of chemical metabolites which may signal specific disorders—or may just signal deviation from an assumed norm. A few disorders detectable by MS/MS were already incorporated on NBS panels, but dozens of new ones were not. A subset of these newly screenable, rare conditions were life threatening and available data suggested they might be effectively treatable. For most, however, it was difficult to assess the reliability of the screening, the meaning for the infant's health of detected abnormalities, or the impact of an early diagnosis, since the natural history of these diseases were only poorly understood (Ross, 2012). When MS/MS first arrived on the market, some states adopted the new technology and vastly increased their screening panels; others did not.

Evolving ethical norms

As state-level NBS programmes in the US struggled to resolve the technical and clinical uncertainties associated with MS/MS technologies, the US Department of Health and Human Services commissioned the American College of Medical Genetics (ACMG) to suggest a uniform screening panel for the US. The ACMG's 2005 final report identified 54 conditions for recommended inclusion on NBS panels across the US: 29 'primary' conditions which ACMG controversially argued might meet conventional norms of reliability and treatability, and another 25 'secondary' conditions which were inexpensively identifiable by MS/MS, but for which treatments clearly did not yet exist.

By laying out new criteria for screening and recommending that secondary conditions be universally included, the ACMG report went far beyond a technical review. It asserted two key normative claims, both substantial shifts from the previous moral and legal foundations for NBS in the US. First, the report portrayed existing interstate variation in the scope of screening panels as unacceptable, rather than as a reflection of reasonable state-level differences in assessments of MS/MS technology. Second, the report asserted that 'benefits to family and society' ought to be considered in determining whether screening was appropriate for any given condition. This second assumption was the key rationale for identifying and reporting secondary conditions (ACMG, 2006).

The ACMG report had an immediate impact. Within two years after its publication, virtually every state had incorporated MS/MS into its newborn screening programme. The average number of conditions in NBS panels grew from 10 in 2005 to 33 in 2007 and 43 by 2009, putting the US far beyond other nations with respect to the range of mandatorily screened conditions (Cornel et al., 2014).

Public health officials, however, remained divided about secondary conditions. By 2009, states diverged widely with respect to how many of these conditions they announced they were screening for on their panels (Grob, 2011a). The decade 2001–2010 was thus characterized by great change and persisting controversy for US NBS policy. Similarly, in Canada, some provinces offered broad panels to parents on a voluntary basis while others maintained much more restricted ones. As a result, Canada also experienced—and continues to experience—substantial geographic variation in NBS: as of September 2015, the Canadian province with the most expansive panel (Manitoba) screened for almost six times as many conditions as the province with the least expansive panel (Newfoundland).

Newborn screening in the United States: crafting a public narrative

The first decade of the twenty-first century was also a period of increasingly mobilized advocacy for NBS expansion. Parents of children who died of screenable (though not always treatable) conditions, or who were successfully treated after screening, raised their voices most loudly and persistently. They were also sought after by other actors eager for expansion, including private labs and some state legislators. These parents testified at public hearings, joined advisory committees making decisions about NBS expansion, and became regular resources for the media (Grob, 2011a). Formal advocacy groups also proliferated. Some of these focused exclusively on newborn screening (e.g., Save Babies Through Screening), others on conditions members wanted included in NBS panels (e.g., Hunter's Hope, CARE), and still others on genetic disorders more generally (e.g., the Genetic Alliance, the National Organization of Rare Disease) or on children's health (e.g., March of Dimes).

One core 'urgency narrative', however, was used consistently by parents and advocacy groups alike. As documented elsewhere (Grob, 2011b), the heart of this narrative is tragic stories of children who died or were disabled by a screenable condition. Its moral is that simple, inexpensive tests at birth save lives. Moving vignettes reiterating this story garnered considerable media coverage, and reporters often focused on interstate disparities in the number of conditions covered—or 'newborn roulette', as one article described the phenomenon of babies 'living or dying' based on which side of a state line happened to be their birth place. (Grob, 2011b).

Ironically, the rise of a consolidated public story about newborn screening as a life-saving necessity coincided with NBS expansion to many untreatable conditions. As a result, direct benefit to screened infants actually became a decreasingly prominent feature of the programme. Almost half of the ACMG's 54 recommended conditions had no known treatment, and many had high rates of false positive results or unclear consequences (i.e., an abnormality was detected but its significance in terms of the infant's health was uncertain). Yet even as private experiences with NBS continued to become more diverse and diffuse (Timmermans and Buchbinder, 2010; Grob, 2011b), the urgency narrative's power in public discourse persisted. It also extended to an increasingly broad range of conditions for which only experimental treatment—which could actually be dangerous to infants— existed (Ross, 2012; Lantos, 2011).

By representing NBS as a uniformly life-saving procedure with no downsides, the crafted public narrative skewed the ethical debate over newborn screening in favour of expansion. For advocates, the ethical issues all lined up in favour of expanded screening and notification: they proclaimed interstate variation in NBS to be ethically indefensible and argued that states' failure to screen for secondary conditions and then notify parents was inappropriately paternalistic and impeded science (Grob, 2011b). Advocates rejected ethicists' concerns that the case for expanding NBS to create new knowledge made it a form of research, for which parents ought to be giving informed consent, rather than having their infants subjected to mandatory screening (Botkin et al., 2006).

The remainder of this chapter uses data from a survey of newborn screening directors and from an analysis of NBS media coverage to explore the impact of NBS's public narrative. It demonstrates that parental advocacy, as measured by frequency of citations in media reports, was associated with substantial differences in the content of coverage. Further, states in which media coverage incorporated more parental influence from 2000 to 2005 adopted a broader panel of secondary conditions in the years that followed.

Research methods

The primary data explored here was generated by the authors via two interconnected studies: qualitative interviews with directors of NBS programmes across the US, and a content analysis of NBS media coverage in the US and four Commonwealth countries over four decades.

Media analysis

This study analysed all newspaper coverage of NBS in the US between 1965 and 2007. In total 189 articles were identified from databases of stories in periodicals and television coverage using the search terms 'newborn screening', 'perinatal screening', and 'infant screening'. The bulk of these (109) were published during the peak of media attention around the 2005 ACMG report.

Using conventional techniques of grounded theory, the project began with a conceptual schema regarding media coverage based on previous NBS research, which was then revised inductively as the content of the articles was coded. The refined schema contained 158 distinct codes, grouped into perceived benefits of NBS (16 codes), perceived costs (17 codes), drivers of expansion (8 codes), issues related to implementation (31 codes), ethical considerations (22 codes), types of evidence (15 codes), audience depiction (15 codes), and presentation format (22 codes). Two graduate students coded each article; inconsistencies in coding were adjudicated by the authors.

For comparison, 130 articles on newborn screening were similarly coded from four Commonwealth countries: the United Kingdom (UK), Canada, Australia, and New Zealand. These countries constitute suitable international comparisons for several reasons. First, they are all English-speaking. Second, their media coverage has historically been skewed—like the American media—to present new medical technology in a favourable light (Rachul and Caulfied, 2015; Jensen, 2012). Finally, they have a similar constellation of stakeholders striving to influence NBS policymaking, including parent and disease advocates (Potter, Avard, and Wilson, 2008). Due to database limitations, Commonwealth country review was restricted to 1990–2007, but since there was so little coverage of NBS in the US prior to 1990 (four articles) the cross-national comparisons were not unduly affected.

Newborn screening programme director interviews

To explore how public narratives about NBS and media coverage shaped NBS practices, NBS programme administrators from throughout the US (N = 48) were interviewed. The interviews, which lasted from 45 to 90 minutes, were taped, transcribed, and coded using a schema designed to parallel that used for the media analysis, albeit with appropriate adaptations. The interviews included both open-ended questions and specific probes. Foci included how expansion debates were influenced by various actors, ethical issues raised in state-level discourse, and reflections on the use of narratives and other forms of evidence in policy debates.

Findings

Views from the field: NBS programme interviews

The first source of evidence about the impact of crafted narrative comes from the interviews with NBS programme administrators. As Figure 23.1 highlights, more than half of all respondents identified 'advocates' and/or 'parents' as central drivers of NBS expansion in their state. Many of these described the impact of the urgency narrative on policy deliberations. As one administrator put it, a mother who lost her child to the metabolic disorder Medium-Chain Acyl-coa Dehydrogenase (MCAD) 'became very active in trying to get expansions in [our state].... Actually his death certificate had said SIDS and she had gotten on the Internet and done some research and had his body exhumed and tested and he was tested positive for MCAD'. Other respondents describe how 'emotional testimony' from parents about 'their poor dead baby' made it impossible for others to testify at public hearings. Respondents also emphasized how 'a baby that was born and presented clinically with one of the disorders and didn't have a very good outcome' carried tremendous weight and captured public attention during state-level policy debates.

DRIVERS OF NBS EXPANSION

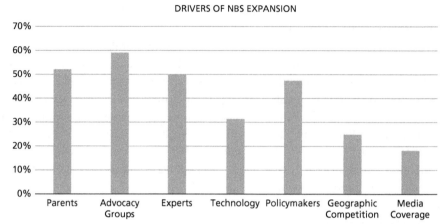

Figure 23.1 Drivers of NBS expansion. Percent of NBS programme directors in US reporting that each factor influenced expansion of screening panels.
Reproduced courtesy of the authors.

Media representation of these narratives was also influential, both directly and indirectly. Eighteen percent of respondents explicitly identified media coverage as a pressure for NBS expansion, and a half dozen described it as an important driver. 'The media played a big role,' said one administrator, ' … a big role in terms of saying whether we were screening for 28, 29 or 67 … [conditions and in creating] the interest of that [influential] parent and legislation in order to expand'. Others described media coverage of signing ceremonies for new expanded screening panels as significant. The complex interactions between advocacy and media coverage were also cogently captured, as highlighted by this excerpt.

> Well, as soon as the ACMG came out with their report, March of Dimes immediately said that that was their recommendation too and supported that, so our [state] chapter immediately contacted us and wanted to know what we were doing and they wanted to be in the media. They set up a whole media outlet … with the governor when he signed the bill.… And, every year they would call us and … push forward to be [more] comprehensive.

Another dozen respondents directly identified interstate competition as a powerful driver of NBS expansion (Figure 23.1). We believe that this in large part reflected an indirect influence of media because parents and advocates were characterized as leveraging differences in screening panels among neighbouring states to generate media attention to the case for expansion. Administrators noted that stories of babies who died because they were born on the wrong side of a state border resulted in 'a lot of pressure' on states not screening for all possible conditions because they were used to 'shame, shame'. Another described NBS as 'very much in the news', with extensive 'publicity about being slow to jump on board' that made it very hard to avoid rapid expansion.

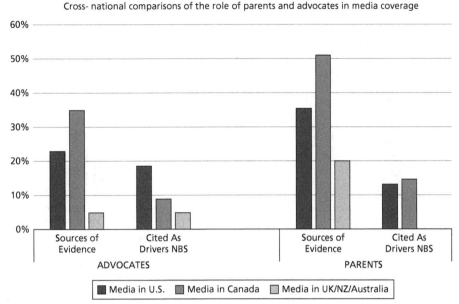

Figure 23.2 Cross-national comparisons of the role of parents and advocates in media coverage. Percentage of media articles that favorably mention parents or advocates.
Reproduced courtesy of the authors.

Sources of information and coverage differences: media analysis

The hypothesis underlying this media analysis was that mobilization in response to NBS interstate disparities would mean US parents/advocates had a more substantial impact on NBS media coverage and policy discourse than counterparts in the Commonwealth countries. Analysis of media content suggests that this prediction was only partly correct; parent voices appeared even more influential in Canada.

Advocacy differences reflected in media across countries

The presence of parents and other advocates in media stories was assessed using two metrics: how often in each article they were (1) cited as a source of evidence in the article and (2) described as an important 'driver' of NBS expansion. Parents were cited three times as often as sources of evidence in US media compared to the UK, New Zealand and Australia, and advocates three times as often (Figure 23.2). Furthermore, parents were described as important drivers of NBS expansion in 13% of US coverage, but never in the other three countries. Other advocates were depicted as influencing NBS policies in the UK, New Zealand, and Australia, but less than a third as often as in US coverage.

Media coverage in Canada was far *more* likely to cite parents and advocates as was coverage in the US. Although other advocates in Canada were only half as likely as in US media to be identified as drivers of NBS expansion, parents were slightly more often depicted as drivers in Canadian than in US coverage.

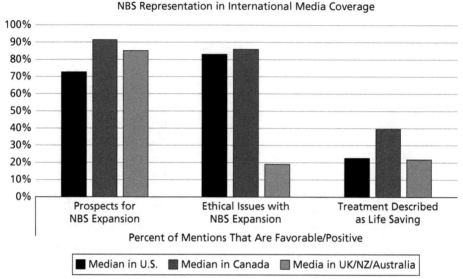

Figure 23.3 Cross-national comparisons of media coverage of NBS impact. Percentage of media articles that favorably mention these three topic areas.
Reproduced courtesy of the authors.

The origins of these patterns are too complex to be fully investigated here, but one influential factor appears to be geographic variation in NBS practices. In Canada, as in the US, NBS policies are set at a subnational level. This variation was reflected in media accounts. Outside of North America, geographic variation in practices was identified as a concern in only 17% of all coverage. In the US and Canada, it was mentioned in 55% and 67% of articles, respectively.

Cross-national differences in media content

To assess the impact of differences in the sources of evidence on public discourse over NBS, the study analysed three aspects of media content: the extent to which (1) articles describe NBS in positive or questioning terms, (2) the ethical issues associated with NBS are presented as favouring or constraining expansion, and (3) the benefits of NBS are presented as life-saving. Each of these measures are represented as proportions in the results presented here (Figure 23.3): the proportion of implications that are positive, the proportion of ethical issues that favour expansion, and the proportion of benefits represented as life-saving.

Given the frequency with which parents and other advocates are cited in this coverage (figure 23.2), one would expect that if advocates were the most influential over media content, the coverage in Canada and the US should look similar—and both more positive than in the other Commonwealth countries. If parents are the most impactful sources, however, one would expect content in Canadian coverage to be skewed even more positively or more focused on life-saving benefits than in the US.

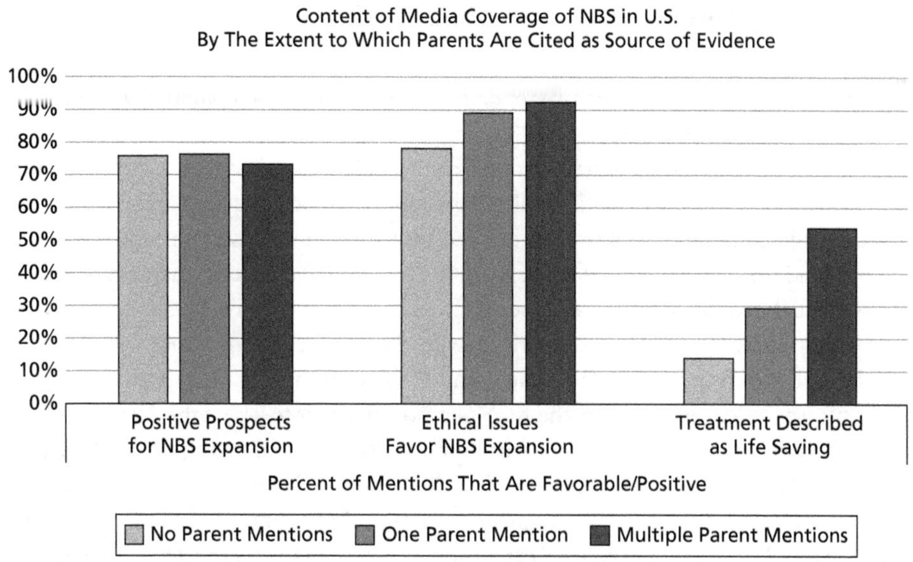

Content of Media Coverage of NBS in U.S.
By The Extent to Which Parents Are Cited as Source of Evidence

Figure 23.4 Media coverage of NBS impact in the US, by parent representation. Percentage of media articles that favorably mention these three topic areas.
Reproduced courtesy of the authors.

Findings suggest that parents do, in fact, have the most consequential impact. Canadian coverage is persistently more positive than in the US, especially with respect to the frequency with which NBS benefits are described as life-saving, which happens twice as often in Canada as in the US (Figure 23.3). By contrast, the one metric for which other Commonwealth countries look markedly different than either the US or Canada is balance of reported ethical issues: these are 80% positive in North American coverage, but only 20% positive in the UK, New Zealand, and Australia.

Differences in coverage within the United States

Cross-national comparisons are useful, but complicated by other differences in culture and attitudes across countries, including the public's embrace of medical technology (Kim, Blendon, and Benson, 2001). By looking at coverage within a single country (the US), these other factors can be held constant. This was done here by comparing the content of articles where: (1) no parents were cited as evidence, (2) parents were cited once, and (3) parents were cited two or more times.

Here the pattern is mixed, but with some striking differences (Figure 23.4). Citing parents is not associated with the overall representation of NBS in positive or negative terms, but when parents are more frequently cited as evidence, NBS's ethical issues are presented in more positive terms. Most notably, treatment is described in life-saving terms four times as often in articles with multiple parental citations as in those with none.

Does media content shape NBS policy-making?

These findings document an association between the use of the crafted urgency narrative in media coverage and more positive reporting about newborn screening. But is this relationship causal or coincidental?

To address this question, media coverage prior to 2005 was linked to NBS practices after the 2005 ACMG report, when NBS policy debates focused on the adoption of 'secondary', non-treatable conditions. States were divided into three tiers based on how many secondary conditions they adopted through 2009. To assess the urgency narrative's impact on policy-making, the measures of parent/advocate voice in the pre-2005 media were organized into three strata of US states: those with no media citations, those with less than half the evidence from parents/advocates, and those with more than half such evidence. The focus was on coverage before the ACMG report in order to assess the extent to which that crafted narrative laid the groundwork for a subsequent policy response rather than reflecting celebration of a policy position (e.g., state X's panel expanded and then parents/advocates were cited in the media to justify or praise that course of action). Since other factors certainly also influenced NBS expansion, this 'test' of media impact should be seen as more suggestive than definitive.

The patterns emerging from this analysis are striking (Figure 23.5). Where media coverage prior to 2005 had no evidence drawn from parents or advocates, the states' 2009 NBS practices were divided evenly between those with limited, moderate, and substantial

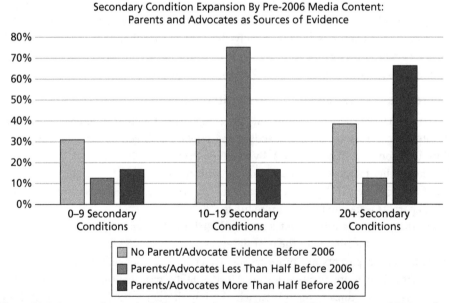

Figure 23.5 Percent of states including secondary conditions in NBS panels, by pre-2006 media coverage. For three types of prior coverage, distribution of states' NBS panels.
Reproduced courtesy of the authors.

adoption of secondary conditions. By contrast, in states where parents/advocates had offered less than half the evidence in media coverage, the vast majority (75%) were sub-sequently expanding in the middle tier. Most notably, in states where previous media coverage had more than half its evidence drawn from parents/ advocates, by 2009 two-thirds were in the highest tier for secondary condition reporting.

When public and private narratives diverge: lessons and implications

The urgency narrative—at least in its current form—emerged in the US at a time when some states where slow to adopt the new MS/MS screening technology and therefore failed to screen for conditions that were truly life-saving. The passion of that crafted rep-resentation of parental experience resonated with journalists' efforts to find stories that moved their readers, making the storyline powerful, particularly in countries like the US and Canada that situate NBS policymaking at the state or provincial level where the more localized scale of policy action makes personal stories feel more salient. Perhaps even more crucially, comparisons across states or provinces also created a powerful moral ar-gument for advocates and particularly poignant personal narratives.

The urgency narrative's more lasting and troubling legacy, however, was its persistence long after every American state had adopted screening for all of the ACMG's 29 primary (treatable) conditions. The crafted narrative's mantra 'NBS saves lives, NBS saves lives' retained such a powerful hold in the public domain that parents' increasingly diverse narratives about experiences with expanded screening remained largely sequestered in the private one (Grob, 2011a; Ross, 2012; Lantos, 2011). As this chapter shows, this skew was evident both in the media and in NBS policy debates. As one NBS programme leader interviewed put it when describing public hearings in his state, ' … after hearing the hor-rible stories and the parents saying … "we need this, we needed it years ago", the com-mittee person [asked] … is there anyone in opposition? At that point, there was virtually nobody willing to speak.'

Narratives are a uniquely textured and valuable form of evidence. They can and should be used to enrich public discourse, guide health practices, and inform policy debates. But when narratives evolve from informal stories to qualitative data put to use in the public domain, that use must be guided by standards of practice just as rigorous as those em-ployed for quantitative data. At the very least, this means actively eliciting stories from maximally diverse sources, rigorously analysing them in aggregate, and striving to en-sure that public narratives align as closely as possible with private ones. It also means keeping in check public narratives that silence other stories. Clearly the story of how the use of narratives can iteratively enrich system change and public discourse is still being written; it will be crafted most fully if it is informed by many voices.

References

American College of Medical Genetics (ACMG), 2006. Newborn screening: toward a uniform screening panel and system. *Genetics in Medicine*, **8**(Suppl) (Accessed 10 November 2009) https://www.acmg.net/resources/policies/NBS/NBS_Main_Report_00.pdf

Barry, C., Brescoll, V., and Gollust, S., 2013. Framing childhood obesity: how individualizing the problem affects public support for prevention. *Political Psychology*, **34**(3), 327–349.

Botkin, J., Clayton, E. W., Post, N., Burke, W., Murray, T., Baily, M. W., Wilfond, B., Berg, A., and Ross, L. F., 2006. Newborn screening technology: proceed with caution. *Pediatrics*, **114**, 1793–1799.

Burke, W., Olsen, A. H., Pinsky, L. E., Reynolds, S. E., and Press, N. A., 2001. Misleading presentation of breast cancer in popular magazines. *Effective Clinical Practice*, **4**(2), 58–64.

Cornel, M. C., Rigter, T., Weinreich, S. S., Burgard, P., Hoffmann, G. F., Lindner, M., Gerard Loeber, J., Rupp, K., Taruscio, D., and Vittozzi, L., 2014. A framework to start the debate on neonatal screening policies in the EU: an expert opinion document. *European Journal of Human Genetics*, **22**(1),12–17.

Deyo, R. A. and Patrick, D. L., 2005. *Hope or hype: the obsession with medical advances and the high cost of false promises.* New York: AMACOM.

Dresser, R., 1999. Public advocacy and the allocation of federal funds for biomedical research. *The Milbank Quarterly*, **55**(2), 257–274.

Grob, R., 2011a. A house on fire: newborn screening, parents' advocacy, and the discourse of urgency. In: B. Hoffman, N. Tomes, R. Grob, and M. Schlesinger, eds. *Patients as policy actors.* New Brunswick, NJ: Rutgers University Press. pp. 231–156.

Grob, R., 2011b. *Testing baby: the transformation of newborn screening, parenting, and policymaking.* New Brunswick NJ: Rutgers University Press.

Jamison KH, Hardy B. (2011). The Effect of Media on Public Knowledge. In: R. Shapiro and L. Jacobs, eds. *The Oxford Handbook of American Public Opinion and the Media.* New York: Oxford University Press. pp. 236–250.

Jensen, E., 2012. Mediating subpolitics in US and UK science news. *Public Understanding of Science*, **21**(1), 68–83.

Kim, M., Blendon, R., and Benson, J., 2001. How Interested Are Americans In New Medical Technologies? *Health Affairs*, **20**(5), 194–201.

Kim, S. H., Tanner, A. H., Foster, C. B., and Kim, S. Y., 2015. Talking about health care: news framing of who is responsible for rising health care costs in the United States. *Journal of Health Communication*, **20**(2), 123–133.

Lantos, J. D., 2011. Dangerous and expensive screening and treatment for rare childhood diseases: the case of Krabbe disease. *Developmental Disabilities Research Reviews*,**17**(1). 15–18.

Potter, B. K., Avard, D., Wilson, B. J., 2008. Newborn blood spot screening in four countries: stakeholder involvement. *Journal of Public Health Policy*, **29**, 121–142.

Rachul, C. and Caulfield, T., 2015. The media and access issues: content analysis of canadian newspaper coverage of health policy decisions. *Orphanet Journal of Rare Diseases*, **10**, 102.

Rose, S., 2013. Patient advocacy organizations: institutional conflicts of interest, trust and trustworthiness. *Journal of Law, Medicine and Ethics*, **41**(3), 680–687.

Ross, L. F., 2012. Newborn screening for lysosomal storage diseases: an ethical and policy analysis. *Journal of Inherited Metabolic Disease*, **35**(4), 627–634.

Seale, C., 2003. Health and media: an overview. *Sociology of Health & Illness*, **25**(6), 513–531.

Timmermans, S. and Buchbinder, M., 2010. Patients-in-waiting: living between sickness and health in the genomics era. *Journal of Health & Social Behavior*, **51**(4), 408–423.

Illness narratives in the media

Chapter 24

Pregnancy 2.0

A corpus-based case study for the analysis of illness narratives online

Eleonora Massa and Valentina Simeoni

The narrativization of pregnancy

This paper proposes a narrative, linguistic, and socio-pragmatic analysis of a corpus of 300 posts written by 20 mothers-to-be between 2010 and 2015 and posted either as 'public' or as 'shared with friends' on their Facebook (FB) profile during pregnancy and/or shortly after giving birth. Roughly aged between 25 and 40, almost all of them are Italian and live in Italy.

The aim of this analysis is to understand why and how pregnancy is increasingly being narrated on FB and in what way this social network can be thought of as a narrative device.

Both the offline and the online culture of pregnancy are characterized by a continuous interlacing of subjectivity and social values: no pregnancy is like another, and yet they all seem to have very much in common.

On one hand, every woman lives and experiences her own pregnancy as unique and involving, especially the first one. In order to be understood and woven into the fabric of her personal biography, pregnancy is usually narrated repeatedly to herself and to others, mirroring the plots and formulas available in her social environment. This is why, on the other hand, such a narration will often be shaped in order to be socially acceptable and respond to the criteria of a recognizable pregnancy profile. Pregnancy roughly develops through similar stages that pave the way to a sharable experience. This experience has been charged with deep socio-cultural meanings and representations across times and cultures (Duden, 1993; Davis-Floyd and Georges, 1996). It remains the focus of intense social discourses, political negotiations, and ritual practices (Mead and Newton, 1967; Chodorow, 1978; Rich, 1977; Kitzinger, 1980; Jordan and Davis-Floyd, 1993[1978]; MacCormack, 1994; Ammaniti, 1995; Tremayne, 2001; Bonfanti, 2012), that is systems of expectations that frame feelings and behaviours and constitute culturalized ways of becoming a mother.

These socially recognized paths are usually layered through collective and trans-generational narratives, which, at least in the Italian context, are influenced by socio-cultural factors such as a peculiar view of family and motherhood (Fiume, 1995), the ideological pressure of the Catholic Church, and the linear organization of time typical of Western cultures (Lauer, 1981; Brislin and Kim, 2003). Pregnancy is thus associated with the idea of waiting, the pregnant woman is often depicted in the grip of either nausea or cravings (Angelini and Trinci, 2000), becoming mother is considered a blessing, if not the perfect fulfilment of a woman's life, and expressing positive feelings towards pregnancy and the unborn is a sort of emotional must. Contemporary aspects of the local culture of pregnancy include its increasing commodification in terms of babies' furniture, clothes, games, and accessories and a countertendency towards its re-naturalization (home birth-giving, lotus-birth, etc.).

The inherently temporal dimension and the partial sharability of the psycho-physical status of being pregnant actually make pregnancy one of the most narrated experiences in a woman's life and the perfect plot for a prototypical story. In fact, on both levels— the subjective and the social—storytelling comes in as one of the most powerful strategies of sense making that allows the mother-to-be to organize her personal experience into structured paths, and emplot it within culturally recognized narrative frames that borrow their language from different sources, e.g., tradition, religion, common sense, biomedicine, the Internet.

Nowadays, pregnancy is acquiring an increasing relevance as a narrative theme on social networks. Statistics show that women are, on average, more on FB than men and, especially when pregnant with their first child, they show a strong tendency to structure quite standardized—and yet not totally expectable—narratives of their pregnancy, using FB as a 'story-making device' in very interesting ways that deserve closer examination. In fact, what used to happen offline, among people and across generations, is now developing online as well: the sharing of the pregnancy experience on social networks in the specific modalities analysed here, in particular, is producing something very close to a narrative community (Massa and Simeoni, 2014) that builds, cultivates, and shares what might be called a 'tradition'.

The online storytelling of pregnancy partly replicates offline verbal storytelling and partly makes active use of the specific codes provided by the platform. This chapter argues that on FB, in particular, mothers-to-be follow specific, yet culturally and narratively shaped, strategies for announcing, telling, and sharing the whole process, thus experiencing it as a socially-mediated story.

Posting as a form of storytelling: the case of Facebook

The narrative construction of the social and cultural world expresses itself as the modality of weaving, i.e., structuring experience into habitudinary plots of content (Massa and Simeoni, 2014). In the daily practice of assigning a sense to the flux of perceptions and events, nothing is really newly 'invented' but instead is more likely to follow formats of action and knowledge which are commonly accepted within one's culture. Humans inhabit the world by telling stories, i.e., by constantly reconfiguring pre-experienced, routinized, conventional interpretations of reality which mostly confirm identities, be-haviours, and perspectives (Bruner, 2004; Mitchell, 1981; Polkinghorne, 1988; Ricoeur, 1981; cf. also Brown, 2001; Haiman, 1997; Johnstone, 1994).

Currently, this continuous relationship between individuality and intersubjectivity finds a particularly fertile ground of expression within the online spaces of social networks. As concerns FB, the possibility of narrating experience begins where users are requested to create an own personal (either true or fictitious) profile or, in exquisitely narrative terms, a 'diary', which functions as a primary instrument stimulating the biographization of ex-perience. If, as Ricoeur's 1984 work suggests, the relationship between narrative and the chronologization of experience is of crucial significance, then the platform confirms its fundamentally narrative structure in that it suggests, and de facto offers to its users, a chronological configuration of the posted contents. Moreover, FB allows its audience to use versatile tools of interaction (asking other users for friendship, greeting friends on their birthday, celebrating the anniversary of a friendship on FB), thus expanding the individual's subjective profile to the social dimension (Montemagno and Ruggeri, 2009; Borgato, Capelli, and Ferraresi, 2009). The possibility of sharing the posted contents with a selected audience, who in turn will respond to the input and thus contribute to its fur-ther construction, constantly pushes FB users to shape an individual space of social action that replicates and amplifies offline standardized practices.

Through the repetitive actions it spurs—the scrolling down of the home page, the visu-alization of other users' diary, the commenting and 'liking' of their posts— FB prompts its community to shape a highly routinized space of action (Volli, 2003), which can some-times even lead to addiction. In turn, the experiential domains configured within it are mainly plots of habitual content, i.e., scripts or frames (Ghidoli, 2010) wherein prototyp-ical roles co-act and 'practices of microcelebrity' are promoted (Shank, 1995; Herman, 2005; Horning, 2012).

The possibility of attributing a usual, common, and commonly accepted sense to ex-perience is in fact particularly dense on FB. For instance, the verbal code—one of the most significant tools for constructing a common-sense (Schutz, 1964; Bégout, 2005) of reality in the offline environment (Massa and Simeoni, 2014; Massa, 2016)—used in its written form leads to a reconfiguration of the traditional categories of orality and writing (Martini, 2005): graphical aids like punctuation and emoticons are in fact mostly used to boost the expressive power of the communication. A crucial semiotic role is played by the visual code, which alternates or even replaces the verbal one (Alexander and Levine, 2008). Therefore, a single post, which can be considered as the narrative unit in FB, is often exclusively made of images and/or memes. This complex semiotic potentiality makes FB a powerful space of re-semantization of experience since it constantly stimu-lates the opportunity of attributing it a consuetudinary sense. This happens, for instance, in the 'guided memories', through which users are invited by the platform to re-share pre-viously posted contents and thereby to reconfigure and partially innovate their meaning. As Rosen (2010) puts it, 'The web means the end of forgetting' (on the relationship be-tween narrative and collective memory, cf. also Halbwachs, 1992 [1925])).

Because of all these aspects, posting on FB unveils as a narrative praxis which follows, as well as amplifies, offline narrative processes of sense-making. This chapter will now investigate in more detail the role of FB as a story-making device through the analysis of a corpus of online narratives of pregnancy.

Analysing pregnancy narratives on Facebook: the case study

Pregnancy is an excellent example of a biographical experience physiologically developing as a linear process that lends itself to a structured account and finds in storytelling its perfect dimension (see The narrativization of pregnancy). Nowadays social networks, and FB in particular, are becoming the privileged spaces wherein the narration of pregnancy is cultivated and shared. Hence, an approach that draws partly from netnography (ethnography conducted on the Internet as a 'field') and partly from corpus-based linguistics: this chapter treats FB as a source and users (in this case, pregnant women) as informants (for privacy concerns, we have changed their names and are not going to reveal any of their sensitive data).

Thanks to the constructional power of FB's interface (see Posting as a form of storytelling), each post—whatever its form—constitutes a further node in the texture of a story which can be analysed on at least three interlaced levels.

From a global narratological point of view: what temporal frameworks are adopted to narrate pregnancy? Can any recurrent plot and/or prototypical role be identified in the posts? How is the 'pregnant body' narratively shaped?

Almost every online narrative of pregnancy weaves a plot constructed through the three main steps of any good story: a beginning (the 'incipit'), constituted by the announcement of pregnancy, an internal development paced by events such as echographies, check-ups, or the discovery of the sex, and a possibly happy end (the 'epilogue'), usually constituted by a reference to birth-giving.

As regards the incipit, for example, pregnancy can be explicitly announced ('Me and E. have got pregnant!' [Tatiana]), just hinted at ('Waiting for the stork … ' [Rosa]), visually shown either through a picture stressing the growing belly or by posting the first echography which sometimes even substitutes the mother-to-be's profile picture. Other secondary announcements—e.g., the just-discovered sex of the baby—structure the overall storytelling of pregnancy; the most exploited subplots to narrate the course of pregnancy are the count of time already gone by ('5 months of you' [Rosa]) and the countdown to birth-giving, this being often celebrated through photos that allude to the new-born rather than clearly show him/her: a picture of the mum's, dad's, and new-born's hands holding each other is a good example of such an allusion.

Some recognizable narrative patterns, clearly borrowed from the offline culture, contribute to giving such narratives a specific structure: among them, the tendency to describe pregnancy as a time of waiting (*dolce attesa*), and the connected development of the nesting process, i.e., the progressive configuration of a domestic environment dedicated to the baby-to-be: in this case, the narration is constructed through pictures of, or links to, the furniture for his/her future bedroom, the clothing, the equipment for the baby's transportation, and related accessories. In such a narrative format, the whole family management is projected into the future and the woman seems to stop cultivating any other aspect of her life to prepare for the child and make herself up as a 'mother'. In other cases, on the contrary, pregnancy is presented as a path of personal growth, with the woman progressively acquiring a better awareness of her becoming a 'mother', in a sort of parallel gestation: 'Delivering was the most revolutionary act in my life. Doors have shut that I feel will never open again. I came out of it totally transformed' (Jenny).

The model of pregnancy as a mission and/or its celebration as a gift or a blessing, usually expressed by a religious language or system of representations, is also particularly widespread in the corpus, as when Silvia writes the prayer 'Always bless my family' on a meme picturing the Virgin Mary.

The woman's body undergoes a complex narrative shaping as well: while some users insist on the negative aspects of pregnancy, such as nausea and cravings, others never even hint at this dimension, preferring to stress the emotional and existential ones instead; the mother's increase in weight is often socially approved through the interplay of posts and comments.

The online storytelling of pregnancy often borrows its characters from already-established narrative plots, thus making it even more tellable and shareable.

It is the case of what we have labelled 'the pregnancy tale': a story in which protagonists assume prototypical roles, with the father often presented as a hero or protector, the newborn as a little prince/princess, and the mother-to-be's friends assimilated to aunts: Rosa, for instance, posts the image of a pregnant belly, tied up in a blue ribbon, with the caption 'Waiting for a handsome little prince', while Maria writes 'Little prince I. has arrived!!!' under the first picture of the just-enlarged family. 'The pregnancy tale' tends to conclude with a happy ending represented by the child's birth and the beginning of an exciting family life.

'The pregnancy saga', on the contrary, puts on stage the listing of continuous adventures, misadventures, ups-and-downs of a mother-to-be: the struggle with nausea, the need to rest or avoid certain foods, the night cravings, the troubles in negotiating the name for the baby with the partner and/or other family members. Giorgia's profile is particularly telling in this sense:

> Acidity … leave my stomach! … Nausea, leave this body! … I'm hungryyyyyyy! Having to be content with boiled spinach and some vegetables is just not fair! … Giorgia, don't think about food, don't think about sandwiches, toasts, bruschettas, pizzas and the like … don't think about hamburgers, hot dogs and kebabs … just concentrate! Don't think! Remind yourself that they will harm you, harm you a lot! Think of the day you will just sit down and eat as many sausages as you wish …

In most cases, such outbursts stimulate supportive replies by her FB friends, whose comments contribute to the story as much as the original post does.

As is evident from these examples, online pregnancy narratives are often characterized by a shared and distributed authoriality, confirming what Alexander and Levine (2008, p. 40) state about Web 2.0 storytelling: 'stories now are open-ended, branching, hyperlinked, cross-media, participatory, exploratory, and unpredictable'. If on one side they are necessarily linear—an aspect imposed by the platform design—on the other these stories are also distributed among posts, comments, replies, and quotations and have become 'more like environments than classic tales' (Alexander and Levine, 2008, p. 46). Such nature of FB narratives is enabled and promoted by the structure of the site itself and is especially evident in the case of pregnancy: here, the teller's story interlaces with other mothers giving her reassurances and suggestions (e.g., 'Sleep while you still can') or even recalling their own experience, thus multiplying the narrative levels.

The choice of FB as a medium for pregnancy narratives affects their structure in complex ways: the platform partly organizes them according to a linear temporalization, and partly leaves the user free to select her audience, the contents posted, and code used to post. Standardized formulas and traditional narrative patterns—clearly mirroring the usual offline word of mouth, which forms the traditional culture of pregnancy—interact with personal strategies of re-semantization and agency and undergo a continuous pluralization, negotiation, and dynamic interplay with other—similar and/or different—stories.

As concerns the second analytic level: by means of which semiotic modality do such stories take place on FB? How are the contents illustrated and discussed so far constructed through the platform?

The role played by the visual code in the shaping of 'good stories' is particularly evident in the incipits: breaking-the-news posts are in fact often made of images, mostly photographs of the belly that exploit the semantic potential of the changing body. Even when the verbal code is used, only rarely do sentences explicitly contain the substantive 'pregnancy' or the adjective 'pregnant'. Allusions to elements belonging to the typical offline stories of pregnancy are much more frequent: Arianna writes 'Everything's fine on the Blue Coast ... but in restaurants they don't serve any dish with cooked vegetables!'; Amelia wonders 'Was this nausea ever to end?'. Sometimes verbal and visual resources can intersect in the captioning of the pictures: here the semantic fields mostly alluded to refer to 'life', 'love' and 'tenderness', 'novelty', and 'waiting': 'A new life in a new office' is Elena's caption to the picture of herself in her new workplace; in Maria's story, instead, the visual content (herself smiling with two friends) is introduced by the sentence 'Waiting for the sweet I'. The comments stimulated by the announcement often assume very similar forms, which, from time to time, combine lexemes referring to the field of 'greetings', smiling emoticons, heart images, and shorter or longer series of exclamation marks. Sometimes the appreciation of the just-started story can be expressed by the community through the mere 'liking' of the post.

The development of the story of pregnancy usually unfolds as some kind of narrative of the assurance: the semiotic practice counts again mostly on the meaning evoked by the 'growing belly', this being shown on photographs by 60% of the informants at least once during the months following the announcement. When it comes to verbal storytelling, the post often informs about the good clinical progress, i.e., positive evolution, of the pregnancy. Here the semantics of the 'passage of time' is particularly exploited, as in the 'countdown' to giving birth: some rare occurrences of use of the clinical terminology of pregnancy appear in such cases, for instance when it comes to the good news about the 'echography'. The semantization of further related narrative fields corroborates the 'good story' previously started: the 'love for the partner', primarily, pulls up to the meanings already configured at the beginning of the story such as those of 'love', 'novelty', and 'waiting'. An additional example can be found in the metalinguistic domain of the 'naming' of the baby-to-be, within which, for instance, photographs showing a flower which bears the same name as the future child are shown, as in Elena's story. The comments raised by such posts extend a 'semantics of excitement': they often invoke meanings related to 'beauty' and even to 'wonder'. As in the incipits, they mostly assume the form of 'chunks' of both verbal and graphical nature: roughly the same words and emoticons, icons, punctuation, and their sequences are used by the community to express such meanings (e.g., ☺, ♥, !!!!!!!!!!!!!), as the event of delivery leads to the narrative climax.

The news of the birth is in fact often announced by means of a photograph which finally concludes the process of personification of the baby: the zoom of his/her little hands and feet is particularly recurrent (e.g., in the stories by Arianna, Marta, Sara, Cristina, and Ludovica). Scenes of physical contact, and even of breastfeeding are sometimes portrayed (e.g., in the stories by Sandra, Silvia, and Mara). The verbally semanticized contents refer again to 'wonder' and 'welcoming', often intersected with lexical choices exploiting the affective register: our informant Lucia, for instance, posts: 'I just didn't think we'd do it today … Indeed on 17 October 2013 she has arrived', and similarly, Rosa posts: 'Welcome to the world, sweet child of mine'. Even the natural pain of delivery is recalled in a positive, assuring sense: different women of the sample have posted the same link to a poem that celebrates it, both visually and verbally, as a necessary step for the rebirth of the woman as a mother and heroine: an interpretation that had already been anticipated by other references during the development of pregnancy (this specific practice of posting a link to further Internet sites and contents can be understood as a 'technique of quotation').

By means of the continuous relation between subjectivity and collectivity, on one side memories are constructed on FB, on the other they unveil as the reconfiguration and adaptation of previous interpretations of reality. This constant 'semiotic game', as Wittgenstein (1958 [1953], p. 5) puts it, is already approaching the construction of new fields of meaning, and therefore the telling of new stories, such as the one of 'being a mother' and of the 'new family life'.

Finally, the socio-pragmatic level of storytelling on FB has to do with the authorial and relational dimension of these narratives: pregnancy stories are always produced by a specific subject and addressed to an audience with the aim of communicating a message or producing social effects. Posting is a complex narrative practice and, as such, it does not just respond to the platform norms but also represents an expression of agency and creativity.

Despite being extremely autobiographical, these stories are not necessarily ego-centric: on the contrary, as pregnancy advances, greater numbers of posts are actually dedicated—if not directly addressed—to the coming baby and projected into the future. As confirmed by the use of echographies or visual memes replacing the woman's profile picture, her personal identity is often progressively mixed, and finally wholly identified, with that of the unborn baby.

What many pregnancy narratives carry out, in this perspective, is the gradual construction—we might even say the narratively mediated 'gestation'—of the socially acceptable profile of a 'mother': posting her own 'typically motherly' steps in everyday life makes a woman feel legitimized as a 'good (future) mother'.

Through the storytelling of their pregnancy the authors seem to mirror themselves in specific patterns of motherhood. Among these, the following (at least) were identified: a) the 'traditional mother', who posts exactly what 'normal' mothers would be expected to post and displays typical motherly feelings (e.g., love, happiness, fear); b) the 'natural mother', who wants to have the complete control over her pregnancy: typically vegan and hyperinformed, she promotes natural nutrition, home delivery, and breast-feeding; and c) the 'successful mother', who does not want to completely renounce her own life path and thus continues to work until the very end of pregnancy, cultivates her passions, and assumes an intellectual attitude toward her free time.

On the relational side, the privacy settings and the 'politics' of sharing are quite significant as well: most of the contents which contribute to conquering the social approval of the author's forming motherhood are shared publicly, a smaller percentage only with friends. In this sense, during gestation the social value of pregnancy is negotiated not only in the woman's main narrative, but also in this continuous play between posts and comments, whereby she asks more experienced women for advice and searches for a legitimation and justification of her decisions and behaviours.

Posting on FB gives way to a shared authorship and a continuous pluralization of the narrative levels, especially where posts are enriched by comments. These, in turn, intersect with other comments entailing questions, suggestions, and memories, thus making up for a collective storytelling experience: a narrative community of feeling and interpretation.

The storytelling of pregnancy on Facebook: preliminary conclusions and open questions

Pregnancy is a deeply physical and psychological experience developing on both an individual and a social level. Charged with complex cultural expectations and always framed within the local representations of body, family, and motherhood, on the woman's side it stimulates a continuous need of sense-making which finds an ideal form in storytelling (Staton Savage, 2001).

Thanks to its particular interface and settings, FB constitutes the perfect narrative environment wherein to weave and share such sense: by telling her story of pregnancy on the platform while resorting to well-known narrative patterns, as well as through various forms of agency and re-semantization, the mother-to-be gradually shapes her future motherly profile, while finding her place in a specific narrative community of feeling and practice. Social networks are, in fact, becoming increasingly similar to off-line communities, thus fostering the collectivization of experience through practices of sharing that—although guaranteeing the space for individual variation—tend to reinforce common plots and formulas.

The approach proposed in this chapter insists on the importance of considering story telling as an integral part of any human practice of sense-making, especially when it comes to the understanding and managing of illness and similar experiences such as pregnancy (Kleinman and Kleinman, 1991; Kleinman, 1988; Giarelli et al., 2005).

Analysing a written corpus produced for a virtual social environment has provided both the aspects that are specific to the medium and those which these narratives have in common with our everyday stories, there being an important continuity between the two.

Online storytelling practices of this kind should be studied at least on three levels: a global narratological, a linguistic-rhetorical, and a socio-pragmatic one. As emerges from this analysis, pregnancy stories on FB tend to reproduce inherited cultural narrative patterns, exploit specific semantic fields, and produce socially significant effects, partly reinforcing and partly enriching those of offline storytelling. If the most exploited plots in the posts tend to replicate those of everyday narration, peculiar to these stories is the resort to both verbal and visual codes, the shared authorship, and a pluralization of the narrative levels. Further analyses of FB narratives of pregnancy should thus focus on such aspects.

These narratives are a precious source of knowledge about how people perceive and construct experience through storytelling, not only in general, but in the particular linguistic dimension offered today by social media.

References

Alexander, B. and Levine, A., 2008. Web 2.0 storytelling. Emergence of a new genre. *EduCAUSE Review*, **43**(6), 40–56. Available at: <http://www.educause.edu/ero/article/web-20-storytelling-emergence-new-genre>. (Accessed on 11 June 2016)

Ammaniti, M., 1995. *Maternità e gravidanza: studio delle rappresentazioni materne.* Milan: Raffaello Cortina.

Angelini, M. and Trinci, M., 2000. *Le voglie: l'immaginazione materna tra magia e scienza.* Rome: Meltemi.

Bégout, B., 2005. *La découverte du quotidien.* Paris: Allia.

Bonfanti, S., 2012. Farsi madri. L'accompagnamento alla nascita in una prospettiva interculturale. *Quaderni di Donne & Ricerca*, **27**, 1–75.

Borgato, R., Capelli, F., Ferraresi, M., eds., 2009. *Facebook come. Le nuove relazioni virtuali.* Milan: Franco Angeli.

Brislin, R. W. and Kim, E. S., 2003. Cultural diversity in people's understanding and uses of time. *Applied Psychology*, **52**(3), 363–382.

Brown, P., 2001. Ripetizione/Repetition. In: A. Duranti, ed. *Culture e discorso: un lessico per le scienze umane.* Rome: Meltemi. pp. 313–318.

Bruner, J. S., 2004. Life as narrative. *Sociological Research*, **71**(3), 691–710.

Chodorow, N., 1978. *The reproduction of mothering: psychoanalysis and the sociology of gender.* Berkeley, CA: University of California Press.

Davis-Floyd, R. and Georges, E., 1996. On Pregnancy. In: D. Levinson and M. Ember, eds. *Encyclopedia of cultural anthropology*. New York: Holt. pp. 1014–1016.

Duden, B., 1993. *Disembodying women. perspectives on pregnancy and the unborn*. Cambridge, MA: Harvard University Press.

Fiume, G., 1995. *Madri. Storia di un ruolo sociale*. Venice: Marsilio.

Ghidoli, D., 2010. *Facebook e la celebrazione della Quotidianità. Semiotica del social (media) networking*. PhD Dissertation. Università degli Studi di Torino, Turin.

Giarelli, G., Good, B. J., Del Vecchio Good, M. J., Martini, M., and Ruozi, C., eds., 2005. *Storie di cura. Medicina narrativa e medicina delle evidenze: l'integrazione possibile*. Milan: Franco Angeli.

Haiman, J., 1997. Repetition and identity. *Lingua*, 100(1), 57–70.

Halbwachs, M., 1925/1992. *On collective memory*, trans. L. Coser. Chicago, IL: University of Chicago Press.

Herman, D., 2005. Narrative as a cognitive instrument. In: D. Herman, M. Jahn, and M. L. Ryan, eds. *Routledge encyclopedia of narrative theory*. London: Routledge. pp. 349–350.

Horning, R., 2012. Fragments on microcelebrity. *The New Inquiry*. 1 October. Available at: <https://thenewinquiry.com/blog/fragments-on-microcelebrity/>. (Accessed 1 November 2016).

Johnstone, B., ed., 1994. *Repetition in discourse: interdisciplinary perspectives*. Vol. 2. Norwood, NJ: Ablex.

Jordan, B. and Davis-Floyd, R., 1978/1993. *Birth in four cultures. a crosscultural investigation of childbirth in Yucatan, Holland, Sweden, and the United States*. 4th edn. Long Grove, IL: Waveland Press.

Kitzinger, S., 1980. *Women as mothers: how they see themselves in different cultures*. New York: Vintage.

Kleinman, A., 1988. *The illness narratives. Suffering, healing and the human condition*. New York: Basic Books.

Kleinman, A. and Kleinman, J., 1991. Suffering and its professional transformation: toward an ethnography of interpersonal experience. *Culture, Medicine, and Psychiatry*, 15(3), 275–320.

Lauer, R. H., 1981. *Temporal man: the meaning and uses of social time*. New York: Praeger.

MacCormack, C. P., 1994. *Ethnography of fertility and birth*. Long Grove, IL: Waveland Press.

Martini, O., 2005. Raccontare dentro i media. Riflessioni sulle forme e dimensioni del racconto nella società dell'informazione e della comunicazione. *Tecn Did*, 34(1), 43–47.

Massa, E., 2016. Stories of words, words as stories. Some lexico-statistically based reflections on the meaning unit in spoken language. *Linguistik Online*, 75(1), 103–142.

Massa, E. and Simeoni, V., 2014. Once upon a tale. On the foundational role of narrative in constructing linguistic and social experience. *COMPASO*, 5(1), 71–96.

Mead, M. and Newton, N., 1967. Cultural patterning of perinatal behavior. In: S. Richardson and A. Guttmacher, eds. *Childbearing: its social and psychological aspects*. Baltimore, MA: Williams and Wilkins. pp. 142–244.

Mitchell, W. J. T., 1981. *On narrative*. Chicago, IL: University of Chicago Press.

Montemagno, M. and Ruggeri, M., 2009. *Alla conquista del web*. Milan: Mursia.

Polkinghorne, D. E., 1988. *Narrative knowing and the human sciences*. Albany, NY: State University of New York Press.

Rich, A., 1977. *Of woman born: motherhood as experience and institution*. London: Virago Press.

Ricoeur, P., 1981. Narrative time. In: W. J. T. Mitchell, ed. *On narrative*. Chicago, IL: University of Chicago Press. pp. 165–186.

Ricoeur, P., 1984. *Time and narrative*. Vol. 1. Trans. K. Mclaughlin and D. Pellauer. Chicago, IL: University of Chicago Press.

Rosen, J., 2010. The web means the end of forgetting. *The New York Times*, 21 July. Available at: <http://www.nytimes.com/2010/07/25/magazine/25privacy-t2.html?pagewanted=all&_r=0>. (Accessed 1 November 2016).

Schutz, A., 1964. The dimensions of the social world. In: **A. Brodersen**, ed. *Collected papers II: studies in social theory*. The Hague: Martinus Nijhoff. pp. 20–63.

Shank, R. C., 1995. *Tell me a story: narrative and intelligence*. Evanston, IL: Northwestern University Press.

Staton Savage, J., 2001. Birth stories: a way of knowing in childbirth education. *Journal of Perinatal Education*, 10(2), 3–7.

Tremayne, S., 2001. *Managing reproductive life: cross-cultural themes in fertility and sexuality*. London: Berghahn Books.

Volli, U., 2003. Azioni e tipologie di siti. Versus. Quaderni di studi semiotici, 94–95–96, 271–282.

Wittgenstein, L., 1953/1958. *Philosophical Investigations*. Oxford: Basil Blackwell.

Chapter 25

Changes in authenticity

Perceptions of parents and youth with ADHD of the effects of stimulant medication

Erez C. Miller and Amos Fleischmann

Introduction

> *This above all: to thine own self be true ...*
> *Thou canst not then be false to any man ...*
> *Shakespeare, Hamlet, I,iii, 78, 80*

Attention Deficit Hyperactivity Disorder (ADHD) is a common neurodevelopmental condition that begins in childhood and may continue through adolescence and adulthood (APA, 2013). It is defined as a persistent pattern of inattention and/or hyperactivity-impulsivity that impairs an individual's functioning and development (APA, 2013). The recommended treatment for ADHD may be educational, nutritional, psychological (Sonuga-Barke et al., 2013), and/or pharmacological. Psychopharmacological treatment (e.g., Ritalin) is the first and most common treatment for ADHD (Millichap, 2010).

The use of these medications has been strongly debated because medications may alter an individual's sense of authenticity and even affect their free will (Comstock, 2011). This can seriously compromise young people's adherence to medication management (e.g., Charach and Fernandez, 2013; McCarthy, 2014). Although some attempts have been made to understand the factors that may affect medication adherence generally (e.g., Charach and Fernandez, 2013), and the extent to which ADHD medications affects sense of authenticity particularly, the matter warrants further examination. In addition, when considering a treatment that may change an individual's sense of psychological authenticity, ethical issues should be borne in mind.

This chapter discusses a study that examined online forums of young people's narratives about experiences with ADHD medications and their sense of control over the use and effects of the medications on authenticity.

Effect of medications on youth with ADHD

ADHD among youth often hampers the individuals' functioning at school, home, and work (APA, 2013). It is often associated with oppositional and aggressive behaviours, depression, anxiety, low self-esteem, and learning disorders (Sonuga-Barke et al., 2013).

Studies that examine the attitudes of youngsters with ADHD and their parents toward the disorder and its psychopharmacological treatment reveal widely divergent attitudes. Some of those who have ADHD understand it as a neurobiological condition and accept medication as an effective neurobiological treatment; others frown on the use of medication, believing that it impairs their functioning and fearing its burden (Bussing et al., 2012; Walker-Noack et al., 2013).

Pharmacological treatment has been documented for decades as improving the functioning of individuals with ADHD by reducing impulsiveness and hyperactivity and enhancing attention (Charach and Fernandez, 2013). Indeed, research on the experiences of young people with ADHD in using medication suggests that they credit the medication for improving their academic attainments and social relations (Charach et al., 2014; Singh, 2013; Walker-Noack et al., 2013). Aside from recognized side effects of the medication (e.g., loss of appetite, headaches), however, some youth report adverse psychological and behavioural effects such as depression, nervousness, overly subdued personality, and impairment of social conduct and relations. These psychological effects modify their sense of authenticity (Avisar and Lavie-Ajayi, 2014; Charach and Fernandez, 2013; Walker-Noack et al., 2013) and, possibly, their willingness to adhere to the use of medication for treating their ADHD (Charach et al., 2014; McCarthy, 2014).

Online forums as research tools

Millions of people around the world are increasingly using the Internet as a source of health information. Online forums offer support communities for those in need. These types of forums may provide people with disabilities or their families with a sense of belonging and a platform where they may explore and construct their identity, interact with others who have similar experiences and concerns, or consult with professionals. These online interactions are an important venue that could help individuals with disabilities construct their personal narratives.

When a narrative is constructed while its author is adjusting to an illness or a disorder, it may help invest the individual's struggle with the illness and the hardships of treatment with meaning (Frank, 1995). Internet forums might serve as significant tools in creating such narratives (Fleischmann and Miller, 2013). Sharing personal narratives with others also includes individuals sharing their understanding of the condition and its implications. This understanding could be a resource of support for others (Cole et al., 2011; Eysenbach, 2008). These forums facilitate social interaction and allow individuals to disclose their experiences, concerns, and opinions regarding health and disability issues.

However, communication in these forums can be dominated by other participants, by professionals, or by both (Cole et al., 2011; Mackey and Schoenfeld, 2016; Orr, Baram-Tsabari, and Landsman, 2016), and that type of control over the discussion may represent hidden agendas reflecting the medical model, rather than a more humanistic approach to treatment of ADHD.

Authenticity and the aim of the study

'Authenticity' is an accepted term that describes an individual's true essence (Varga and Guignon, 2016). Wood and colleagues (2008) empirically tested a model that was based on Barrett-Lennard's (1998, p. 82) definition, which described authenticity as a tripartite construct that involves 'consistency between the three levels of (a) a person's primary experience, (b) their symbolized awareness, and (c) their outward behavior and communication.' This study asserts that an ethical medical treatment is one that allows its recipients to maintain their authenticity. An indication of the maintenance of one's authenticity during medical treatment and, in turn, of the ethicality of the treatment, may be obtained by examining the possibility of applying free will and investigating the meaning of the treatment in the individual's life (Newson and Ashcroft, 2005).

In recent years, online forums have been documenting the way youth with ADHD view the effects of medications on their authenticity and personal narratives, and the advice provided to them by professionals. Thus, these forums may help social researchers to examine the opinions of professionals on safeguarding these young people's authenticity. The goal was to examine how the safeguarding of authenticity is discussed and constructed both by young people with ADHD or their parents and by professionals.

Method

The study investigated four Hebrew-language online forums dedicated to ADHD issues. Most people who participated in them were interested in receiving some form of consultation on various aspects of ADHD. In each forum there was a group of professionals responding to questions posted by participants, although some responders were not professionals. The following forums were monitored; the dates of monitoring are shown in parentheses:

- Tapuz (Orange), for support of persons with attention disorders (5 November 2013–20 September 2016).
- Kamoni (Like Me) (5 November 2013–20 September 2016).
- BeOK for Attention Disorders, You Have a Question (1 September 2013–17 April 2014).
- Ynet Forum for Children with ADHD (1 September 2011–8 January 2012).

Data selection criteria

The forum sites include hundreds of pages of Q&A and discussions. These were filtered for narratives that focused on personal experiences with ADHD treatment and, especially, psychopharmacological treatment. A second criterion for selection was the presence of some evidence of age (12–25 years old).

Data analysis

An ethnographic-discursive approach (Montaki and Frigerio, 2016) was applied to all posts in order to examine forms of interaction agreement and disagreement among participants and professionals. This inquiry is instrumental for understanding the power relations that evolve between participants and professional respondents.

In the first stage of the data analysis, each researcher read the discussions and posts individually and profiled various themes that focus on psychopharmacological treatment (Saladana, 2012). In the second stage, commonalities and differences among the posts in the forums were identified and the themes were combined into categories. In the third stage, the responses were sorted in an attempt to uncover the different narratives from the text (Potter, 2004).

Rigour

Both researchers are experienced in qualitative research on narrative inquiries relating to ADHD (e.g., Fleischmann and Miller, 2013). One of them is a licenced school psychologist who evaluates and treats youth with ADHD, and the other is a father of a young adult with ADHD; these close connections to young people with ADHD allowed them to judge the authenticity of the various discussions in the forums.

The researchers analysed the data individually. Agreement was usually high. Disagreements were resolved by discussing and re-examining the data.

To strengthen the validity of the conclusions, an integrated method was used that examined the categories raised in various discussions and applied a discourse analysis that focused on the essence of the responses to various topics in the forums (Montaki and Frigerio, 2016).

Ethical aspects of the study

The proposal for the study was examined and approved by an institutional review board (IRB). Online content, such as that posted on Internet forums, may serve as research data if the forum is considered part of the public domain and has no restrictions or requirements for registration (Buchanan, 2011), giving it a status equivalent to published material in other media. None of the selected forums had restrictions on use or access.

Finally, the study strove for maximum authenticity in quoting the participants (the translation from Hebrew to English attempted to maintain the spirit of the original post). All details in the forum that might have identified participants and respondents were omitted to maintain anonymity.

Results

Discussions in online forums on ADHD treatment suggest a clash between two competing narratives. The first is expressed by young people with ADHD and their parents. The other narrative is presented by professionals often holding a medical view of treating ADHD (henceforth the 'respondents'). Participants (youth or their parents) viewed the effects of ADHD medications as sometimes having dramatic effects on their authenticity.

Comments about medication-induced changes

Changes in authenticity

Some forum participants stated clearly that the medication was causing them to change. One girl explained that she became a more efficient person with the medication but also one that had a different sense of authenticity: 'It turns me into another person'. Another female teenager stated that the medication affected her priorities:

> Right now I'm treated with Concerta and I feel that my friends don't interest me anymore, my ADHD friends don't suit me when I'm on Concerta, my parents do suit me when I'm on Concerta, and my boyfriend does not suit me when I'm on Concerta, one subject [at school] suits me and another doesn't.

Another female adolescent felt that she was two different people in her performance capacity and that her inner feelings had changed: 'I feel that I live a double life [with the medication and without it]'. This 'split' could have an important impact on the development of her personal narrative.

The narratives of parents echoed similar sentiments. One mother explained that her son did not wish to take medication for ADHD because he did not want to change:

> Now he's in ninth grade, and he strongly refuses to take it because the medication changes him [it makes him unsociable] and it took him time to become socially accepted. In the meanwhile, he doesn't study. He can't study without the medication and we're getting calls from his teachers left, right and center.

The nature of participants' reports about changes in authenticity

The changes induced by methylphenidate hydrochloride (MPH), the active ingredient in stimulant medications used for treating ADHD), are usually described when participants ask the forum for help in coping with side effects associated with taking it, such as nausea, headaches, lack of appetite, and stomach aches. The terms used imply that the medication induces deep psychological changes, and included 'always (under drug effects) being offended', 'angry', 'anxious', 'asocial', 'cowardly', 'cries a lot', 'depressive', 'fatigue', 'feeling down', 'feeling like a pressure cooker', 'irritability', 'needy', 'not happy', 'not smiling', 'not wanting to meet friends', 'outbursts', 'rage', 'robot', 'serious', 'stressed out', 'total lack of concentration', 'turned-off character', 'unusually quiet', 'weird discomfort', 'hypersensitive to noise', and 'zombie'.

Effects on mood and activities

Many participants in the forums stated that the medication compromised their mood and willingness to perform tasks, e.g., 'Is there a type of Ritalin that doesn't give you a sense of depression or lack of desire to talk and do things? That's a shame because this [medication's] disadvantage is very meaningful to me'; 'She says that the medications suppressed her feelings and that she was acting like a robot'; 'While the medication influences him, he turns from a happy, chatty, and smiling teenager to a solemn, unsmiling teenager'.

Social impact

Several participants described the medication as affecting their social functioning for the worse. Two examples follow:

> My daughter is in high school and in the middle of last year she decided that the medication was hurting her in terms of her mood, her skills, and her social contacts. She claims … that her grades are less important to her than her functioning as a human being.

> In 7ᵗʰ grade she [his daughter] stopped taking the medication because it was affecting her socially. This [treatment with medication] makes her feel less happy, moody, and it badly affected her socially.

Responses to reports about changes

When participants raised questions implying that medication affected them psychologically, they received responses ranging from partial confirmation to total disagreement.

Partial confirmation. Usually the respondents (i.e., professionals who participated in the forums and responded to posts and/or served as administrators of the forums) agreed somewhat with participants who implied that MPH had some effect on their authenticity. One way they chose to attenuate their agreement was 'correction'. Some, for example, agreed that the medication may have some unwanted psychological effects but attributed these effects to incorrect use. The correct dosage or the right medication, they stated, would prevent undesirable psychological effects. Here are two examples:

> It would be a good idea to go back to your doctor and consult with him so he could offer you another suitable treatment. There are some side effects such as lack of appetite, feeling like a zombie, and depression.

> This [decline in *joie de vivre*] might be connected to the medication. (It's certainly possible that it's due to a dosage that's too low). It might be connected to the beginning of a decrease in the level of medication in the body.… Different ways of absorbing the medication may dramatically affect the way the active ingredient acts or the side effects. (Therefore, one needs to choose the right drug.)

Sometimes respondents who were forum administrators agreed in part with the participants' narrative that medication could cause significant psychological changes but thought that the changes affect only some young people. The following examples demonstrate that the respondent's view of the medication and its effects is not suitable for everyone:

> After meeting with hundreds of children, I could responsibly say that there are children whose anxiety increases after taking Ritalin, while with other children the Ritalin's impact was a positive one—since it's very personal, the only way to know its impact is through trial and error.

> Based on my experience, the most important thing is not to be afraid!! If the child responds well to Ritalin that's wonderful, because he could then fulfill his potential.… Every child responds differently so there's no need to get stressed out.

Suggestions about taking less medication. Some responses demonstrate that the experts agreed with the participants about undesired effects of medication but doubted the narrative on changes in authenticity as unbearable. Two examples follow:

> Look for whatever it is that improves your life significantly and has bearable side effects.

> If there were one medication that's effective and has no side effects, we would have thrown all the other medications out. There's no telling … Don't look for an ideal medication: One that does not have any side effects and that will change your life forever—there's no such thing. (So you should be satisfied that the medication you're currently taking helps you [Respondent's comment]).

One of the side effects that often prompted participants to stop using medication was lack of *joie de vivre*. It was particularly apparent in highly active youngsters who suddenly seemed to be 'switched off'. Still, these youth often functioned much better on medication even when they felt like 'zombies'—a combination supportive of the argument that taking medication should be accepted. Since the experts considered side effects inevitable, they suggested that the medication be taken only when needed. Here are two examples:

> It's possible that you haven't figured out completely for yourself when you should or should not take the medication …

> Based on my own family experience with adults who've been taking Ritalin since childhood, you should look into when you should take Concerta and when you shouldn't. Since it's not a medication that builds up inside your body, you can skip it on the day you think it isn't necessary …

This approach appears to uphold the right of the individual with ADHD to decide when and how to use the medication.

Disagreement

A physician who participated in the forum agreed that medication has an emotional effect on youngsters but disputed the statement that it hampers their authenticity, and even hinted that (in his opinion) the medication helps them *bring out* their identity, thus suggesting that many youth do feel that it changes who they are:

> Ritalin is not a panacea; it just enables the child to have a better quality of life and to fulfill his true abilities. Often I hear children saying 'With Ritalin I'm not myself' and I tell them: 'With Ritalin you're exactly yourself, just with better abilities'.

This suggests that many youth do feel that MPH changes who they are.

Freedom of choice: taking medication based on needs. Due to some of the aforementioned side effects—impaired social activity in particular—many young people preferred to medicate themselves on a need-only basis. Here are several examples:

> [I've been] in a relationship with MPH of various forms for four years. I don't take it regularly but based on my need at the time.

> During the year she [her daughter] took medication only on days when she had to study intensively (because the medication badly affects her social life).… She takes [ADHD] medications according to how she assesses the days and the tasks ahead of her. Her social situation is great.

Responses to discussions on freedom of choice

Some responses reflect agreement with the action or choice of an individual who used medication. When an adolescent who used to medicate stopped doing so on the grounds that it hampered his ability to make social connections, other laypersons in the forum tended to endorse her exercise of free will. Here are some examples:

> It's no wonder that a normal girl would prefer her social life to her studies and would therefore refuse to take any medication …

> We should respect their need for social life (and therefore not to use any medication), which is especially important in this age, to maintain a healthy, mature relationship, etc.…

> The side effects that your daughter describes [Ritalin hampering her social capabilities] are definitely worthy of attention, and I think her claim that the emotional and social damage is greater than the academic benefit is a worthy claim …

> Of course, it's possible that she's inflating the social cost that she's paying as part of the rebelliousness that Z [the female professional] describes, but it's not certain at all, and if I were in your place I'd take the opposite view—assuming that she [the girl] is the only one who can judge how it affects her.… No one but her can judge it. She's the only one who lives inside her skin and feels the impact [of the medication] …

Some professionals agreed with participants who implied that since the medication has side effects, the participant or their child with ADHD uses it infrequently and only when needed:

> As you said, there's no problem with taking the medication only on specific days. It won't compromise your health and it shouldn't worry you. Some people need to take it regularly and some do not …

> There's no problem taking Ritalin on days when one feels it's necessary, or even only once a week …

Objection to the use of medications

Some participants in the forums phrased their questions a way that doubted the legitimacy of using MPH. A therapist, for example, claimed that the medication may inflict physical and emotional damage on adolescents. Other participants thought homeopathic remedies should replace MPH because they, unlike methylphenidate, 'have no side effects and do not affect youngsters psychologically'.

Responses to objections to the use of medications

One respondent answered the person who objected to using medication by asking, 'Why do you hate it [the medication] so much'? Another young respondent wrote:

> After watching the clips that you've attached to your previous postings, I now understand some very important things about you. I'd like to ask you: Why don't you present yourself as who you really are??? You could be a holistic therapist, but your worldview is one of a Scientologist. So if we're into clips, here's an illuminating clip about Scientology.

When a participant claimed that MPH has drug-like and possibly sedative effects on young people, they received the following angry response:

> At first I thought you meant well. I read what you wrote all the way to the end and almost all the way through I thought you meant well, until I got to the ugly words 'drugging children needlessly'. Shame on you.

One of the respondents, a professional, explained the forum's policy in response to a participant who expressed surprise about not being answered contemptuously when she claimed that a food additive helped her son:

> If you wrote that after your successful experience you concluded that Ritalin is a bad thing and shouldn't be used, that anyone who takes Ritalin isn't doing the right thing or is just a sucker, and that mothers who give their children Ritalin are anything but good mothers ... then yes, it's forbidden to write in our forum anything bad about Ritalin, or about who gives it to children, or who uses it themselves.

The professional went to explain that since the participant had merely praised a food additive and did not vilify the use of medication, her opinion was not silenced.

Discussion

The regnant perspective on ADHD in many countries (including Israel) is the medical model, which views the condition as a disorder (Hinshaw et al., 2011). Accordingly, the medical and educational establishments put forth the following narrative: Individuals with ADHD are treated with medication in order to cope with the symptoms of ADHD and subsequently to improve the individuals' functioning. Hence, the treatment enables students to fulfill their academic potential (Hinshaw et al., 2011). Nevertheless, it is crucial to find the most effective dosage and type of medication in order to avoid side effects as far as possible (McCarthy, 2014). The professionals in the examined forums appear to have adopted this narrative, i.e., they encouraged participants who sought to continue the use of medication and attempted to help them mitigate its adverse effects. Thus, participants who complained about unwanted psychological side effects were advised to consult with physicians. Some of these professionals, aware that sometimes negative side effects cannot be avoided completely, agreed with the participants that side effects exist but encouraged them to continue using the medication, suggesting that its benefit outweighs its cost. This convergence of views, however, ceased when participants denied the legitimacy of using medications.

The medical model of ADHD has faced serious criticism in recent years (Bailly, 2005; Comstock, 2011; Furman, 2008). The critics propose a contrasting narrative that does not see ADHD as a disorder (Bailly, 2005; Comstock, 2011; Furman, 2008). The critics charge that the educational and medical establishments support the use of medication for the purpose of changing individuals who exhibit challenging behaviour into submissive individuals who lack free will and are easier to control and manage (Bailly, 2005; Costmock, 2005). The results of the present study, however, do not support such a narrative. They indicate that young people who participated in the forum used their judgment when using medication. While some of them reported a modification of authenticity under the influence of medication, it appears that they were aware of the medication's effects. Therefore, they put the medication aside when they thought it important to remain spontaneous for social interaction. Furthermore, professionals who provided consultation in the forums usually supported the participants' perspective of using the medication on the basis of need. Lay respondents similarly supported calculated decisions by youth to stop taking the medication altogether when the change that it induced in participants' authenticity hampered their social life.

Summary and conclusions

Questions and answers in online forums yield narratives that point to a struggle for the preservation of authenticity. Youth who opted to improve their functioning by means of psychopharmacological medication reported changes in their authenticity and responded by using discretion to limit these changes. Some professionals agree with these young people's perspectives, suggesting that the changes may be kept in check by using the medication selectively. In the authors' opinion, the debate over whether or not ADHD is a disorder is secondary in importance to the question of how youth with ADHD who are treated with medication negotiate and construct their personal narratives as they struggle to express their free will and maintain their authenticity. Constructing and negotiating these narratives is particularly difficult as it clashes with the medical perspective of ADHD and its treatment. On the one hand, to promote affirmative discussions in online forums and the construction of healthy personal narratives of youth with ADHD, young people must be well informed about the benefits of the medication as well as its potential effect on their authenticity. On the other hand, these young people should be made aware that the medical perspective presents a professional narrative. To help their child maintain their authenticity and avoid unethical conduct, adults at home and at school should discuss with these young people the various aspects and implications of making an informed decision about using medication, thus helping them negotiate what ADHD means for them and the best ways for them to manage its consequences.

References

American Psychiatric Association (APA), 2013. *Diagnostic and statistical manual of mental disorders*. 5th edn. Arlington: American Psychiatric Publishing.

Avisar, A. and **Lavie-Ajayi, M.**, 2014. The burden of treatment: listening to stories of adolescents with ADHD about stimulant medication use. *Ethical Human Psychology & Psychiatry*, **16**, 37–50.

Bailly, L., 2005. Stimulant medication for the treatment of ADHD: evidence-b(i)ased practice? *Psychiatric Bulletin*, **29**, 284–287.

Barrett-Lennard, G. T., 1998. *Carl Rogers' helping system: journey and substance*. London: Sage.

Buchanan, E. A., 2011. Internet research ethics: past, present, and future. In: **R. Burnett, M. Consalvo**, and **C. Ess**, eds. *The Handbook of Internet Studies*. Oxford: Wiley-Blackwell. pp. 83–108.

Bussing, R., Koro-Ljungberg, M., Noguchi, K., Mason, D., Mayerson, G., and **Garvan, C. W.**, 2012. Willingness to use ADHD treatments: a mixed methods study of perceptions by adolescents, parents, health professionals and teachers. *Social Science & Medicine*, **74**, 92–100.

Charach, A. and Fernandez, R., 2013. Enhancing ADHD medication adherence: challenges and opportunities. *Current Psychiatry Reports*, **15** (7), 1–8.

Charach, A., Yeung, E., Volpe, T., and Goodale, T., 2014. Exploring stimulant treatment in ADHD: narratives of young adolescents and their parents. *BMC Psychiatry*, **14**, 110. doi: 10.1186/1471-244X-14-110.

Cole, J., Nolan, J., Seko, Y., Mancuso, K., and Ospina, A., 2011. GimpGirl grows up: Women with disabilities rethinking, redefining, and reclaiming community. *New Media & Society*, **13**(7), 1161–1179.

Comstock, A. J., 2011. The end of drugging children: toward the genealogy of the ADHD subject. *Journal of the History of the Behavioral Sciences*, **47**, 44–69.

Eysenbach, G., 2008. Medicine 2.0: social networking, collaboration, participation, apomediation, and openness. *Journal of Medical Internet Research*, **10**(3), e22.

Fleischmann, A. and Miller, E. C., 2013. Online narratives by adults with ADHD who were diagnosed in adulthood. *Learning Disability Quarterly*, **36** (1), 47–60.

Frank, A., 1995. *The wounded storyteller: body, illness and ethics*. Chicago, IL: University of Chicago Press.

Furman, L. M., 2008. Attention-deficit hyperactivity disorder (ADHD): does new research support old concepts? *Journal of Child Neurology*, **23**(7), 775–784.

Hinshaw, S. P., Scheffler, R. M., Fulton, B. D., Aase, H., Banaschewski, T., Cheng, W., Mattos, P., Holte, A., Levy, F., Sadeh, A., Sergeant, J. A., Taylor, E., and Weiss, M. D., 2011. International variation in treatment procedures for ADHD: Social context and recent trends. *Psychiatric Services*, **62**, 59–64.

Mackey, T. K. and Schoenfeld, V. J., 2016. Going 'social' to access experimental and potentially life-saving treatment: an assessment of the policy and online patient advocacy environment for expanded access. *BMC Medicine*, **14**(1), 17–26.

McCarthy, S., 2014. Pharmacological interventions for ADHD: How do adolescent and adult patient beliefs and attitudes impact treatment adherence? *Patient Preference and Adherence*, **8**, 1317–1327.

Millichap, J. G., 2010. Medications for ADHD. In: J. G. Millichap, ed. *Attention deficit hyperactivity disorder handbook: A physician's guide to ADHD*. (2nd ed.) New York: Springer. pp. 121–123.

Montaki, L. and Frigerio, A., 2016. An ethnographic-discursive approach to parental self-help groups: the case of ADHD. *Qualitative Health Research*, **27**(7), 935–950.

Newson, A. J. and Ashcroft, R. E., 2005. Whither authenticity? *American Journal of Bioethics*, **5**, 53–55.

Orr, D., Baram-Tsabari, A., and Landsman, K., 2016. Social media as a platform for health-related public debates and discussions: the polio vaccine on Facebook. *Israel Journal of Health Policy Research*, **5**, 34. doi: 10.1186/s13584-016-0093-4.

Potter, J., 2004. Discourse analysis as a way of analysing naturally occurring talk. In: D. Silverman, ed. *Qualitative research: theory, method and practice*. (2nd ed.) London: Sage. pp. 144–160.

Saladana, J., 2012. *The Coding Manual for Qualitative Researchers*. Thousand Oaks: Sage.

Singh, I., 2013. Not robots: children's perspectives on authenticity, moral agency and stimulant drug treatments. *Journal of Medical Ethics*, **39**, 359–366.

Sonuga-Barke, E., Brandeis, D., Cortese, S., Daley, D., Ferrin, M., Holtmann, M., Stevenson, J., Danckaerts, M., van der Oord, S., Döpfner, M., Dittmann, R. W., Simonoff, E., Zuddas, A., Banaschewski, T., Buitelaar, J., Coghill, D., Hollis, C., Konofal, E., Lecendreux, M., Wong, I. C., Sergeant, J.; European ADHD Guidelines Group, 2013. Nonpharmacological interventions for ADHD: systematic review and meta-analyses of randomized controlled trials of dietary and psychological treatments. *American Journal of Psychiatry*, **170**, 275–289.

Varga, S. and Guignon, C., 2016. Authenticity. In: E. N. Zalta, ed. *The Stanford Encyclopedia of Philosophy* (Summer 2016 Edition). Available at: <https://plato.stanford.edu/archives/sum2016/entries/authenticity>. (Accessed 17 October 2017).

Walker-Noack, L., Corkum, P., Elik, N., and Fearon, I., 2013. Youth perceptions of attention-deficit/hyperactivity disorder and barriers to treatment. *Canadian Journal of School Psychology*, **28**, 193–218.

Wood, A. M., Linley, P. A., Maltby, J., Baliousis, M., and Joseph, S., 2008. The authentic personality: A theoretical and empirical conceptualization and the development of the Authenticity Scale. *Journal of Counseling Psychology*, **55**(3), 385–399.

Chapter 26

Illness narratives in political communication

Instrumental, institutional, and social functions of political actors' public illness accounts

Matthias Bandtel

The problem: stigmatized political bodies

Public interest in politicians' affliction with illness is not a new phenomenon, as evidenced by the pathographies of Woodrow Wilson, Franklin D. Roosevelt, or John F. Kennedy (L'Etang, 1970; Vandenberg, 1991). Politicians, however, used to conceal illness during their time in office or even for their whole lifetime in order to protect their identity, and their institutions, from the damage inflicted by the stigma of physical or psychological suffering (Goffman, 1990a).

Today, by contrast, pathological health records of political actors often become public as soon as they start running for office. It is no longer exclusively investigative journalism, physicians' indiscretion, or rumours leaking from the entourage that publicly expose politicians' illnesses. Rather, the political actors themselves approach the media and talk about their health history. In some instances, the politician's self-account on his or her physical or mental condition comes out rather as a reaction to some kind of external force. For example, politicians have to provide acceptable legitimizations if they have skipped or missed public events for a longer period of time. Moreover, if rumours about a political actor's health problems break ground, he or she might want to take the lead in the enfolding discourse by talking openly about the situation. Last but not least, visible signs of an illness simply cannot be concealed (Goffman, 1990a, pp. 64–67).

But there are also several cases among the German politicians studied in this chapter where factors other than those mentioned seem to trigger the illness account. For example, demissions are often justified with impairments to health. Obviously, there is no need for a resigning political actor to go into detail. Furthermore, while it is widely believed that discussing someone's 'fitness for office' during electoral campaigns is harmful for the candidate, some political actors pro-actively issue statements on their illnesses.

This chapter explores how politicians contribute proactively and reactively to media discourses about their (potential) illnesses, how images of compromised corporeality are thereby presented, and to what extent the presentation of pathologies contributes to the construction of politics in the media. In a first approach, the focus lies on three body functions: the political body as the hinge between the individual and society, the institutional representation and strategic self presentation of mediated bodies, and the presentational constraints and potentials of the sick body. These theoretical basics constitute the foundation for an empirical analysis of two German state ministers' illness accounts.

Intertwining of political, mediated, and sick bodies

The sociology of the body is approaching the connection of politics and the body from two directions. Structural theory identifies the body as a product of social order: '[T]he body of the individual is regulated and organized in the interest of population' (Turner, 2008, pp. 40–41). Structuration theory argues that discourses about the body actively influence social structures and thus have the ability to reproduce, transform, and negate institutional settings: '[T]he theoretical objective is to move from body to self to society' (Frank, 2001, pp. 47–48.). This transition from individual bodily needs and desires to societal power structures notably takes place in face-to-face-interactions. In situations of physical co-presence of two or more actors, the interaction partners make sense of their respective actions and reactions. Hereby, social aspirations, as expressively negotiated in the face-to-face interaction, constitute an interaction order and are preserved in what Goffman calls 'face' (1990b, 2005). According to Goffman, face is an image of self that is created in the mutual interaction during an encounter of two or more actors if the positive social values that one of the interaction partners claims for him/herself are approved and shared by the other (Goffman, 2005, pp. 5–15). Hence, the meticulously cultivated 'impression management' (Goffman, 1990b, pp. 203–230) contributes to the replication of a social order that is shaped by body practices during a face-to-face encounter.

For this reason, the body is of central importance for political representation (Diehl, 2010, p. 254; Raab, 2008, pp. 236–237; Raab et al., 2001, p. 193): the body of a politician symbolizes political values, principles, and institutions; personal appearances by political actors, pictures of their bodies, and body discourse convey these political dimensions and make politics tangible. Against this backdrop, media images of political actors' bodies impaired by illness seem to cut against the grain of the representative features of the political body.

In his study *Stigma: notes on the management of a spoiled identity* (1990a), the interaction theorist Erving Goffman examines strategies that are employed by individuals to control their body expression in face-to-face interactions. His main focus is on sick bodies. Goffman (1990a) understands illness as stigma because deviations from bodily norms as perceived or ascribed in the cultural practice imply a devaluation of social status and personal identity of a human being.

Goffman distinguishes between two perspectives of stigmatized individuals: if the stigma is clearly visible and known by others, he speaks of a discredited person. If the stigma is unknown by others and can be disguised, the person is discreditable and can

try to avoid open discreditation. Both types see themselves confronted with social demands of different kinds. Discredited individuals have to manage tensions that particularly emerge in interactions with the 'normal', who lower their status expectations for the
counterpart due to the stigma (Goffman, 1990a, p. 13). The discreditable person, however,
has to manage information. Hence, the task is to develop techniques that direct the knowledge over the so far undiscovered flaw according to her or his interests (Goffman, 1990a,
pp. 113–124).

Illness narratives reflect in a particularly illustrative manner on the embedding of the
corporeality and materiality of the body in cultural practices and social expectations.
They present 'styles of body usage' (Frank, 2001, p. 53), practices the storyteller exploits
to deal with the fundamental problems of the sick body (Frank, 2001, pp. 51–56; 1995,
pp. 27–40). A reconstruction of these practices not only sharpens the awareness for institutional and discursive requirements that generate specific bodies. It also points to the
potential to transform a society's understanding of the body.

For this reason, illness accounts of political actors can be analysed as contributions to
a discourse that reifies, actualizes, and transforms the social significance of illness, the
body, and politics. A discourse-analytical approach to the mediated illness narratives by
two German state politicians helps uncover the ways in which the sick body is depicted
and how the social and institutional contexts are reflected upon.

'Stigmatizing the body' and 'normalizing the disability': a case study of two German state ministers' illness narratives

The term illness narratives is used here with reference to the definitions of personal stories
by patients as coined by Kleinman (1988, p. 49), Hawkins (1994, p. 1), and Frank (1993,
p. 42). In the context of the study at hand, the concept comprises autobiographical and
biographical texts that are published in different mass-media outlets and that publicly
stage the meaningful processing of illness experiences of political actors (Bandtel, 2014;
2016). As it is often the case with private stories told by patients, political actors' illness
narratives, too, evolve slowly over time. But in contrast, the latter not only comprise of
contributions of the actors involved. Usually, comments from third parties like journalists and the public come into play. Last, but not least, scientific accounts like the study
at hand also constitute additional texts that contribute to a specific illness narrative. In
this regard, for analytical purposes it is crucial to differentiate between certain speaker
roles and various types of texts. In the case study here, autobiographical statements from
the affected political actors are taken into account as well as comments by public figures
and media texts. Altogether, these fragments constitute a public discourse that takes the
form of an illness narrative. To put it another way, political actors' illness narratives are
co-constructed; they are based on the accounts of the afflicted politicians themselves, but
their relevance and meaning is disputed by voices from other actors as well.

The following case study aims to contrast the illness narratives of two German state
ministers, Monika Hohlmeier and Malu Dreyer. The material is taken from a sample of

189 self-thematizations of illnesses by 36 then-active German politicians at state and federal level, published during the investigation period from 2008 to 2012. The accounts of Hohlmeier and Dreyer are worth a closer look as they illustrate two typical, albeit contrasting, courses of political actors' illness narratives. The written and visual media presentations of both politicians' illnesses reflect different discourse positions on the significance of body, illness, and politics. By contrasting these two accounts, it is possible to reconstruct the political body that is discursively created in the respective illness narrative. Furthermore, a certain understanding of social order can be identified that is symbolically embodied in political actors' illness thematizations.

Monika Hohlmeier, member of the conservative Christian Social Union in Bavaria, had been minister for education and cultural affairs in the German federal state of Bavaria from 1998 until 2005. In the year of her resignation, Hohlmeier gave an interview to the German people magazine *Bunte*, in which she made her affliction with an autoimmune disease public (Hohlmeier, 2008, p. 208). Her autobiography (Hohlmeier, 2008) vividly describes symptoms like viral infections, kidney failure, pancreatitis, muscular atrophy, and weight loss.

Maria Luise 'Malu' Dreyer was state minister for social issues, labour, health, and demographics in Rhineland-Palatinate from 2002 to 2013. Afterwards, the social democrat became minister president of this same state. In 2006, she disclosed her battle with multiple sclerosis to the press (Löwisch, 2013). At times, she relies on a wheelchair.[1]

The following sections discuss instructive sequences of Hohlmeier's and Dreyer's illness accounts in greater detail. To begin with, the different strategies in handling the public exposure of the illnesses will be of interest.

Body practices to cope with 'spoiled identity'

The normative expectations regarding socially accepted body presentations are reflected in illness narratives (Frank, 2001, 1995). In this respect, the illness narratives by the former state ministers primarily point to institutional requirements targeting the body of political actors. The autobiographical texts and quotations by Mrs Hohlmeier and Mrs Dreyer tell about the experience and fear of having opponents and internal-party challengers interpret visible physical impairments as a symbol of weakness and political defeat (see, for example, Hohlmeier, 2008, p. 81). Repeatedly the fear is expressed that admissions of fragile health could be used as a point for strategic attacks:

> When the moment came that I wanted to reveal my illness (or whatever I wanted to call it back then—I didn't know at that time) to fellow party members, I suddenly lost my courage to confess the whole truth. [...] Why did I want to avoid public controversy about my illness? On the one hand, I was afraid of the consequences and on the other hand, I refused to accept reality despite the severe symptoms. I had reached the peak of my political career and I wanted it to stay that way (Hohlmeier, 2008, pp. 107–108; trans. M. B.).

This type of statement is very common in political actors' illness accounts. Illness is regarded to be contradictory to the perceived normative expectations and institutional requirements politicians are expected to meet. Especially in text fragments from the affected politician, the physical stigma is typically presented as the root for refused recognition and as the basis for discrimination. Because body and identity are inextricably intertwined, the patients in political actors' illness narratives argue for the necessity to either control the bodily expressions or to reveal the stigma.

Control of 'discreditable' political bodies

According to Goffman's dichotomy of stigma (Goffman, 1990a, pp. 57–58), the politicians' illness narratives retrospectively illustrate the plight of the discreditable. The accounts of Hohlmeier and Dreyer both tell the story of how the politicians had initially chosen the typical strategy of the discreditable person to cover the respective stigma symbol (Goffman, 1990a, pp. 125–128). In an instructive text fragment of Dreyer's illness narrative, a newspaper reporter discloses how the then-minister for social affairs and health had initially avoided the wheelchair in order to conceal her multiple sclerosis:

> There had been reason to suspect something even before that day [of Mrs Dreyer's revelation to the press; M. B.], walking became more and more difficult for her, sometimes she stumbled. She had been minister for social affairs and health for four years at the time, when she spoke in front of a big audience of neurologists and she was thinking, now someone should take notice. But nobody did (Widmann, 2012b, p. 3; trans. M. B.).

Hohlmeier's autobiography describes the plight of the discreditable in even greater detail. The perceived risk of exposure culminates in an episode at a party event in which a journalist made the derogatory interpretations of a body expression that is considered a deviation from the norm explicit:

> The attack came out of nowhere and consisted of one word: anorexia. It struck me in the evening of 22 July 2004, a Thursday, in the Munich Hofbräukeller. [...] While I ignored the palpably nosy looks in my back and had a conversation with some colleagues and journalists, suddenly a representative of the press unapologetically interrupted and asked bluntly since when I was suffering from anorexia. Everyone around me held their breath (Hohlmeier, 2008, pp. 7–8; trans. M. B.).

In Monika Hohlmeier's account, the dramatic implications of such an insinuated exposure are located at the level of personal identity as well as in the political dimension. In her autobiography, Hohlmeier pointedly seems deeply emotionally hurt by the journalist's infringement. Apart from that, she repeatedly expresses her concern about her political reputation (Hohlmeier, 2008, p. 9).

This example of body control demonstrates that the strategy of hiding the stigma does not solve the plight of the discreditable. Even the most meticulous control of the body expression still bears the risk of getting 'exposed'.

Negotiating the meaning of 'discredited' political bodies

A way out of the contingent situation of the discreditable is the full disclosure of the stigma. Disclosure of oneself implies a radical shift from information management to the management of uneasy situations—from a discreditable person into a discredited one (Goffman, 1990a, p. 122).

One strand of Malu Dreyer's illness narrative revolves around the conditions and implications of such a confession. Based on interview statements by the state minister, media reports present a strategy to manage the tensions within the new social situation (see Löwisch, 2013). In the press, Mrs Dreyer's revelation received overwhelmingly positive acclaim; from the political actor's point of view, this approach can therefore be regarded as rather successful.

Close reading of the relevant media texts reveals three preconditions for disclosing the stigma without spoiling the politician's identity. First, they reflect upon how the political actor managed to stay ahead of the course of the public discourse.

> In 2006, the SPD [Social Democratic Party of Germany; M. B.] gets re-elected [in the state of Rhineland-Palatinate, M. B.], even wins the absolute majority. Dreyer is in a safe position. October 4, she holds a press conference, she tells it in a cabinet meeting, she tells it to her staff, she tells it to members of the parliamentary faction, all in one day. She was in control of the communication. 'That has been organized very well', she says satisfied, looking back from today (Löwisch, 2013, np; trans. M. B.).

As this sequence suggests, it is advantageous to reduce the risks of depreciating attributions to the illness by maintaining the prerogative of interpretation over the media discourse.

Second, Dreyer's illness account proposes a technique to indirectly balance the stigma by compensating the qualities that have been denied by others due to the stigma with special achievements in just those areas (Goffman, 1990a, pp. 45–56). In the media texts contributing to Dreyer's illness narrative, a press trip is described that the then-minister for social affairs had arranged for journalists. Against the backdrop of knowing about Dreyer's political ambitions, the German newspaper *Süddeutsche Zeitung* retrospectively makes sense of this PR stunt by calling it a demonstration that Dreyer was 'fit for office' (Widmann, 2012b, p. 3). The article implies that Dreyer had wanted to prove her physical fitness in front of press representatives and the media audience.

This strategy can often be observed in political actors' illness narratives. Sicknesses that in cultural interpretation are associated with physical frailty and psychological stress are compensated with the demonstration of an ability to perform and mental strength.[2]

But political actors rarely succeed in reinterpreting the stigma symbol as a sign of a different characteristic other than the flaw (Goffman, 1990a, pp. 148–150). In Malu Dreyer's illness narrative, however, it is ironically her wheelchair that several text fragments stylize into the symbol of the graceful handling of the experience of physical contingency:

> On this day [of the press trip; M. B.] the journalists witnessed a premiere: [Dreyer; M. B.] presented herself in the wheelchair for the first time. When it came to long walks, she let herself slide into her 'wheelie' and had her press secretary or a consultant push her to the destination. She laughed so gleefully that one thought could not be dismissed: If all people could be as happy as this woman in a wheelchair, nobody would wonder about the constantly grumbling Germans anymore (Widmann, 2012a, p. 5; trans. M. B.).

Third, Malu Dreyer's illness narrative also suggests that the confession is not only associated with new social challenges, but also that it promises a moral victory to add to her personal biography and social identity (Goffman, 1990a, pp. 148–150). In accepting and respecting their own situation, the stigmatized can gain reputation and status.

Construction of political bodies in illness narratives

In Frank's reception of Goffman's interactionist approach as 'structuration theory of the body and society' (Frank, 2001, p. 48), our common understanding of the body is not only the outcome of social discourses and institutions. In their practical use, body techniques can transform the cultural contexts in which bodies are conceived (see Intertwining of political, mediated, and sick bodies). Rather than adapting the corporeal presence to a prevailing perception of normalcy, a dissociation from this same conventional image of what is normal can be pursued. In particular, when the fight of stigmatized people for recognition gains broader public attention, a modification of normalcy perceptions can be the result (von Engelhardt, 2010, p. 136). Moreover, the stigmatized individual can achieve 'secondary gains' (Goffman, 1990a, p. 20) by rejecting social categories that fall within the accepted norm. For example, what is often taken unquestioned as 'normal' can become open to debate when the situation of discredited people attains more attention. Taking a standpoint in controversies like this by confession to what is widely regarded as stigma can become a crucial aspect of one's personal identity. In addition, as discussed next, the stigma can be used strategically to legitimize individual actions (Goffman, 1990a, pp. 19-21).

Legitimization of political action through illness

Political actors' illness narratives hint at how political decisions can be reinterpreted retrospectively by different observers against the backdrop of the illness. As Parsons has shown, accepting the 'sick role' (Parsons, 1951, p. 438) allows an individual to legitimately suspend his or her usual societal expectations to a certain extent (see Intertwining of political, mediated, and sick bodies). Hence, referring to an illness generates acceptance for violations of tasks delegated to political actors.

This approach of dealing with the stigma can be found in an episode of Monika Hohlmeier's illness narrative. In her autobiography, she excuses political misconduct that was attributed to her in retrospect with reference to her health issues (see Hohlmeier, 2008, pp. 76–77): by pointing to her health crisis, she tries to brush aside media criticism along the lines of staying passive in an election fraud scandal.[3]

Turning the stigma into a personal advantage by retrospectively using the illness to suspend responsibility and to legitimize political (non-)action displays a typical form of the strategic use of illness thematization by political actors as, for example, medical historian Hugh L'Etang (1970) has pointed out. However, the retrospective explanation of political decisions using the argument of health impediments is always open to scrutiny. When political action is made subject to retrospective revisions based on impaired health in the respective illness narratives, a political body is constructed that is overshadowed by perceptions of the illness. The following analysis of a media text contributing to Monika Hohlmeier's illness narrative will shed light on the discourse process creating this type of political body. Furthermore, Hohlmeier's case serves as an instructive example for polit ical consequences such a body construction may yield.

Initially, the politician herself suggested in her autobiography that in hindsight some of her actions should be relativized against the backdrop of her illness (see Hohlmeier, 2008, pp. 76–77). In the course of the evolving illness narrative, this interpretation transcends different text types, as the video analysis of the media discourse reveals (on methodology, see Dörner et al., 2015, pp. 65–95). In particular, one year after the publication of her autobiography, Monika Hohlmeier appeared in the popular German political TV talk show *Anne Will* (Anne Will, 2010). In a key sequence of this TV interview with talk show host Anne Will, Hohlmeier verbally claims to have overcome her illness. But on the TV screen, in a total camera perspective, the political actor is only shown in the background of the studio while she delivers this statement of her restitution. Simultaneously, in the foreground of the TV picture, archive images of Hohlmeier, showing her body marked by visible signs of her illness, are presented to the audience on a monitor set up in front of the stage.

This particular studio setting and audiovisual *mise en scène* serve as an external comment on the interplay of politics and illness that has been constructed before in Hohlmeier's own written account. Remember that in her autobiography Hohlmeier urged her readers to le-gitimize certain political (non-)actions through her illness. That way, Hohlmeier herself has cast doubt if her political decisions will stand against possible future revisions. In the sequence of the TV show described here, this notion is visually mirrored and reinforced at the same time. No matter how thoroughly Hohlmeier verbally reaffirms her recovery (in the background), the stigma symbol of being underweight (in the foreground) visually remains connected with the personal identity of the allegedly fully recovered politician. In this regard, the image composition suggests that all of Hohlmeier's statements should be interpreted against the backdrop of her illness. Hence, in the unfolding illness narrative, Hohlmeier's political body cannot emancipate itself from depreciating attributions.

The 'secondary benefit' that a stigmatized individual gains from using the illness to retrospectively rationalize personal failure thus comes at the price of keeping the stigma symbol front and centre with respect to body perception. Clearly, the construction of a political body that is subject to illness-related contingencies is problematic for Monika Hohlmeier's image as an accountable and trustworthy politician. So it is barely surprising that the media response to Monika Hohlmeier's autobiography is characterized by sus-picions that publishing the illness account was primarily driven by strategic calculation (see, for example, Volkert, 2010).

Identity-creating processing of the illness experience

In Malu Dreyer's illness narrative, a completely different approach in terms of the body confronting social normalcy expectations is presented. Rather than using the illness to excuse political action, the illness experience is portrayed as meaningful for the political work. Instead of having the political body retreat behind the sick body, in Malu Dreyer's illness narrative a positive image is built upon the basis of the stigma. This section investigates what aspects contributed to the widely positive response to Mrs Dreyer's illness account.

An article on German weekly newspaper's website *Zeit Online* reflects on the image of Rhineland-Palatinate's first female premier minister (Rosenfeld, 2013). The discourse fragment herein rejects the cultural practice to determine identity and status solely on the basis of the stigma. Instead, the illness account articulates the claim of people with deviant characteristics to a fully recognized identity (see also von Engelhardt, 2010, p. 136). Additionally, the negative connotations of the stigma symbol are reinterpreted as a resource for the development of a positive identity concept. Discursively, the illness account creates a political body that has special potential simply because of the experienced impairment:

> This is one of the goals that Malu Dreyer has worked towards in past years: That old people do not necessarily have to go into nursing homes [but live in self-organized communities instead; M. B.]. 'I do live in such a housing project myself', said the state minister. She is living in Schammatdorf in downtown Trier, a residential project where disabled people and people who are not, the old and the young, live together much like in a small village and take on 'responsibility for each other', as Malu Dreyer puts it. So, she is a state minister who is living her own politics, which definitely makes a clear difference when it comes to the passion with which she talks about her initiatives [...]. (Widmann, 2012a, p. 5; trans. M. B.)

In this contribution to Dreyer's illness narrative, two 'secondary gains' are ascribed to the political body emerging from this self-conscious reflection of social normalcy expectations: the illness experience opens access to political issues from the standpoint of those impacted. On the one hand, this ability to capture a perspective is presented as a requirement for responsible, target group-oriented political decisions. On the other hand, it makes political action sensually tangible in the media presentation. In this sense, the illness narrative constructs the image of a politician who in particular draws strength from her illness in order to overcome her own as well as others' impairment through political action.

A photo-portrait of Malu Dreyer delivers a visual confirmation of this discursive construction of the political body. The image accompanying the *Süddeutsche Zeitung* article (Widmann, 2012a, p. 5) shows Dreyer sitting in her wheelchair. This stigma symbol, surprisingly, is covered by six white geese in the foreground of the picture.

This picture, and especially the positioning of the fowl, deserves closer examination. The geese situate the scenery in the inclusive housing project, which the article describes as Dreyer's private setting but also as her exemplary political cause. Therefore, the geese symbolize the unity of private and political body. Moreover, they can be interpreted as a metaphor for the moral career that Dreyer has undergone from initially keeping her illness a secret to her fully exposing it (see Negotiating the meaning of 'discredited' political bodies). They hint to the children's book *The Wonderful Adventures of Nils* by Swedish author Selma Lagerlöf (1920), which is very popular in Germany. The story is about an initially feeble boy of deficient character, who on his fabulous trip with wild geese develops physical strength and a sense of social responsibility Along the same lines, the geese in Malu Dreyer's photograph depict her moral victory, which comes along with the acceptance of a stigma and the open confession (Goffman, 1990a, p. 123).

Hence, due to their metaphorical connotation and their placement in the picture, the geese allow the wheelchair to blend into the background of the body presentation. Symbolically, Dreyer's physical impediments are declared insignificant. As a result, the image confirms the tenor of the written body discourse: by openly dealing with her illness, Malu Dreyer has found a way to seamlessly integrate the illness into her private life as well as into her political agenda. This coherent identity construction levels potential obstacles in the way of her political ambitions.

Furthermore, the practices of body presentation described in the illness narrative take on model character for people who suffer from similar impediments and who are affected by social marginalization. The exemplary confrontation of body presentation with traditional normative expectations in media coverage and through the sponsorship of famous political advocates is helpful to provide the stigmatized with orientation and to reaffirm their sense of normalcy (Goffman, 1990a, pp. 35–56). In this context, political actors' illness narratives attain a special social relevance. For once, the effect is directed inwards by supporting comrades of fate when learning different techniques to control information about the stigma (see Legitimization of political action through illness), especially by modifying derogative attributions through body practices (see Identity-creating processing of the illness experience). Secondly, illness narratives also emanate outwards by reflecting and scrutinizing identity attributions and cultural expectations of what is normal. In this way, they contribute to modifying stereotypical expectations (Goffman, 1990a, pp. 38–44). In an interview with German tabloid *Bild am Sonntag,* Malu Dreyer explicitly confronts the conventional image of 'normal' corporeality in politics. Here, she refers to the former German finance minister Wolfgang Schäuble, who is paralyzed as the result of an assassination attempt:

> Cripple is a term from bygone times that I would not want to use. Minister Schäuble is a great role model: it is generally accepted that he is a very effective minister with great responsibilities while naturally moving around in his wheelchair. By doing so, he has done a lot for the normalization concerning the interaction with the disabled (Eichinger and Hellemann, 2013, np; trans. M. B.).

In contrast to Monika Hohlmeier's case (see Legitimization of political action through illness), Malu Dreyer's illness narrative hence constructs a political body that receives 'secondary gains' from the specific way of dealing with the stigma. First, Dreyer can point to positive effects for her image due to the disclosure of the stigma. Second, the described coping strategy with the illness experience takes on a role model function.

Illness narratives in political practice

Political actors' illness narratives represent the culminations of embodied presentations of politics in the media democracy. First of all, disclosed illness narratives reflect the phenomenological, discursive, and institutional prerequisites of corporeality in the social present. Because politicians' illness narratives put bodies in the centre of attention, the otherwise intangible sphere of politics becomes comprehensible for wider audiences. That way, abstract values, decisions, and power structures are presented as actions by bodies on bodies. Hence, politicians' illness narratives make politics sensually tangible in their medial representation. They connect the challenges of political order with the aspect of physical integrity. Additionally, politicians' illness narratives demonstrate various practices to present bodies on a continuum of identification with and in contrast to normalcy standards. Thus, politicians' illness narratives update and reproduce the prevalent cultural interpretations of body and illness. As shown in the analysis of Malu Dreyer's account (see Identity-creating processing of the illness experience), politicians' illness narratives can argue for change and differentiation of traditional perceptions of normalcy. Thereby, political actors' public illness accounts might contribute to alter our understanding of illness and disability.

Political actors' illness accounts always have an instrumental dimension. Illness narratives can serve as a means for identity construction. With a reference to illness, political action can be legitimized or delegitimized (see also Bandtel, 2014). From a mediated illness experience, politicians can derive special competency for particular areas of politics (see also Bandtel, 2016). A political actor's open confession of an illness can contribute to the creation of an authentic image and provoke emphatic resonance (see also Bandtel, 2012).

In view of the mediated illness narratives by two state politicians analysed in the case study (see 'Stigmatizing the body' and 'normalizing the disability'), not only different styles of body use become apparent. In addition, two fundamentally different types of political bodies are constructed in the course of the unfolding illness narratives. Hohlmeier's autobiography revolves around the topic of control. Illness is described as the loss of control; the ultimate objective is its re-establishment. Therefore, the body is interpreted to be subordinate to institutional requirements of politics and conventional medicine. As a typical style of body use, in this illness narrative the adaptation to normalcy concepts is being promoted, in particular by hiding stigmatized characteristics.

By contrast, in Malu Dreyer's illness narrative a political body is constructed that fully consents to the illness experience. Narratively, Dreyer is credited with a high degree of empathy for those who suffer. Hence, not the restitution of normalcy, but the acceptance of contingency and the reciprocal assumption of responsibility are elevated to become the political message.

The results of the study presented in this chapter suggest that politicians' illness narratives form discursive transit points, where expressive body presentations are thickened into a political order and vice versa. In the media, illness narratives by political actors construct bodies that offer practical coping strategies for individual issues. Since all bodies are facing similar challenges, illness narratives connect to people's day-to-day realm of experiences. However, to what extent the body practices proposed in the course of politicians' illness narratives are adopted and accepted, modified or neglected by various audiences, is open to further research.

Notes

1. Monika Hohlmeier's illness narrative is included in the case study with three discourse contributions; Malu Dreyer's illness account is reconstructed using six discourse contributions. The methodological approach to the material is outlined in Dörner et al. (2015, pp. 65–95). On the research programme of discourse analysis in the Sociology of Knowledge see Keller (2011a; 2011b).
2. Regarding this result, also compare my analysis of former German minister of the environment Jürgen Trittin's public handling of his heart attack in Bandtel (2014).
3. In 2002, newspapers discovered election manipulation in a Munich CSU-chapter. Hohlmeier denied any involvement, but resigned from her district chair and her post as minister of education (*Der Weg in die Krise* 2010).

References

Anne Will, 2010. Aus dem Labor auf den Tisch—aber ist Bio wirklich besser? Season 1 episode 129. [TV programme]. ARD, 24 October 2010.

Bandtel, M., 2012. Authentizität in der politischen Kommunikation. Mediale Inszenierungsstrategien und authentifizierende Selbstdarstellungspraktiken politischer Akteure. In: **A. Weixler**, ed. *Authentisches Erzählen. Produktion, Narration, Rezeption*. Berlin: De Gruyter. pp. 215–238.

Bandtel, M., 2014. Die mediale Inszenierung von Pathologien politischer Akteure. Krankheit in der politischen Kommunikation der Moderne. In: **R. John** and **A. Langhof**, eds. *Scheitern—Ein Desiderat der Moderne?* Wiesbaden: VS. pp. 167–195.

Bandtel, M., 2016. Aporien politischer Körper in der Mediendemokratie. Zur Inszenierung verkörperter Politik in Pathographien politischer Akteure. In: **P. Hubmann, M. Frick**, and **M. Gronau**, eds. *Politische Aporien. Akteure und Praktiken des Dilemmas*. Vienna: Turia + Kant. pp. 199–228.

Der Weg in die Krise (2010). Süddeutsche.de. 11 May, np. Available at: <http://www.sueddeutsche.de/muenchen/2.220/chronologie-der-weg-in-die-krise-1.744947>. (Accessed 30 September 2017).

Diehl, P., 2010. Zwischen dem Privaten und dem Politischen. Die neue Körperinszenierung der Politiker. In: **S. Seubert** and **P. Niesen**, eds. *Die Grenzen des Privaten*. Baden-Baden: Nomos. pp. 251–265.

Dörner, A., Vogt, L., Bandtel, M., and **Porzelt, B.**, 2015. *Riskante Bühnen. Inszenierung und Kontingenz—Politikerauftritte in deutschen Personality-Talkshows*. Wiesbaden: VS.

Eichinger, R. and **Hellemann, A.**, 2013. Malu Dreyer: Der Rollstuhl gibt mir Freiheit. *Bild.de*. 20 January, np. Available at: <http://www.bild.de/politik/inland/malu-dreyer/der-rollstuhl-gibt-mir-freiheit-2-28172466.bild.html>. (Accessed 30 September 2014).

Frank, A. W., 1993. The rhetoric of self-change: illness experience as narrative. *Sociological Quarterly*, **34**(1), 39–52.

Frank, A. W., 1995. *The wounded storyteller: body, illness, and ethics*. Chicago, IL: University of Chicago Press.

Frank, A. W., 2001. For a sociology of the body. An analytical review. In: **M. Featherstone, M Hepworth**, and **B. S. Turner**, eds. *The body. Social process and cultural theory*. London: Sage. pp. 36–102.

Goffman, E., 1990a. *Stigma: notes on the management of spoiled identity.* London: Penguin.

Goffman, E., 1990b. *The presentation of self in everyday life.* London: Penguin.

Goffman, E., 2005. *Interaction ritual: essays in face to face behavior.* New Brunswick, NJ: AldineTransaction.

Hawkins, A. H., 1994. *Reconstructing illness. Studies in pathography.* West Lafayette, IN: Purdue University Press.

Hohlmeier, M., 2008. *Meine mageren Jahre sind vorbei!* Munich: Nymphenburger.

Keller, R., 2011a. Wissenssoziologische Diskursanalyse. In: R. Keller, A. Hirseland, W. Schneider, and W. Viehöfer, eds. *Handbuch sozialwissenschaftliche Diskursanalyse.* Wiesbaden: VS. pp. 125–158.

Keller, R., 2011b. *Wissenssoziologische Diskursanalyse. Grundlegung eines Forschungsprogramms.* Wiesbaden: VS.

Kleinman, A., 1988. *The illness narratives: suffering, healing, and the human condition.* New York: Basic Books.

L'Etang, H., 1970. *The pathology of leadership.* New York: Hawthorn Books.

Lagerlöf, S., 1920. *Wunderbare Reise des kleinen Nils Holgersson mit den Wildgänsen.* Munich: Albert Langen.

Löwisch, G., 2013. Ministerpräsidentin Malu Dreyer—Die eiserne Prinzessin. *Cicero Online.* 7 January, np. Available at: <http://www.cicero.de/berliner-republik/ministerpraesidentin-malu-dreyer-die-eiserne-prinzessin/53065?print>. (Accessed 30 September 2017).

Parsons, T., 1951. *The social system.* Glencoe, IL: Free Press.

Raab, J., Grunert, M., and Lustig, S., 2001. Der Körper als Darstellungsmittel. Die theatrale Inszenierung von Politik am Beispiel Benito Mussolinis. In: E. Fischer-Lichte, C. Horn, and M. Warstat, eds. *Verkörperung.* Tübingen: Francke. pp. 171–198.

Raab, J., 2008. Präsenz und mediale Präsentation. Zum Verhältnis von Körper und technischen Medien aus Perspektive der phänomenologisch orientierten Wissenssoziologie. In: J. Raab, J. Dreher, M. Pfadenhauer, B. Schnettler, and P. Stegmaier, eds. *Phänomenologie und Soziologie. Theoretische Positionen, aktuelle Problemfelder und empirische Umsetzungen.* Wiesbaden: VS. pp. 233–42.

Rosenfeld, D., 2013. Ihr großer Schritt. *ZEITonline.* 16 January, np. Available at: http://www.zeit.de/2013/03/Ministerpraesidentin-Marie-Luise-Dreyer (Accessed 30 September 2017).

Turner, B. S., 2008. *The body and society. Explorations in social theory.* Los Angeles: Sage.

Vandenberg, P., 1991. *Die heimlichen Herrscher. Die Mächtigen und ihre Ärzte. Von Marc Aurel bis Papst Pius XII.* C. Munich: Bertelsmann.

Volkert, L., 2010. Das verpatzte Comeback. *Süddeutsche.de,* 17 May, np. Available at: <http://www.sueddeutsche.de/bayern/2.220/csu-monika-hohlmeier-das-verpatzte-comeback-1.702155>. (Accessed 30 September 2017).

von Engelhardt, M., 2010. Erving Goffman: Stigma. Über Techniken der Bewältigung beschädigter Identität. In: B. Jörissen and J. Zirfas, eds. *Schlüsselwerke der Identitätsforschung,* pp. 123–40. Wiesbaden: VS.

Widmann, M., 2012a. Die Siegerin. *Süddeutsche Zeitung,* 29 September, p. 5.

Widmann, M., 2012b. Die Gute. *Süddeutsche Zeitung,* 4 December, p. 3.

Biographies

Manna Alma is senior researcher at the Department of Health Sciences at the University Medical Center Groningen, University of Groningen. She is trained as a human movement scientist and has been involved in several projects focusing on understanding of personal health experiences. As an experienced qualitative researcher, she is currently working as coordinator of the Dutch DIPEx research group PratenOverGezondheid. Furthermore, she is Director of the Board of DIPEx International.

Yong Ik Bak is a research professor at the Department of Medical Humanities, University of Konyang in Daejeon, Republic of Korea. His research interests are dialogue analysis, narrative analysis, and human-orientated medical communication.

Matthias Bandtel is director of the educational programme kompass at Mannheim University of Applied Sciences. He obtained degrees in Political Science, Media and Communication Studies, and Philosophy from University of Mannheim. At the Universities of Wuppertal and Marburg, he has conducted multiple research projects at the intersection between media sociology, sociology of the body, and political sociology. His latest publications comprise studies on political satire and on illness in politics.

Jens Brockmeier is a professor at The American University of Paris. With a background in psychology, philosophy, and language sciences, his interests are in the cultural fabric of human identity, mind, and language, which he has examined in a variety of sociocultural contexts and under conditions of health and illness. He also is a Visiting Professor of Psychology at the University of Manitoba, Canada, and an Honorary Professor at the University of Innsbruck, Austria.

Martina Breuning is a psychologist and research assistant at the Department of Rehabilitation Psychology and Psychotherapy at the University of Freiburg, Germany. Since 2008 she has been conducting qualitative research and teaching qualitative methods. She is a member of the international collaboration, DIPEx International, which is engaged in the collection, analysis, and application of patients´ narratives worldwide.

Sabine Corsten is a Professor of Therapy and Rehabilitation Sciences (Speech and Language Therapy) at the Catholic University of Applied Sciences, Mainz, Germany. Trained as an academic speech and language therapist, she has worked as an assistant researcher at the Department of Neurology, University Hospital Aachen, Germany. Quality-of-life-orientated intervention in case of chronic illness, especially in case of neurologically based communication difficulties, is the topic of her current research projects.

Amos Fleischmann is a Class A Senior Lecturer at the Graduate School of Education at Achva Academic College. Throughout his research career, he has dealt with questions relating to coping with helplessness and ways to enhance individuals' control of the conditions that they face. In recent years, he has conducted qualitative research to examine how people with disabilities cope with their hardships.

Peter Frommelt, MD, is a board-certified specialist in neurology and rehabilitation medicine. He is in private practice for neurorehabilitation in Berlin. Before, he was head of neurorehabilitation in the inpatient hospital Asklepios in Schaufling, Bavaria. Co-editor (with Hubert Lösslein) of *NeuroRehabilitation* (3rd ed., Springer, 2010), he is interested in context-sensitive and narrative approaches to rehabilitation after neurotrauma. Since 2013, he has been co-organizer (together with Jens Brockmeier and Maria Medved) of the annual Berlin Symposium on Narrative Medicine.

Rachel Grob is Director of National Initiatives, Clinical Professor at the Center for Patient Partnerships, and Senior Scientist at the Department of Family Medicine and Community Health at the University of Wisconsin–Madison. She is a sociologist who uses qualitative and mixed methods to elicit, synthesize, and amplify patients' diverse voices, with a special focus on their experiences with health and healthcare. She is happiest working at the cusp where innovative research meets applied projects.

Elisabeth Gülich was chair of Romance Languages and Linguistics at the University of Bielefeld (1981–2002). Her current research interest is in medical communication, working with interdisciplinary research teams on patients' illness descriptions and narratives. The principal aim of her projects is to contribute to differential diagnosis.

Hille Haker holds the Richard McCormick, S. J., Endowed Chair of Moral Theology at Loyola University Chicago. She is the co-director of the Research Project 'Medical Ethics in Health Care Chaplaincy', and was the President of Societas Ethica, the European Society for Research in Ethics from 2015–2018. From 2005–2015, she was a member of the European Group on Ethics in Sciences and New Technologies (EGE) to the European Commission. Trained in theology, literature, and philosophy, her works are in the fields of bioethics, social ethics, feminist ethics, and ethics and literature.

Friedericke Hardering is senior researcher at the Institute for Sociology, Goethe-University, Frankfurt. She received her doctorate in political science in 2010 at RWTH Aachen University. She has worked in research projects at different institutions and was co-operation partner in the narraktiv research project. Since 2014, she manages a research project on meaningful work. Her main research areas are sociology of work, identity and work, work and health, and qualitative research methods.

Chris Heape is a Design Research Consultant with SDU Design, University of Southern Denmark. His research interest is in social design with a focus on the micro-interactions of how people get things done in professional healthcare practice to inform change in that practice. His work focuses on chronic pain with an understanding of chronic pain as a social, rather than an individual phenomenon and the dilemmas GPs can face when interacting with patients who have existential or broken life narrative issues.

Cornelia Helfferich is professor of Sociology at the Protestant University of Applied Sciences (EH), Freiburg i.Br., Germany, and senior lecturer at the University of Freiburg. Trained in Medical Sociology, she is head of SoFFII (Institute for Social Science Research on Gender) as a department of FIVE (Research and Innovation Group at EH Freiburg), a university institute for research in Social Work, Care and Civil Society. She focuses on qualitative research methods, life course/biography, family, and violence.

Wolfgang Himmel is sociologist and professor of Health Sciences at the Department of General Practice of the University Medical Center Göttingen. His current scientific interests include health services research, the doctor–patient relationship, research methods, and the role of the Internet for patients. As a member of the German DIPEx group, he was responsible for the diabetes, inflammatory bowel disease, and ADHD modules. Orcid-ID: http://orcid.org/0000-0003-3523-5486

Lisa Hinton is a medical sociologist and director of applied research for the Health Experiences Research Group, University of Oxford. She specializes in women's health (infertility, maternal morbidity, pre-eclampsia) and experiences of neonatal and adult intensive care medicine.

Christine Holmberg is Professor of Social Medicine and Epidemiology at the Medical School Brandenburg Theodor Fontane. She was trained in anthropology at Humboldt University Berlin and Harvard Medical School and in epidemiology at the University of Illinois at Chicago. Her research interests include the influence of medical and statistical technologies on patient narratives, experiences, and decision making. She is co-editor of the recently published *The politics of vaccination: a global history* (Manchester University Press).

Lars-Christer Hydén received his PhD in Psychology from Stockholm University, Sweden. His current position is full Professor of Social Psychology at Linköping University. His research concerns how people living with dementia interact, use language, and tell stories. He has published articles in international journals and books, including *Health, Culture and Illness: Broken Narratives* (together with Jens Brockmeier, Routledge, 2008), and *Entangled Narratives: Collaborative Storytelling and the Re-Imagining of Dementia* (Oxford University Press, 2017).

Yeonok Jeoung is a professor at the Department of Nursing, University of Kyungdong in Gangwon-do, Republic of Korea. Her research interests are nursing management, nursing communication, and qualitative research.

Ernst von Kardorff is Professor Emeritus of Rehabilitation Sciences at Humboldt University of Berlin; he was and is still project leader in the fields of vocational rehabilitation, return to work, ways into early pension, and working with disabilities. Trained as a sociologist and psychologist he has worked on different topics, including qualitative research and evaluation, social psychiatry, stigmatization, the doctor–patient relationship, social support networks, medical sociology, and vocational rehabilitation.

Alexander Kiss is Professor for Psychosomatic Medicine at the Faculty of Medicine in Basel, Switzerland. He studied medicine in Vienna and Heidelberg, was trained in internal medicine at the Medical University of Vienna and obtained his psychoanalytic training at the Vienna Psychoanalytic Society. He is interested in qualitative research in medicine and communication skill training in oncology. He is responsible for the mandatory Medical Humanities Program for medical students in Basel.

Janka Koschack is a psychologist and was senior researcher at the Department of General Practice of the University Medical Center, Göttingen until 2015. She now works as a clinical psychologist with inpatients with traumatic disorders and drug addiction. Her scientific interests focused on the patient perspective in evidence-based medicine. As a former member of the German DIPEx group, she was responsible for the diabetes and inflammatory bowel disease modules.

Joyce Lamerichs is assistant professor and senior researcher at the department of Language, Literature & Communication at VU University in Amsterdam. She is trained as a researcher in Science and Technology Studies and moved to discursive psychology and conversation analysis to study the ways in which people interact in different health settings. Her research interests lie in exploring peoples' accounts of health and illness, with a special interest in issues to do with mental health and settings that involve young people as interactional partners talking to a health professional.

Henry Larsen is Professor of Participatory Innovation with SDU Design, University of Southern Denmark. His research interest focuses on understanding social interaction as transformative and as a complex process of relating. In collaboration with professional actors, he engages communities of inquiry by using improvised theatre to engender new conversations and to identify new themes that encourage a reflexive understanding of the micro-interactions in which those involved find themselves engaged.

Dr Maya Lavie-Ajayi is a senior lecturer at the Spitzer Department of Social Work at Ben-Gurion University of the Negev, and the chair of the Israeli Center for Qualitative Research of People and Societies. She wrote her doctoral thesis on the social representations of anorgasmia and women's experiences of it. Today her research focuses on professional discussion about sex and sexuality, subjective experiences of health and illness, and inequality in healthcare.

John Lavis is Professor and Canada Research Chair in Evidence-Informed Health Systems at McMaster University in Hamilton, Ontario. He is the founder and director of the McMaster Health Forum, and co-director of the WHO Collaborating Centre on Evidence-Informed Policy. His passion is developing and evaluating ways to harness research evidence, citizen values, and stakeholder insights to strengthen health and social systems and get the right programmes, services, and products to the people who need them.

Susan Law is Director of Research and scientist at the Institute for Better Health in Mississauga Ontario, and Associate Professor at the Institute for Health Policy, Management and Evaluation at the University of Toronto. She has held leadership positions in research and management in the UK and Canada. Her research focuses on patient and family experiences of illness, patient engagement and co-design, and she directs the Canadian Health Experiences Research Program.

Louise Locock was appointed Professor of Health Services Research at the University of Aberdeen in October 2017. She was previously Director of Applied Research at the Health Experiences Research Group, University of Oxford. Her background is in social policy. She specializes in qualitative research into patient experience, quality improvement, and patient involvement.

David Loutfi is a PhD candidate in the Department of Family Medicine at McGill University studying social networks and HIV prevention. He has a Master's degree in community health from the University of Montreal. He has worked as a research assistant on health experiences research projects in Canada.

Gabriele Lucius-Hoene is a retired professor and psychotherapist at the Department of Rehabilitation Psychology, Institute of Psychology, University of Freiburg. Her research interests are narrative and conversational analysis of life stories, especially illness narratives, and the ways people construct their identities and cope with challenges and suffering by telling their stories.

Paula McDonald is a GP in Brighton, UK and has worked as a Teaching Fellow and Senior Teaching Fellow at Manchester and Brighton medical schools. She is also trained in Public Health Medicine and worked as a Consultant in Public Health for several years. She has a research interest in narrative medicine and creative writing.

Eleonora Massa gained her PhD in General Linguistics at the University of Rome (2013). Her research focuses on storytelling as a device of shaping of socio-cultural forms and on the semiotic praxes through which such a device finds expression: among these, in particular, on the spoken use of verbal language. More recently, she has extended her interest to the narrative practices on online settings. She is currently a language teacher and an independent researcher based in Rome.

Maria I. Medved is Professor of Psychology at The American University of Paris, adjunct Professor of Psychology at the University of Manitoba in Canada and a licensed clinical psychologist with a specialty in rehabilitation and neuropsychology. Her research interests include narratives of risk and resilience as told by people dealing with illness, injury, and disability in various contexts and cultures. Her primary focus is neurotrauma narratives.

Thorsten Meyer is Professor of Rehabilitation Sciences and has recently become a member of the Faculty of Public Health at the University of Bielefeld, Germany. Trained as a psychologist, he has worked in different health research departments (social psychiatry, social medicine, rehabilitation) in Germany and Switzerland. He currently serves as a speaker of the Qualitative Research Working Group with the German Network on Health Services Research.

Erez C. Miller is a senior lecturer of Psychology and Special Education at Achva Academic College, Israel. Trained as a school psychologist, he has worked in various public psycho-educational services and in private practice in Israel and specializes in working with children and young people with disabilities. He currently serves as the Chair of the Department of Education at Achva Academic College.

Ora Nakash, PhD, is an associate professor at the Baruch Ivcher School of Psychology at the Interdisciplinary Center in Herzliya, Israel, and School for Social Work, Smith College, Northampton, MA. Her research focuses on the study of the effects of social and cultural factors on mental health, with specific interest in mental health disparities with the goal of improving the access, equity, and quality of these services for disadvantaged and minority populations.

Ilja Ormel is a PhD student in the Department of Family Medicine at McGill University. She completed her MSc (Public Health) at the London School of Hygiene and Tropical Medicine. She worked in humanitarian settings before becoming the Research Program Coordinator for the Canadian Health Experiences Research team. Her thesis research is based in Haiti and explores the use of participatory research and co-design to inform humanitarian service improvements in response to the cholera epidemic.

Alexander Palant is sociologist and health science researcher at the Department of General Practice of the University Medical Center, Göttingen. He finished his PhD in 2017 on peoples' experiences with inflammatory bowel disease. His current scientific interests include health services research, the doctor–patient relationship, research methods, the role of the Internet for patients, and children's health. As a member of the German DIPEx group, he was responsible for the inflammatory bowel disease and ADHD modules.

Christian Roesler is Professor of Clinical Psychology at the Catholic University of Applied Sciences in Freiburg/D, lecturer of Analytical Psychology at the University of Basel/CH and visiting professor to the Kyoto University, Japan. He is a Jungian psychoanalyst in private practice in Freiburg and member of the faculty of the C. G. Jung–Institutes in Stuttgart and Zurich. He specializes in working with couples and families and interpretive research methods. His research and publications focus on analytical psychology and contemporary sciences, couples therapy, postmodern identity construction, narrative research, and media psychology.

Merja Ryöppy is currently a PhD research fellow with SDU Design, University of Southern Denmark. Trained as an engineer (MSc) and an actress (BA), she currently runs Theatre Lab where improvised theatre is used as a means to explore inquiries into the human interaction of social relations, e.g., in doctor–patient communication. Her PhD study lies at the intersection of theatre and design with a focus on understanding objects as material and relational entities in social interaction.

Mark Schlesinger is Professor of Health Policy at Yale University. He is trained as an economist, but is often mistaken for a political psychologist, organizational sociologist, or clinical therapist. He applies innovative research methods—most notably Internet-based survey experiments—to study how people experience healthcare and respond to those experiences. He is happiest working in interdisciplinary teams and on projects that translate diverse individual experiences into policy discourse.

Victoria A. Shaffer is an associate professor in the Department of Psychological Sciences at the University of Missouri in Columbia, Missouri. She is a quantitative psychologist with a background in decision theory and behavioural economics. Her research has broadly focused on identifying and testing methods to improve the quality of decisions about healthcare, with her most recent work devoted to the study of patient narratives and decision support tools for both patients and healthcare providers.

Valentina Simeoni is a social anthropologist, language teacher, and copywriter based in northeastern Italy. Specialized in the anthropology of storytelling, after her fieldworks in the diné reservation (USA) and the Southern Caucasus (Georgia), she gained her PhD at the University of Bergamo (2012) and has since then continued to conduct independent research on the dynamics of online storytelling communities through an approach that combines netnography and corpus-based linguistics.

Claudia Steiner is trained in biology and social anthropology and worked in the fields of primatology and in museum education before joining the Psychosomatic Department, University Hospital of Basel, Switzerland as a research associate. She is interested in the effect of mindfulness interventions on patients with chronic deceases and qualitative research in medicine and medical education. She coordinates the Medical Humanities Program for medical students in Basel.

Margret Xyländer is a sociologist and health science researcher at the Faculty of Public Health at the University of Bielefeld, Germany. Her current scientific interests include qualitative healthcare research and research methods. Her research focuses are, inter alia, patient orientation and participation and patients' view on counselling centres. She is a member of the Qualitative Research Working Group with the German Network on Health Services Research.

Sue Ziebland is a professor of Medical Sociology and director of the Health Experiences Research Group (HERG) in the Nuffield Department of Primary Care Health Sciences at the University of Oxford. Her work specializes in qualitative research methods for understanding health experiences. Sue was a founder member of the DIPEx project, which publishes narrative interview studies on a public-facing multimedia website (Healthtalk.org in the UK). This has stimulated similar projects in 13 other countries who are members of dipexinternational.org.

Brian J. Zikmund-Fisher is associate professor of Health Behavior and Health Education and Research Associate Professor of Internal Medicine at the University of Michigan, as well as Associate Editor of the journals *Medical Decision Making* and *Medical Decision Making: Policy and Practice*. Trained in decision psychology and behavioural economics, he researches health risk perceptions, meaning-rich methods of communicating health data, and the power of narratives in health communication.

Author Index

Subject Index

Notes

Abbreviations used can be found on page xi

vs. indicates a comparison

Tables, figures and boxes are indicated by an italic *t, f* and *b* following the page number.